UNDERSTANDING HEALTH POLICY

Also available in the series

Understanding global social policy (second edition)

Edited by Nicola Yeates

"Nicola Yeates has brought together an impressive, coherent collection of contributors providing comprehensive coverage of developments in global social policy across a wide range of policy areas. The relationship between globalisation and social policy is one that is rapidly evolving and differentiated." Patricia Kennett, Department of Applied Social Sciences, The Hong Kong Polytechnic University

PB £21.99 (US$36.95) ISBN 978 1 4473 1024 2 HB £65.00 (US$85.00) ISBN 978 1 4473 1023 5
368 pages March 2014
E-INSPECTION COPY AVAILABLE

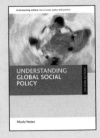

Understanding crime and social policy

Emma Wincup

"An engaging, wide-ranging and up-to-date introductory text for students and practitioners who wish to get to grips with the interconnections between criminology as the study of crime and social policy as the study of human well-being." Dr Ros Burnett, Centre for Criminology, University of Oxford.

PB £21.99 (US$36.95) ISBN 978 1 84742 499 0 HB £65.00 (US$85.00) ISBN 978 1 84742 500 3
224 pages May 2013
E-INSPECTION COPY AVAILABLE

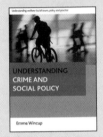

Understanding research for social policy and social work (second edition)

Edited by Saul Becker, Alan Bryman and Harry Ferguson

"Becker and Bryman did a masterful job ... North American public policy students could learn a lot from this book and methodology instructors could have their load considerably eased if URfSPP was more widely read". Kennedy Stewart, Associate Professor, Simon Fraser University School of Public Policy and Member of Parliament for Burnaby-Douglas

PB £24.99 (US$42.95) ISBN 978 1 84742 815 8 HB £65.00 (US$89.95) ISBN 978 1 84742 816 5
448 pages March 2012
E-INSPECTION COPY AVAILABLE

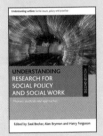

Understanding health and social care (second edition)

Jon Glasby

"This is an ambitious and wide ranging book which provides a valuable historical perspective, as well as a forward looking analysis, based on real experience. It will be a valuable tool for leaders, policy makers and students." Nigel Edwards, Policy Director, The NHS Confederation

PB £21.99 (US$34.95) ISBN 978 1 84742 623 9 HB £65.00 (US$85.00) ISBN 978 1 84742 624 6
224 pages February 2012
E-INSPECTION COPY AVAILABLE

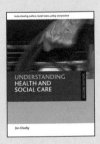

For a full listing of all titles in the series visit www.policypress.co.uk

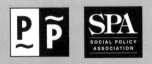

www.policypress.co.uk

INSPECTION COPIES AND ORDERS AVAILABLE FROM:

Marston Book Services • PO BOX 269 • Abingdon • Oxon OX14 4YN UK
INSPECTION COPIES
Tel: +44 (0) 1235 465500 • Fax: +44 (0) 1235 465556 • Email: inspections@marston.co
ORDERS
Tel: +44 (0) 1235 465500 • Fax: +44 (0) 1235 465556 • Email: direct.orders@marston.c

UNDERSTANDING HEALTH POLICY

Second edition

Rob Baggott

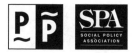

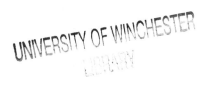

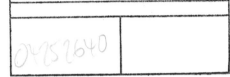
First published in Great Britain in 2015 by

Policy Press
University of Bristol
1-9 Old Park Hill
Bristol
BS2 8BB
UK
t: +44 (0)117 954 5940
pp-info@bristol.ac.uk
www.policypress.co.uk

North America office:
Policy Press
c/o The University of Chicago Press
1427 East 60th Street
Chicago, IL 60637, USA
t: +1 773 702 7700
f: +1 773 702 9756
sales@press.uchicago.edu
www.press.uchicago.edu

© Policy Press and the Social Policy Association 2015

British Library Cataloguing in Publication Data
A catalogue record for this book is available from the British Library.

Library of Congress Cataloging-in-Publication Data
A catalog record for this book has been requested.

ISBN 978-1-4473-0011-3 (paperback)
ISBN 978-1-4473-0012-0 (hardcover)
ISBN 978-1-4473-1248-2 (ePub)
ISBN 978-1-4473-1249-9 (Mobi)

Cover design by Qube Design Associates, Bristol
Front cover: image kindly supplied by www.alamy.com
Printed and bound in Great Britain by Hobbs, Southampton
Policy Press uses environmentally responsible print partners

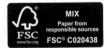

To Auntie Joan Clark and in memory of
Auntie Joan Docker

Contents

Detailed contents

List of boxes

List of abbreviations

ABPI   Association of the British Pharmaceutical Industry
A&E   accident and emergency
APPG   All Party Parliamentary Group
ASH   Action on Smoking and Health
BMA   British Medical Association
BMJ   *British Medical Journal*
BSE/CJD   Bovine Spongiform Encephalopathy/Creutzfeldt Jakob Disease
CAA   comprehensive area assessment
CAG   Comptroller and Auditor General
CAP   Common Agricultural Policy
CCG   clinical commissioning group
C.diff   Clostridium difficile
CHAI   Commission for Health Audit and Inspection (the Healthcare
          Commission)
CHC   community health council
CHCP   community health and care partnership
CHI   Commission for Health Improvement
CHP   community health partnership
CHRE   Council for Healthcare Regulatory Excellence (now Professional
          Standards Authority for Health and Social Care)
CMO   Chief Medical Officer
COREPER   Committee of Permanent Representatives (European Union)
CPP   community planning partnership
CPPIH   Commission for Patient and Public Involvement in Health
CQC   Care Quality Commission
CQUIN   Commissioning for Quality and Innovation
CSR   comprehensive spending review
CSU   commissioning support unit
DCLG   Department for Communities and Local Government
DCMS   Department for Culture, Media and Sport
DECC   Department of Energy and Climate Change
DEFRA   Department for Environment, Food and Rural Affairs
DfE   Department for Education
DFID   Department for International Development
DfT   Department for Transport
DH   Department of Health
DHA   district health authority
DHSS   Department of Health and Social Security

DHSSPS	Department of Health, Social Services and Public Safety (Northern Ireland)
DPH	director of public health
DWP	Department for Work and Pensions
ECJ	European Court of Justice
EDM	early day motion
EEC	European Economic Community
EU	European Union
FAO	Food and Agriculture Organisation (UN)
FHSA	family health services authority
FFT	Friends and Family Test
FOREST	Freedom Organisation for the Right to Enjoy Smoking Tobacco
FPC	family practitioner committee
FT	foundation trust
GM	genetically modified
GMC	General Medical Council
GP	general practitioner
HAZ	health action zone
HIA	health impact assessment
HIV/AIDS	Human Immunodeficiency Virus/Acquired Immunity Deficiency Syndrome
HMO	health maintenance organisation
HOSC	health overview and scrutiny committee
HSCP	health and social care partnership
HSM	health social movement
ICAS	Independent Complaints Advocacy Service
IGC	inter-government coordination
IHSM	Institute of Health Service Management (now Institute of Healthcare Management)
ILO	International Labour Organisation
IMF	International Monetary Fund
IPPR	Institute for Public Policy Research
ISTC	independent sector treatment centre
JASP	Joint Approach to Social Policy
JEC	Joint Epilepsy Council
JHWS	joint health and wellbeing strategy
JSNA	joint strategic needs assessment
LAA	local area agreement
LGA	Local Government Association
LGBT	Lesbian, Gay, Bisexual and Transgender
LHB	local health board

LHW	local healthwatch
LINk	local involvement network
LSP	local strategic partnership
MAFF	Ministry of Agriculture, Fisheries and Food
MAT	modernisation action team
MDGs	Millennium Development Goals
MEP	Member of the European Parliament
MMR	measles, mumps and rubella
MOD	Ministry of Defence
MP	Member of Parliament
MRSA	Methicillin Resistant Staphylococcus Aureus
MSP	Member of the Scottish Parliament
NAO	National Audit Office
NCD	non communicable disease
NGO	non-governmental organisation
NHS	National Health Service
NHSE	National Health Service Executive
NHSTDA	NHS Trust Development Authority
NICE	National Institute for Health and Care Excellence (formerly National Institute for Clinical Excellence)
NPSA	National Patient Safety Agency
NSF	national service framework
OECD	Organisation for Economic Cooperation and Development
Ofsted	Office for Standards in Education (now Office for Standards in Education, Children's Services and Skills)
OMC	Open Method of Coordination
ONS	Office for National Statistics
PAC	Public Accounts Committee
PALS	Patient Advice and Liaison Service
PASC	Public Administration Select Committee
PBC	practice-based commissioning
PBR	payment by results
PCG	primary care group
PCT	primary care trust
PFI	private finance initiative
PMB	Private Member's Bill
PMSU	Prime Minister's Strategy Unit
POPP	Partnerships for Older People Project
PPI	patient and public involvement
PPIF	patient and public involvement forum
PPP	public–private partnership
PQ	parliamentary question

PROMs	patient reported outcome measures
PSA	public service agreement
QIPP	Quality Innovation Productivity and Prevention
QOF	Quality and Outcomes Framework
RAWP	Resource Allocation Working Party
RCN	Royal College of Nursing
RHA	regional health authority
SAP	structural adjustment programme
SARS	Severe Acute Respiratory Syndrome
SDP	Social Democratic Party
SEA	Single European Act
SHA	strategic health authority
SMC	Scottish Medicines Consortium
SNP	Scottish National Party
SPS	sanitary and phytosanitary measures
SSI	Social Services Inspectorate
TB	tuberculosis
TSO	The Stationery Office
TTIP	Transatlantic Trade and Investment Partnership
UKIP	UK Independence Party
UN	United Nations
UNAIDS	Joint UN Programme on HIV/AIDS
UNCTAD	UN Conference on Trade and Development
UNDP	UN Development Programme
UNEP	UN Environment Programme
UNESCO	UN Educational, Scientific and Cultural Organisation
UNHCR	UN High Commission on Refugees
UNICEF	UN Children's Fund
UNODC	UN Office of Drugs and Crime
WEF	World Economic Forum
WFP	World Food Programme
WHO	World Health Organisation
WTO	World Trade Organisation

Preface

I am grateful for the opportunity to produce this second edition of *Understanding health policy* for Policy Press. This is a fully updated edition, which takes account of the politics and policies of the Conservative–Liberal Democrat coalition government 2010–15. At the time of writing, the coalition has recently been replaced by a Conservative government (with David Cameron continuing as Prime Minister). Although this book looks back over the past five years (and indeed beyond), its analysis remains relevant for the future. Most of the policy themes of the recent past will continue and indeed develop further in the coming years. I expect the NHS in England to be subjected to further political pressures to privatise, marketise and increase private funding of health and care services. But at the same time there will be increasing pressures to rationalise and integrate services, while placing greater emphasis on preventing illness. At any rate, health policy will continue to be at the forefront of political debate, despite efforts to take it out of politics.

I would like to thank a number of people for their encouragement and support in the successful completion of this project. My excellent students at De Montfort University have inspired me to write this second edition, against many other competing pressures. Two of my colleagues, Dr Kathryn Jones and Dr Steven Parker, have been particularly supportive and helpful with comments on later drafts. I have received excellent support from the Policy Press, especially Emily Watt, Jo Morton and Laura Vickers. Thanks also to Professor Hugh Bochel for permission to use Table 2.1 from my chapter in his edited volume *Conservative Party and social policy* (Policy Press, 2011).

I would also like once again to express thanks to my family for their patience, unwavering support and encouragement over the years.

Rob Baggott
Leicester
May 2015

Analysing health policy

Overview

This chapter clarifies the meaning of health policy. It also reviews conceptual frameworks that are useful in the study of health policy.

Health policy

The task of defining health policy is difficult, largely because both 'health' and 'policy' are open to different interpretations.

Health can be interpreted in different ways (Aggleton, 1990; Blaxter, 2004). In a narrow, negative sense it can mean the absence of disease or illness. This conventional biomedical approach interprets health as a state of normality disrupted by illness and disease. However, health can be defined in a positive sense, as 'a state of complete physical, mental and social well-being and not merely the absence of disease or infirmity' (WHO, 1946, p 100). The distinction between positive and negative definitions is important for the study of health policy. If one adopts a positive definition, health policy analysis extends beyond health services policy and organisation, incorporating a much wider range of social, economic, environmental and political processes affecting public health and wellbeing.

Policy is also a contested term (Parsons, 1995; Hudson and Lowe, 2004; Cairney, 2012; John, 2012). In broad terms, it refers to a position taken by an organisation or individual in a position of authority. It might refer to a statement, a decision, a document, or a programme of action. A policy is not always the result of positive action, however. It may take the form of inaction or a deliberate attempt to block a decision. The primary focus is usually on *public* policy: how the authoritative positions of governing institutions are determined and how they are put into practice. However, public policy processes involve non-governmental actors, who can be influential. Therefore, their activities should fall within the scope of public policy analysis.

Health policy is difficult to define (Exworthy et al, 2011). However, this has not stopped academics from trying. For example, Green and Thorogood (1998, p 9) define health policy analysis as 'the study of health policy concerns, the origins of that policy, its goals and outcomes.' Blank and Burau (2004, p 17) define it as 'those courses of action proposed or taken by government that impact on the financing and/or provision of health services.' For Walt (1994, p 1), 'health policy is about process and power … it is concerned with who influences whom in the making of policy and how that happens.' According to Buse et al (2005, p 6), 'health policy is assumed to embrace courses of action (and inaction) that affect the set of institutions, organisations, services and funding arrangements of the health system.' Authors acknowledge the wide scope of health policy, including policies in other sectors relevant to health. They also argue that the study of health policy should not be confined to government institutions (Walt, 1994; Buse et al, 2005; Crinson, 2009; Alaszewski and Brown, 2012).

This book adopts the following perspective. It focuses on the political processes that underlie the emergence of health issues, the formulation of policies and their implementation. It is not narrowly confined to NHS policies. It is primarily concerned with institutions and processes of government, but includes the activities of non-governmental organisations (NGOs) such as the media, commercial organisations, professional bodies, pressure groups and voluntary organisations.

Conceptual frameworks

When studying any policy arena, one must be familiar with key concepts of policy analysis. The remainder of this chapter considers the main conceptual frameworks and their relevance to health policy.

Policy as a rational, hierarchical process

This model owes much to Simon's (1945) work on administrative decision-making. He believed that even in a complex environment, rational decision-making was possible. Although decision-makers lacked full information and knowledge, could not know all the consequences of their decisions, and operated within organisations that framed their choices, they should seek to identify the best possible option in terms of their values, based on a comprehensive evaluation of the various alternatives (see Parsons, 1995; Bochel and Bochel, 2004). This meant identifying goals, listing alternative strategies, assessing the consequences of these options and choosing the strategy most likely to achieve these goals. Simon acknowledged that there was 'bounded rationality' in practice, but believed that the scope for rational decision-making could be improved through technology and new management techniques (Simon, 1960).

Others, such as Lindblom (1959), were more sceptical about human rationality within complex policy environments and of the desirability of trying to improve rationality. Lindblom argued that decisions were made in an incremental fashion, and that analysis of options was limited, taking the form of a succession of comparisons rather than a comprehensive analysis. Moreover, for him, values and goals were inseparable from the evaluation of these options. Decisions emerged not from a rational analysis, but by 'muddling through'. Interactions between various participants led to mutual adjustment of competing objectives and, ultimately, compromise (Lindblom, 1965).

Nonetheless, the rational model has been influential. It underpins the 'stagist' approach to policy (see Rose, 1973; May and Wildavsky, 1978; Hogwood and Gunn, 1984; Dorey, 2005), which retains its appeal today. Essentially, the stagist approach breaks the policy process down into distinct parts. Hogwood and Gunn (1984), for example, outlined the following stages:

- deciding to decide – including issue search and agenda setting
- deciding how to decide – deciding how decisions should be made
- issue definition
- forecasting
- setting objectives and priorities
- options analysis
- policy implementation, monitoring and control
- evaluation and review
- policy maintenance, succession or termination.

Although a useful way of thinking about different aspects of policy and the factors that affect them, the model oversimplifies the multidimensional nature of the policy process and imposes artificial rationality on it (John, 2012). In turn, defenders of the stagist approach have acknowledged the dynamics of the policy process and highlighted 'feedback loops' between different stages. For example, the notion of a 'policy cycle' emerged by linking the final stages of the policy process with the initiation of new policies (May and Wildavsky, 1978; Hogwood and Peters, 1983). The stagist approach has also been criticised for failing to provide testable explanations of policy development (Sabatier, 1999). However, its very simplicity enables it to remain attractive as a 'framework for organising our understanding of what happens' (Hogwood and Gunn, 1984, p 4).

Despite criticism of rational, top–down models, there has been much greater emphasis within government in recent decades on how to improve the rationality of policy-making. This has led to efforts to improve policy analysis, including the creation of policy research units within government departments. There has also been an emphasis on policy evaluation and evidence-based policy, as reflected, for example, in the 'what counts is what works' approach endorsed by the former Blair government (Sanderson, 2002). This kind of approach places great faith in pragmatism based on evidence and policy evaluation as drivers of policy development. Unfortunately, however, this is not as simple as it sounds. There is often insufficient, reliable evidence to inform decision-making, and there is often disagreement over the validity of evidence. Moreover, evidence can be manipulated – evidence can be found to justify ideologically driven policies, while negative or cautionary findings are suppressed.

Policy evaluation does not take place in a political vacuum (Taylor and Balloch, 2005). Indeed, it is very difficult to be objective about the success or failure of policies (Bovens and t'Hart, 1996; Bovens et al, 2001; McConnell, 2010). Much depends on interpretation. Furthermore, there are various dimensions of success or failure. For example, it is possible for a policy to be judged unsuccessful in programme terms (it does not meet the stated objectives or is poor value for money), but a success in political terms (it increases the popularity of government or placates a powerful interest group).

The top-down, rational model of policy-making has also been influential over how the process of implementation is understood (Hill, 1997; Hill and Hupe, 2002; Barrett, 2004). Traditionally, implementation was seen as an 'add on' to the process of policy-making. The main focus was on gaps or deficits between the intentions of policy-makers and policy outcomes (see Pressman and Wildavsky, 1973; Hood, 1976; Dunsire, 1978; Hogwood and Gunn, 1984; Marsh and Rhodes, 1992a). An alternative 'bottom-up' perspective was also developed (Barrett and Fudge, 1981; Barrett, 2004) focusing on the processes of negotiation and mediation through which agencies at the periphery (such as local authorities) might modify policy. Others highlighted the discretionary power of frontline professionals and workers or 'street-level bureaucrats' (Lipsky, 1979) and the need to understand their actions in context (Ellmore, 1980). More recently, efforts have been made to transcend this 'top-down' 'bottom-up' dichotomy. Elements from both have been synthesised in order to better understand the dynamics of policy implementation, without the assumption that 'top-down' is necessarily the best way of operating (see Parsons, 1995; Hill and Hupe, 2002; Barrett, 2004).

Nonetheless, recent UK governments, while flirting with localism, have generally adopted a top-down approach through 'managerialism' (see Clarke and Newman, 1997; Newman, 2001). This began with the efforts of the Conservative and Labour governments in the 1960s and 1970s to improve policy and planning. It was followed by reforms to impose stronger performance management on public sector organisations in the 1980s and 1990s. Subsequently, managerialism was evident in New Labour's approach to public services, which was heavily based on centralised targets, performance agreements and audit/inspection regimes to ensure compliance (Newman, 2001). Subsequently, the Conservative–Liberal Democrat coalition, despite championing localism and decentralisation, continued to govern largely with a top-down policy style.

Centralisation and decentralisation

Concepts of centralisation and decentralisation help to make further sense of the implementation process. Deeming (2004, p 60) defined centralisation as where 'significant decisions are taken upstream at the centre of government within a tighter system of control and accountability.' He defined decentralisation as a situation where 'significant decision-making discretion is available at lower hierarchical levels, with the managers and staff who are closer to the people receiving services.' Saltman et al (2007, p 10) similarly define decentralisation as 'the transfer of authority and power from higher to lower levels of government or from national to subnational levels.'

The potential benefits of decentralisation (see Milburn, 2001; Peckham et al, 2008) include greater responsiveness to local service users' needs; enabling local managers to manage services without interference; efficiencies arising from the shedding of bureaucratic tiers and processes; and empowerment of staff leading to greater motivation and service innovation. But decentralisation also has disadvantages, including inequalities between local areas, fragmentation and confusion over accountability (Walker, 2002; Mosca, 2006).

Several writers have identified different types of centralisation and decentralisation (see Pollitt et al, 1998; Peckham et al, 2005; Saltman et al, 2007). For example, Rondinelli (1981) specified three major types of government decentralisation (in addition to privatisation): *deconcentration* – a shift in administrative workload, but not authority, to the regional and/or local offices of an organisation; *delegation* – to semi-autonomous agencies with given powers; and *devolution* – where decision-making and management authority is moved to provincial and local governments.

Decentralisation operates on a number of dimensions. In health and other policy areas, it is possible to centralise some aspects of policy while decentralising others (Pollitt et al, 1998; Dopson et al, 1999; Alvarez–Rosete and Mays, 2008; Exworthy and Frosini, 2008; Peckham et al, 2008; Crisp, 2011). A common theme is that central government delegates functions and even allows greater local autonomy on some issues, but retains strategic control and intervenes in operational matters. Indeed, decentralisation can be seen as a symbolic policy, masking tighter control of local organisations (Mohan, 1995; Ross and Tomaney, 2001; Tallis, 2004). According to Bossert (1998), there are three key aspects of decentralisation in health: the amount of choice transferred from central institutions to those at the periphery; the choices local officials make when given discretion; and the effect these choices have on the performance of the health system.

Partnerships and collaboration

There has been increasing emphasis on building stronger partnerships between agencies in order to maximise the impact of policies and to improve the delivery of public services. It has been argued that such partnerships have a number of benefits (Balloch and Taylor, 2001; Newman, 2001; Sullivan and Skelcher, 2002). These include:

- an integrated, holistic approach to policy and service delivery
- overcoming narrow organisational perspectives ('the silo mentality')
- reducing transaction costs
- reducing overlap and duplication
- improving coordination
- developing innovative approaches
- pooling resources and expertise
- sharing knowledge
- tackling complex issues beyond the capacity of one agency.

Powell and Glendinning (2002, p 3) defined partnership as 'the involvement of at least two agents or agencies with at least some common interests or interdependencies; and would also probably require a relationship between them that involved a degree of trust, equality or reciprocity.' Although such definitions provide a useful starting point, the reality is more complex. Partnership arrangements vary considerably in practice. Even so, there is much consensus about the factors that promote effective partnership working (Hudson and Hardy, 2002; Sullivan and Skelcher, 2002; Cameron and Lart, 2003; Dowling et al, 2004; Cameron et al, 2014). These include: trust; a clearly agreed and realistic purpose; a common vision; joint commitment; leadership and accountability; the longevity of a partnership; previous history of collaboration; good communication and willingness to share information; incentives; monitoring and evaluation (and willingness to learn from this); social capital and a favourable socioeconomic context; and adequate resources. Proximity (for example, co-location of workers from different agencies) and joint training of staff are also often identified as factors conducive to partnership working.

Policy, ideology and political parties

Much attention has been paid to the impact on policy of ideologies, such as conservatism, socialism or economic liberalism. In short, conservatism emphasises the importance of tradition, hierarchy, private property, paternalism and social order. Economic liberalism (or 'neoliberalism' in its modern formulation) stands for the primacy of markets, private property and freedom of the individual. Socialism emphasises equality, state ownership, collective action and social justice (Heywood, 1994). Although these ideologies have shaped policy in a number of ways, a key channel of influence has been the political party system.

Within the vast literature on party politics (Montero and Gunther, 2003) lie two main bodies of theory that aid our understanding of the changes and continuities in health policy. The first concerns the adoption of policy positions by parties. It includes rational choice theories, which conceive parties as positioning themselves on an ideological continuum to maximise public votes and gain office (Downs, 1957). This approach has been superseded by 'soft rational' approaches (see Strom, 1990) which acknowledge the constraints on rational choice and party competition, such as the 'pull' of activists' views and the impact of electoral and parliamentary systems. There is now also greater acknowledgement of political strategy, which incorporates expectations about future election results (Robertson, 1976).

Parties follow public opinion to some extent (Bara and Budge, 2001; Hobolt and Klemmemsen, 2005), and are more likely to respond to public opinion when it is shifting away from them (Adams et al, 2004). Increasingly, party competition in the UK is characterised by 'issue competition'. The key arguments are about which issues should be on the party political agenda rather than between different ideological positions (Green-Pedersen, 2007). As ideology becomes less prominent, voting behaviour depends more on the perceived competence of parties to govern (Green, 2007). Party policies tend to converge as they compete for the public vote, and, correspondingly, are less influenced by activists and core supporters (Bara and Budge, 2001). If necessary, parties will adopt competitors' policies to increase votes, even though this means more policy consensus (Webb, 2000).

The second set of theories explores the impact of changes of parties in office on government policy. According to some, parties have a major impact. Crossman (1972) for example, characterised parties as the 'battering rams of change'. This is seen as particularly true in majoritarian democracies, where governments tend to be run by a single party rather than a coalition (Klingemann et al, 1994). An alternative view is that parties are one of many influences on policy, and that their impact is much weaker (Rose, 1984; Rose and Davies, 1994; Webb, 2000). Incoming governments are constrained by practical factors (such as the time and effort needed to reverse previous legislation as well as the costs of implementing new initiatives), and political factors (such as the power of vested interests, media influence and public opinion). Other events and circumstances also play a part in constraining governments. According to Rose (1984, p 141), 'much of a party's record will be stamped upon it by forces outside its control' and that these constraints produce a 'moving consensus' rather than dramatic policy change.

Furthermore, party policy is influenced by competition and collaboration between parties (Webb, 2000). Parties may borrow ideas from each other in an effort to gain electoral advantage, or to solve an intractable policy problem, although they rarely acknowledge this. Moreover, party policy influences the formation of governing coalitions, although this effect is stronger in some political systems than others (Laver and Budge, 1992). There are circumstances where parties dependent on each other for support (for example, through governing coalitions or electoral pacts) will compromise on policy. The desire for office can overcome policy differences. According to Riker's (1962) theory of minimum winning coalitions, there is an incentive for coalitions to include members only up to the point where they form a majority over their opponents (in order to maximise the benefits of office and to minimise the division of spoils). Research in Europe has found that Riker's theory accurately predicts outcomes in over a third of cases (Laver and Schofield, 1998), a substantial proportion given the possible permutations of coalitions across different countries.

Coalitions are relatively rare in UK national politics, although more common in local government. The Conservative–Liberal Democrat coalition government that took office in 2010 was the first formal national coalition for over 60 years, following an inconclusive general election (Clark, 2012). Scotland, Wales and Northern Ireland, whose devolved assemblies are elected through systems of proportional representation, have shown a greater tendency to produce coalition governments (see Chapter Nine).

For the UK Parliament, party competition has been mainly between three political parties, each with different ideological traditions (see Clark, 2012, and **Box 1.1**). The 'first past the post' system for Westminster elections rewards the two most popular parties (during the post-war period,

Labour and the Conservatives) with a disproportionate number of seats in Parliament. Nationalist parties, whose support is concentrated, can also win a disproportionately greater number of seats than their share of the vote might indicate. It has tended to produce 'majority governments', where the winning party can govern alone. The swing of the political pendulum has allowed each main party the opportunity to bring its own policies to bear on government, often over a number of years, and in some cases (for example, the Conservatives between 1979–97 and Labour from 1997–2010), over a decade. However, there is now less loyalty to the two major parties than was once the case. In recent years other parties have attracted more public support, notably the UK Independence Party (UKIP). As a result, it may become increasingly difficult for single parties to win an overall majority and to form a government alone (though this did not prevent the Conservative Party from forming a government, albeit with a small majority, in 2015).

Box 1.1: The Conservative, Labour and Liberal Democrat Parties

Conservative Party

The modern Conservative Party emerged in the 1830s (Blake, 1985). It is the most successful party, having been in government more often than any of its rivals (Cocker and Jones, 2002, p 123). Since the Second World War the Conservative Party has been in national government on the following occasions: 1951–64, 1970–74 and 1979–97. It was a senior partner in a coalition government with the Liberal Democrats between 2010–15. The Party encapsulates a range of standpoints, although certain principles have been fairly constant. These include an emphasis on individual responsibility, private property and enterprise, and a dislike of the state, public spending and taxation. However, this has been counterbalanced by a 'One Nation' tradition within the Party that emphasises paternalism, social order and the protection of the weak and vulnerable. For most of the postwar period, despite its preference for private ownership and markets, the Party accepted the need for substantial state intervention in the economy and social welfare.

With regard to health policy, the Conservative Party was opposed to the NHS at the outset because it was a nationalised state system, although it acknowledged the need for a comprehensive system of healthcare. When in government, however, it reached an accommodation with the NHS largely for pragmatic reasons, not least of which was the popularity of the service. Under the leadership of Margaret Thatcher, the Party shifted to the right and placed greater emphasis on neoliberal ideas such as privatisation and the increased use of markets. However, it remained publicly committed to the NHS. Since then the Conservative Party leadership has sought to reassure the public of its support for the NHS.

Labour Party

The Labour Party was formed by socialist societies and trade unions in 1900. After a spell as the 'Third Party', it overtook the Liberal Party as one of the two major parties of government. Since the Second World War it has been in government during the following periods: 1945–51, 1964–70, 1974–79 and 1997–2010. Like the Conservative Party, the Labour Party is a broad church, and its policies have shifted over time. Its fundamental principles are rooted in socialism. Broadly, socialism seeks to use the state to improve social justice through redistribution of wealth and the regulation of capitalist enterprise. Although Labour established the NHS as a nationalised service, it allowed the continued provision of private healthcare (even within the NHS itself, in the form of pay beds; see Chapter Two). However, the Party became more hostile to private medicine in the 1970s.

Following general election defeats in the 1980s and 1990s, the Labour Party rebranded itself as 'New Labour', under the leadership of Tony Blair. This involved a more pragmatic approach, which led the Party to embrace policies adopted by previous Conservative governments, such as the use of private finance to build and run healthcare facilities, greater use of private providers to supply care for NHS patients, more patient choice and the use of market forces to allocate resources within the NHS. This continued to some extent, although accompanied by a more traditional Labour rhetoric, under the leadership of Blair's successor, Gordon Brown. Notably, Labour campaigned against the coalition's NHS reforms despite these being an extension of its own policies pursued while in office.

Liberal Democrats

The Liberal Democrats (or Lib Dems) were formed from a merger between the Social Democratic Party (SDP) and the Liberal Party in 1988. The SDP was formed during the early 1980s by a breakaway group of Labour MPs (who were disillusioned with the Party's shift to the left). The Liberal Party had a long tradition in British politics, having formed governments in the 19th and early 20th centuries. However, as support for the Labour Party grew, it was reduced to a small rump of Members of Parliament (MPs). In the postwar period, it built a significant presence in local politics, and also acted as a haven for protest votes against the two main parties, especially at Westminster by-elections. The Liberal Democrats began to make some headway in general elections particularly after 1997, increasing their share of parliamentary seats. Following the inconclusive 2010 general election, the Liberal Democrats formed a coalition with the Conservatives. However, the party suffered a heavy defeat at the 2015 general election.

The Liberal Democrats' policies on health have tended to resemble Labour's traditional policies in several respects (emphasising the importance of the NHS as a public service), while urging greater local accountability. They have also acknowledged the role of patient choice and the need to improve management, flexibility and efficiency in service provision, which are traditionally Conservative policies. In recent years the leadership of the Liberal Democrats has been more disposed to market solutions than its predecessors, and more in tune with the Conservatives' public service reform agenda (Clark, 2012).

The 'doctrine of the mandate', which states that a party victorious at a general election is entitled to carry out its manifesto commitments, has carried considerable weight in the UK (see Birch, 1964). This gives doubtful legitimacy to a government, however. Few people actually read manifestos, which are often vague in their commitments. Furthermore, to vote for a party's manifesto does not mean that one supports the entire range of policies contained therein. Some argue that manifestos have now fallen into disrepute. According to Hilder (2005), for example, '… manifestos have slid towards marketing tools: undemocratic in their compilation, treated cavalierly after elections, they are anyway too general to determine every decision in the years that follow.' Indeed, circumstances can render some manifesto commitments redundant. They may be difficult or impossible to implement for political and technical reasons. Alternatively, by entering a coalition, a party may drop key manifesto commitments (as the Liberal Democrats infamously did in 2010 on the issue of abolishing university fees).

In trying to assess the impact of party politics on health, one is concerned with much more than the formal positions of parties set out in manifestos and other policy documents. Party politics involves a great deal of posturing. A party's stated intentions are not necessarily matched by its actions in office. Moreover, other intended policies may be unarticulated or deliberately understated because of fears of internal party divisions or handing electoral opponents an advantage.

In practice, the ideological breadth of the parties, coupled with the pragmatic nature of British government, has generated substantial consensus on policy matters (Beer, 1965; Addison, 1975). This was certainly the case in the immediate post-war period, but has been true to some extent since, despite the polarisation of the parties during the 1980s. Margaret Thatcher's Conservative Party, strongly influenced by neoliberalism, introduced radical policies such as the privatisation of nationalised industries and the introduction of markets in public services (Marsh and Rhodes, 1992a). However, tensions with traditional Conservative Party values, coupled with the unpopularity of some measures and the difficulties of implementation, diluted this radical programme. As Chapter Two shows, this was particularly true in health policy. Thatcher's successor, John Major, proved more pragmatic, which led to health policies formulated in the 1980s being implemented in a much less ideological fashion than originally envisaged.

Under the 'New Labour' government of Tony Blair between 1997 and 2007, the role of ideology was even less clear. During the 1990s, Labour adopted Conservative policies in an effort to capture votes (Bara and Budge, 2001). Once in government, its policy incorporated elements of both neoliberalism and socialism. This was heralded as the 'Third Way' (Giddens, 1998), drawing heavily on communitarian ideas that involved the rebalancing of individuals' rights and responsibilities while combining choice and enterprise with social justice. The Blair government maintained key elements of policy from the Conservative years – the emphasis on markets to allocate resources, a growing role for the private sector, the centralised performance management of public services and an emphasis on consumerism. The NHS was not exempt from these policy trends.

Chapter Two shows that health policy remains a key issue of party political contention. Health issues are emotive and attract considerable media attention. The NHS is a key area of public expenditure, employs a large workforce, and provides services for the vast majority of the population. Politicians of all parties cannot ignore these factors, and will always strive to gain electoral advantage in this key policy area.

An alternative approach is to see ideological factors as transcending political parties rather than operating through them. According to this perspective, the 'worldview' of those within government is shaped by contextual factors, which, in effect, 'short-circuit' the system of party politics. Politicians and senior bureaucrats find themselves adopting similar positions irrespective of their ideological tendencies. This worldview is intimately connected to ideas about the role of the state, particularly with regard to the economy and social welfare. Indeed, several authors have shown how health policy is shaped by the paradigms of economic and social policy (Klein, 2000) and the context of the welfare state and capitalist economic arrangements (Moran, 1999, 2000; Greener, 2004b).

Policy as the interplay of interests

Policy can be viewed as the product of interplay between different interests with particular goals and values (Bentley, 1967; Baggott, 1995; Grant, 2000). These interests may be organised or diffuse. However, most emphasis has been placed on the participation of organised interests in the policy process, known as pressure groups, defined by Coxall (2001, p 3) as 'any organisation that aims to influence public policy by seeking to persuade decision-makers by lobbying rather than by standing for election and holding office'.

Pressure group theorists see interaction between such organisations and government as central to the policy process. Policy outcomes are determined by the relative influence of groups, which have a range of resources. Groups that have financial resources can mobilise their members and the wider public, have good political contacts with decision-makers, and tend to have more influence over policy. Tactics and strategy also play an important part, and knowledge and understanding of the policy process is crucial. In the British system of government, where policy-making is concentrated in the hands of central government, groups that have good contacts at this level – so-called insider groups – are believed to be in a strong position to influence policy (Grant, 2000). Those that lack this status – outsider groups – are regarded as less influential. However, this simple model has been undermined by three factors: the growing impact of 'outsider' groups, such as the environmental lobby, on agendas and policy decisions (Ridley and Jordan, 1998); the decline in influence of some traditional insider groups, such as trade unions and some professional organisations; and recognition that central government institutions are relatively accessible, which means that relatively few organisations are refused contact if they seek it (Maloney et al, 1994).

The health policy process is host to a wide range of pressure groups: professional and labour organisations, commercial interests and health consumer groups, as well as voluntary organisations and single-issue groups (see Chapter Six). Health policy is also a haven for social movements, which promote particular values among the population, encourage direct action by groups and individuals, and seek to influence policy agendas (see **Box 6.2**).

Any consideration of pressure groups and social movements in health policy must also acknowledge the underlying structural interests relating to capital and labour. Marxists see these as setting the parameters within which issues and policies arise (see O'Connor, 1973; Doyal, 1979; Miliband, 1982; Offe, 1984). For example, with regard to healthcare, Navarro (1978) argued that the capitalist system forecloses certain policy options and facilitates others. Using a different approach, Alford (1975) identified three structural interests in the US healthcare system: the dominant professional interest, the challenging corporate and managerial interest, and the repressed community interest. According to his model, the professional interest maintains its supremacy through underlying power generated by the social structure, and in particular, by an ability to define the values of the healthcare system. His approach has been applied to the UK, with some modification (see Baggott et al, 2005).

Another concept used in the analysis of pressure group politics and government–group relations is the 'policy network' (Richardson and Jordan, 1979; Marsh and Rhodes, 1992b; Smith, 1993). This focuses on relationships between government agencies and NGOs as the key to understanding policy formation and implementation. Marsh and Rhodes (1992b) identified two types of policy network – close-knit and stable 'policy communities', which exhibit a high degree of interdependence between government agencies and NGOs, and 'issue networks', which are more open, less stable and exhibit low levels of interdependence. The policy networks approach has moved beyond describing and categorising different types of relationship towards analysis of the impact of networks on policy (see Smith, 1993; Marsh and Smith, 2000). There has been an increasing interest in the dynamics of policy networks, and in particular, how they change in response to external and internal pressures (see Baumgartner and Jones, 1993; Richardson, 2000). Of particular interest is how governments have applied different approaches to the 'management' of policy networks, how the membership of networks has changed, and how this has affected policy processes and outputs.

Applying the concept of policy networks to health policy facilitates a mapping of the range of government agencies and NGOs involved in this policy arena. It is also useful in posing questions about how changing relationships between government and groups might affect policy formation, implementation and outcomes. Indeed, it appears that the tightly knit 'policy community' that characterised the immediate postwar period, exemplified by the close relationship between the British Medical Association (BMA) and the Ministry of Health, has given way to the looser and more inclusive 'issue network', involving groups representing patients and carers, for example (see Chapter Six).

Policy, institutions and agendas

The so-called 'new institutionalism' revived interest in how political institutions can shape policy. As March and Olsen (1984, p 738) argued, 'the bureaucratic agency, the legislative committee, and the appellate court are arenas for contending social forces, but they are also collections of standard operating procedures and structures that define and defend interests. They are political actors in their own right.' The novelty of this approach has been disputed (Jordan, 1990; Rhodes, 1997; Hudson and Lowe, 2004). Critics maintain that institutions have always been part of policy analysis. Nonetheless, it is acknowledged that new institutionalism has reiterated the importance of institutions in the policy process, and in particular, the way in which they structure interaction between policy actors.

A strand of new institutionalism focuses on the role of institutions in promoting stability and continuity. The path dependency model (David, 1985; Berman, 1998) is based on an assumption that institutions and previous decisions exert a strong influence over current policy-making. The outcome is incremental rather than radical change. This model has been applied to health systems reform (see Immergut, 1992; Wilsford, 1994; Greener, 2006), where divergence between countries has been attributed to institutional factors within each political system. This approach has been criticised for being too deterministic. Radical changes do happen, notably the creation of the UK National Health Service (NHS) in 1948.

Supporters of the path dependency approach, however, deny that today's decisions are automatically determined by past decisions. They believe that their model allows for deviation from the path that previous decisions and existing institutions have set, although only under exceptional circumstances. Wilsford (1994), for example, argued that there are certain factors that can enable decision-makers to break out of the status quo, including the manipulation of incentives within institutions, the development of new technologies and 'conjecture' about future policy options. He also argued that centralised political systems – such as the UK – can be more effective in introducing large-scale reform. However, others argue that centralisation can prevent innovation and the emergence of new policies and practices from the bottom up (Greener, 2006). Path dependency is linked to a broader perspective that seeks to take account of the role of both time and learning in the policy process. Pollitt (2008) argues that we need to learn from the past, and this will enable better policy-making in the future. This appears particularly pertinent to the NHS where successive reorganisations have been implemented with apparently little regard for past experience (see Chapter Seven).

Policy change is closely connected with the setting of agendas and how issues are selected for debate and intervention. Downs (1972) identified an 'issue-attention' cycle, whereby issues attracted public attention, leading to pressure on government to intervene, only for the issue to subside as the costs of intervention became known. Others have noted that the emergence of an issue on the agenda does not necessarily reflect its importance in terms of social impact or cost (Cobb and Elder, 1972). This is more closely related to various 'triggers', such as the issue's ability to attract media attention and the efforts of those seeking to get the issue on to the agenda – including interest groups and even government institutions. It should be noted that political actors vary in their ability to shape agendas (Schattschneider, 1960). Agenda setting is regarded as the 'second face of power' (Bachrach and Baratz, 1962), enabling powerful interests to prevent decisions that adversely affect their interests from being considered. There is also a 'third face' of power – the manipulation of values. Powerful interests, institutions and the media are able to shape perceptions of issues and problems in order to prevent them from being publicly acknowledged (Lukes, 1974).

Related to this is the notion that policy is often a symbolic activity. There may be situations where government cannot solve a problem, or is perhaps reluctant to tackle it for fear of offending powerful interests. The government may devise a symbolic policy in order to maintain its legitimacy and authority. Government engages extensively in 'spin' and media manipulation of policy (see Fairclough, 2000; Jones, 2002), and is not afraid to use 'placebo policies' to convince people that action is taking place, even when it is not (Richardson and Moon, 1984). It is therefore vitally important that policy analysis should take into account the importance of language, discourse and symbolism. Several authors have considered this, notably Edelman (1964, 1971, 1977, 1985), who saw a tendency for government to adopt emotional symbols rather than tangible activities. Indeed, much government activity is concerned with public reassurance – appearing to do something rather than actually solving problems. Such an approach to policy analysis focuses on the role of the media and other policy actors in defining problems and policies. It takes a critical approach to methods used by government and by other participants in the policy process, and sees the underlying purpose of policy-making as a means of reducing public power, avoiding dealing with serious public problems and benefiting powerful interests in society. This is in marked contrast to rational models of policy-making based on normative assumptions of public good.

These concepts are highly relevant to health policy. Health issues are prominent on the political agenda, but some (such as mental health and chronic illness) tend to get less attention and less sympathetic coverage than others (breast cancer, for example). Furthermore, health policy is host to powerful commercial interests (such as the drugs, alcoholic drinks, food and tobacco industries) that seek to influence the perception of health issues. Meanwhile, government itself, which sees health as a highly political issue, is keen to influence the public perception of its management of the health system and its stewardship of public health. It is keen to create an impression that it is actively doing something and is taking the best course of action (Morrell and Hewison, 2013). Moreover, the emotive nature of health issues, and their intractability, increases the scope for symbolic policy-making. These issues are explored further in Chapter Five, in the context of mass media.

Also relevant here is Kingdon's (1984) 'policy windows' model, whereby policy is shaped by a complex interaction between three 'streams':

• *Problem stream*, which comprises problems that the government is considering – this is influenced by measures indicating such problems (such as NHS waiting lists, for example), by events (such as outbreaks of infectious disease) and feedback (on current performance, for example, to what extent health targets have been met).

- *Policy stream*, where ideas about how to deal with problems circulate within policy networks and among 'political entrepreneurs' who play a crucial role in 'selling' policy ideas.
- *Political stream*, which consists of public opinion, organised political forces (such as parties and pressure groups), government and processes of building support and consensus.

Kingdon argues that when these various streams come together (a problem gets on to the agenda, there is a perceived policy solution to this problem, and the political situation is supportive) a 'launch window' opens, enabling policy change to take place.

Policy as an adaptive, learning process

The policy process can be seen as an adaptive process that involves learning about the policy environment, the potential policy options and the political resources of supporters and opponents. One of the best-known exponents of this approach is Sabatier (1987, 1999; see also Jenkins-Smith and Sabatier, 1994), who argues that the key to understanding policy lies in the advocacy coalitions that inhabit 'policy subsystems'. These consist of interest groups, politicians, policy advisers and experts, journalists and commentators as well as professionals, civil servants and service providers, endorsing a particular set of ideas and beliefs about policy in a particular policy subsystem.

Policy change occurs in two main ways. First, external factors, such as socioeconomic conditions or changes in government, can affect fundamental policy positions (known as the policy core). More commonly, however, 'secondary' changes in policy will occur, and this results from policy–oriented learning within advocacy coalitions as well as between them. This policy-oriented learning takes the form of adaptation in the light of experience as advocacy coalitions seek to refashion their strategies and policy ideas. 'Policy brokers' mediate conflicting strategies, aiming to achieve a compromise that will reduce the intensity of conflict. Even so, the model is based on an assumption that policy change can only be understood over a long timespan – a decade or more.

Other models have emphasised the importance of learning within the policy environment. There is a growing literature on the role of experts in policy-making, such as academics, scientists and other professionals (see Collingridge and Reeve, 1986; Fischer, 1990; Barker and Peters, 1993). Although experts do not necessarily determine policy, they can exert influence over policy through legitimacy accorded to their scientific advice. Others may exert influence over the implementation of policy. In the health field, government has relied heavily on medical experts to advise on policy, both individually and via advisory bodies. Government is also dependent on doctors to implement government guidelines and policies, giving the profession considerable leverage (Moran, 1999; Klein, 2000; Salter, 2004).

Another important aspect of policy-oriented learning is 'policy transfer' (Bennett, 1991; Dolowitz and Marsh, 1996; Evans and Davies, 1999; Dolowitz, 2010; Dunlop and Radaelli, 2013) and 'lesson drawing' (Rose, 1991). Policy transfer may involve the movement of policy goals, instruments, institutions, ideologies and ideas, and concepts between other countries or jurisdictions. Lesson drawing is a similar concept that focuses on the process of learning from the policy experiences of other countries/jurisdictions. Policy transfer and lesson drawing may take a stronger form such as direct copying and emulation of policies, or it may be weaker, involving the adaptation of policies from elsewhere, or some form of policy blending from different sources. Policy transfer can take place at various levels: global, national and local, as well as between these levels.

Barriers to policy transfer and policy learning include time constraints, past policies, different political/institutional/structural settings, limited resources and ideological constraints. Facilitators include economic and political pressures to adopt common approaches, consensus on policy problems and solutions, and communication systems and networks that enable the sharing of policy experiences. The key routes for policy transfer include professional networks, political networks, networks of research and expertise, supranational bodies (government and non-governmental), think tanks and policy entrepreneurs. Policy transfer and lesson drawing is important in the health sector. Indeed, NHS reforms such as commissioning, internal markets, privatisation and foundation trusts have been influenced by policies adopted in other countries (see Chapter Ten).

Policy-oriented learning is not confined to policy 'successes', real or apparent. Knowledge and understanding of policy failures and disaster can have an impact on policy debates. Policy learning can occur at the regional and local level (and between different states and territories of a country in federal and devolved systems of government; see Chapter Nine). For example, locally devised policies may have a positive impact on a problem, and this experience could be shared and taken up by other local areas. Alternatively, local experiments and pilot projects may be established in a deliberate effort to inform and encourage future policy development elsewhere.

Health policy analysis

In this book, a 'multiple lens approach' has been adopted (Sabatier, 1999). It does not focus on a single model of the policy process, but is open to the possibility that all models may potentially contribute to our understanding of health policy. Most of the analytical approaches discussed so far are generic. They can be applied to policy processes in any field of domestic or international policy. However, context is important, and any framework of analysis must be sensitive to this. Moreover, it is not only the current context that is important. As Heinz et al (1993), in their study of the policy process in the US observed, policy-making systems have historically situated social structures. Historical circumstance is important in shaping different policy domains such as health, education, criminal justice and so on, which often display different features and policy styles.

Health policy, as defined here, certainly has a number of distinctive features: it is an arena occupied by high-profile political issues; health issues are high on both government and public agendas; government is accountable for a national health service; there are powerful pressure groups involved as well as social movements; it is an area of considerable media interest; it absorbs a significant chunk of public expenditure; and yet it is a field of substantial commercial opportunities. Any approach must be able to capture these key features in a dynamic way, reflecting the weight of historical circumstances as well as contemporary political forces.

The chapters that follow examine different aspects of the health policy process, and are based on secondary sources and primary research. Chapter Two explores the impact of party politics and ideology in national policy. Chapter Three examines the role of central government, and Chapter Four, Parliament. Chapter Five analyses the role of the media in health policy, while Chapter Six looks at the activities of interest groups and external organisations. The following three chapters explore health policy at local and regional level, and in other parts of the UK that possess devolved powers and responsibilities for health. The penultimate chapter considers the international dimension and role of global institutions. Finally, the analysis is brought together to draw conclusions about the nature of the contemporary health policy process in the UK.

Summary

- Health policy is a contested term.
- Health policy can be examined by using several conceptual frameworks.

Key questions

1. What is health policy?
2. What are the main conceptual frameworks for understanding health policy?

Party politics and health policy

Overview

This chapter explores the role of political parties in relation to health policy, focusing primarily on England (Chapter Nine considers party politics elsewhere in the UK in the context of devolution). It explores the salience of health issues in party politics, then goes on to examine the impact of party politics on health policy since the creation of the NHS.

As noted in Chapter One, parties are important political institutions that can shape policy. However, there is disagreement about the extent of their impact. This chapter explores the role of political parties in health policy and assesses their influence. It focuses mainly on UK-wide political parties and health policy in England. Most health policy matters relating to Scotland, Wales and Northern Ireland are devolved to their national governments. The influence of party politics in these countries is explored in the context of devolution in Chapter Nine.

Health policy is often seen as a party political football. It is a major issue of debate between the political parties. Health issues are often prominent at election time, and have been a source of party political conflict (see **Box 2.1**). Issues relating to health and health services are a concern to most people, and so politicians must be ready to take a position and make commitments. Furthermore, the NHS is generally popular and is a major employer, both of which heighten political sensitivity. Moreover, health and the NHS are key areas of government responsibility and public expenditure. They are therefore important in judging the competence of governing parties seeking to retain office (and also in assessing the policies of opposition parties seeking office). Health and the NHS invariably appear among the most salient issues of public importance. This level of public interest is expressed and reinforced by media interest in health matters (explored more fully in Chapter Five).

Box 2.1: Health policies, parties and elections, 1992–2010

Although the NHS has long been a prominent political issue, its emergence as an election issue is a more recent phenomenon (Klein, 2001). The turning point was the 1987 General Election, when the NHS was the Conservatives' weakest issue but Labour's strongest. Labour focused heavily on health in this campaign, featuring cases of patients facing long delays for treatment. The Conservatives responded by defending their record and accusing Labour of hypocrisy, identifying examples where senior party members or their relatives had used private healthcare.

At the 1992 General Election, health was again a key issue. Labour criticised the Conservative government for introducing a 'two-tier' system of healthcare and commercial values into the NHS. During the campaign, a major row was sparked by a Labour political broadcast which portrayed a young girl needing an ear operation, but who remained on an NHS waiting list as her family were unable to afford private treatment. The resulting furore – known as the 'War of Jennifer's Ear' – initially put pressure on the Conservative government. However, Labour was subsequently criticised for exaggerating an actual case, and for involving a child in such a highly charged political arena. Labour was also accused of leaking the identity of the girl, which was strenuously denied. But as the facts of the case were now in dispute, the government was able to sidestep the issue.

Health was again a major issue in the 1997 General Election campaign. Labour campaigned strongly for the NHS, culminating in Tony Blair's declaration that 'the very simple choice that people have in the next 24 hours is this. It is 24 hours to save our National Health Service' (Blair, 1997). Strong public support for Labour's policies on the NHS was regarded as an important factor in the Party's election victory.

Health was also a prominent issue at the 2001 General Election. Controversy surrounded the Labour Party's policy of increasing private provision of NHS services, indicating a shift towards Conservative policies. There was a tense moment for Labour campaigners when Tony Blair, visiting a Birmingham hospital, was ambushed by a woman who challenged him about the problems in her partner's cancer care, in full view of the television cameras (Rawnsley, 2001, pp 488-9). This incident passed with no visible impact on the polls. An interesting twist, however, was the election of an independent MP, Dr Richard Taylor, who was elected due to his campaign against the closure of services at Kidderminster General Hospital. He was also re-elected at the 2005 General Election.

Health was once again high on the agenda at the 2005 General Election. The main issues in this campaign were hospital cleanliness, NHS bureaucracy, the role of the private sector and the distorting effect of government targets. At the 2010 General Election, health was not a prominent issue (Timmins, 2012). This was partly due to increased satisfaction levels with the NHS, which meant that the opposition parties had less traction to criticise the government. Another factor was that Labour now fully embraced Conservative policies such as choice, competition and the use of private providers in the NHS. The Conservatives, meanwhile, had sought to defuse the NHS as a political issue by backing funding increases and scrapping schemes to subsidise private payments for healthcare (Bale, 2010; Timmins, 2012).

Another reason why health has been a key issue in party politics is that it has provided a focus for ideological conflict between the two main political parties. The creation of the NHS fitted neatly with the Labour Party's traditional support for collective responses to social problems, but was at odds with the Conservative Party's essential values of individual responsibility, private enterprise and market forces (see **Box 1.1**). Although the Conservatives subsequently accepted the NHS, they continued to explore ways of increasing individual responsibility and curbing the costs of healthcare expenditure. The 1970s brought conflict over pay beds and public expenditure, and, in the next two decades, attempts to privatise parts of the NHS and to introduce market forces exposed further ideological divisions. The differences became less clear in recent years as Labour endorsed individualist, market-based and private sector-oriented reforms. Nonetheless, the rhetorical elements of ideological debate remained strong. These trends are now explored more closely.

Party politics and health policy 1945–1997

Creation of the NHS

By 1945 there was a broad consensus about the need for a comprehensive health service (Webster, 1988; Klein, 1995; Powell, 1997). This emerged out of dissatisfaction with the fragmented and inequitable health services of the interwar period, the deliberations of the wartime coalition government about social reconstruction, and the experiences of emergency health service planning. Nonetheless, following the collapse of the wartime coalition and Labour's victory at the 1945 General Election, there was much division on how best to proceed with health services reform.

The Conservative Party manifesto of 1945 proposed 'a comprehensive health service covering the whole range of medical treatment from the general practitioner to the specialist ...', and promised that services would be accessible to all irrespective of ability to pay (Craig, 1975, p 118). Although acknowledging the role of the state, the Conservatives emphasised choice and individual enterprise. They wished to retain the voluntary hospital sector, working alongside local authority hospitals. Labour, on the other hand, was committed to public ownership. However, its manifesto gave little detail beyond a declaration that 'the best health services should be available to all' and that 'money must no longer be the passport to the best treatment' (Craig, 1975, p 129).

Once in office, with Aneurin Bevan as Minister of Health, Labour's plans developed further. Despite support within the Party for a local government-run health service, Bevan brought both voluntary and local authority hospitals into a nationalised health service. Local authorities remained responsible for community health services and public health functions. Separate bodies (executive councils) were established to administer the NHS contracts of general practitioners (GPs) and other family practitioners.

Conservative MPs took the unconventional step of opposing the NHS Bill at its Third Reading in the House of Commons (Foot, 1975, pp 155-6). The Conservatives were hostile to hospital nationalisation. However, Labour's large (146 seat) majority in the Commons was sufficient to enable it to achieve its legislative aims. Only minor concessions were granted during the passage of the Bill. Others were made after the legislation had been passed, in order to secure the cooperation of GPs (Webster, 1988).

The partisan debates that surrounded the creation of the NHS were somewhat misleading. They reflected the restoration of peacetime adversarial politics, and gave the parties an opportunity to attack each other. In reality, the creation of the NHS was more the product of a continuing and developing consensus rather than the clash of party ideologies (Webster, 1988; Klein, 1995).

It was intended that the NHS would be free at the point of use. However, the cost of the service was higher than expected. This created pressures for greater economy. In 1949, the Labour government acquired powers to levy prescription charges, but this was not implemented. However, in 1951, after narrowly winning the General Election of the previous year, the Labour government decided to impose charges, including fees for dental treatment and ophthalmic services. This led to Bevan's resignation (who had, by now, moved to another department) and two other ministers, including the future Prime Minister, Harold Wilson. Later that year, another general election was called, from which the Conservative Party emerged victorious.

Consensus years?

Given that the creation of the NHS was seen as the post-war Labour government's 'most intrinsically socialist proposition' (Foot, 1975, p 104), one might expect it to have been a target for the incoming government. However, it had become an issue of considerable cross-party agreement. By 1958, the Conservative Minister Iain Macleod was able to claim that, with the exception of charges, health was 'out of party politics' (quoted in Klein, 1995, p 29). But there was even continuity on that issue, as in 1952 the Conservatives introduced health service charges that Labour had previously proposed. At times, however, the consensus was fragile. The Conservative government established a review of the NHS, seen as an attempt to curb expenditure and to restrict the scope of the service, although the review identified a shortfall in funding, and strengthened the case for the NHS to continue in its present form (Committee of Inquiry into the Cost of the National Health Service, 1956). As Rivett (1998, p 114) observed, henceforth 'it became impossible for governments to attack the NHS'.

Later in the 1950s, the Conservative government considered proposals that might have undermined consensus (Webster, 1988, 1996). These included extending charges to cover boarding costs for inpatients (a proposal later explored by Labour), ending free NHS dental services, and imposing fees for GP consultations. Alternative ways of funding the NHS, through a compulsory insurance scheme, were also explored. But these plans never materialised. First, the level of public support for the NHS kept ideological tendencies in check. The Conservatives were reluctant to introduce reforms that might be interpreted by the public as reducing entitlement to health services (Lowe, 1993). To have done so might have given the Labour Party greater electoral support. Even fairly minor proposals, such as small increases in prescription charges, were highly sensitive. When Enoch Powell, as Conservative Health Minister during the early 1960s, decided to raise charges and cut services, he faced fierce public criticism, giving the Labour opposition much political ammunition (Webster, 1996, p 88).

The second reason why the Conservatives did little to disturb the consensus on the NHS was that many of its leading MPs subscribed to 'One Nation' Conservatism, which emphasised the protection of the weak and vulnerable in society, and stressed the importance of civic values and social responsibility (see **Box 1.1**). Furthermore, many new Conservative MPs entering Parliament in the 1950s held these views (Webster, 1988, p 187). This shaped the political character of the Conservative Party in Parliament, and provided some protection against threats to the NHS from the right wing of the Party.

The 1960s and 1970s: reorganisation of the NHS and pay beds

The extent of party political consensus on the NHS was further revealed by the reorganisation of the service (see Chapter Seven). Party ideology had a marginal role in the proposals, first developed under a Labour government in the late 1960s, and then legislated for by the Conservatives in 1973, and finally implemented by another Labour government in 1974 (Klein, 1995). Although the parliamentary debates on the NHS Reorganisation Bill were characterised by adversarial rhetoric (Ingle and Tether, 1981), this posturing had little impact on the eventual outcome.

The 1974 NHS reorganisation was probably the high point of the postwar consensus. The years that followed brought more conflict, and increasingly the rhetoric was matched by real policy differences. The first signs emerged in the mid-1970s in the form of the pay beds controversy (see Klein, 1995; Webster, 1996). The Labour government had a manifesto commitment to phase out beds for private patients in the NHS. The medical profession sensed a broader threat to private practice, and remained unconvinced by assurances from the minister responsible for the NHS (Barbara Castle) that she did not intend to outlaw private treatment. The doctors threatened industrial action. The crisis escalated when trade unions representing ancillary workers, who were in favour of getting rid of pay beds, took direct action, withdrawing services from some private wards. The government moved to placate the doctors, while seeking to reassure the trade unions and the left wing of the Labour Party. A compromise was reached to reduce pay beds, a policy reversed subsequently by the incoming Conservative government.

According to Klein (1995), the pay beds conflict was constrained by the underlying consensus. This consensus survived further challenges in the late 1970s, in the form of an economic crisis, public expenditure constraints and further industrial action. However, in the following decade, it faced a more severe test, with the election of a 'New Right' Conservative government whose ideology challenged the principles of the post-war welfare state on which the NHS was based.

Thatcherism

The Thatcher government, elected in 1979, was strongly influenced by the philosophy of neoliberalism. Neoliberalism consisted of ideas drawn from liberal economists, political scientists and philosophers (see, for example, Friedman, 1962; Olson, 1965; Hayek, 1976) who called for a much smaller state bureaucracy and less government intervention, a reduction in the power of organised labour, a bigger role for the private sector and market forces in the allocation of resources, greater individual responsibility and choice, more voluntary effort and self-reliance among individuals (Green, 1987). However, the Thatcher government was not purely neoliberal in outlook. It blended neoliberalism with traditional Conservative values such as strong government, hierarchy, maintenance of social order and paternalism (see Gamble, 1994).

Under Thatcher, the post-war settlement began to unravel. Industries such as gas, telecommunications and electricity were privatised, and there was deregulation of industry and commerce. Meanwhile, in the welfare state, social security entitlements were cut, and the long-standing commitment to full employment was dropped. Public services faced financial restraint in light of the government's aim to reduce public expenditure and taxes. The NHS could not escape these powerful trends. The Thatcher government encouraged private medicine (through tax incentives), introduced private sector management ideas into the NHS, allowed private companies to tender for NHS support services such as laundry, catering and cleaning, and extended and increased charges for prescriptions and other NHS services.

However, compared with other policy areas (such as the privatisation of nationalised industries and social housing, for example) the impact of neoliberal ideas on health policy was relatively small. Thatcher (1993, p 606) declared that although she wanted to see a flourishing private sector of health, the NHS and its basic principles was always a 'fixed point' in her policies. It is certainly true that she was an astute politician. Thatcher realised that health policy raised sensitive political issues that could lose votes. Instinctively she wanted to increase private health insurance, but acknowledged that the NHS was popular and that the public needed reassurance (Ham, 2000). When early in Thatcher's premiership a leaked report from a government think tank outlined the scope for privatisation of welfare, including the NHS, the Prime Minister was forced to declare that 'the NHS is safe with us' (Thatcher, 1982).

Public support for the NHS remained strong during the 1980s, which reduced the Thatcher government's room for manoeuvre (Fowler, 1991). But following a third electoral victory in 1987, Thatcher unleashed her NHS internal market reforms. The tone was radical. NHS bodies would become either purchasers or providers of specified health services. GPs would be given their own budgets to purchase care, while hospitals would be given a new self-governing status as NHS trusts. Resources would be allocated on the basis of contracts negotiated between purchasers and providers, the latter, in effect, competing for business. But this market ideal never fully materialised, and the plans were diluted, partly for practical reasons and partly due to a change of leadership.

The Major government

In 1990 Mrs Thatcher was replaced by John Major, regarded as a more genuine supporter of the NHS. In his first Party conference speech after becoming Conservative Party leader, he reiterated his commitment to the NHS, and ruled out further health service charges and the privatisation of healthcare. Nonetheless, his government continued to implement Thatcher's internal market, although in a much more cautious way than its original architects envisaged. The Major government also endorsed a greater role for the private sector in providing NHS support services and capital funding (see Chapter Seven).

Major did not share the ideological stance of Thatcher, and was more pragmatic. Although privatisation of support services and marketisation of the NHS continued under his stewardship, the expansion of private healthcare stalled (partly due to a prolonged economic recession). Major's pragmatism was also reinforced by political circumstances. The reformed Labour Party became more of an electoral threat. Moreover, after the 1992 General Election, Major's majority in Parliament was significantly reduced by by-election defeats and backbench rebellions.

The Major government also introduced *The patient's charter* (DH, 1991), an attempt to set out what service users might expect from the NHS. A similar idea was promoted by other parties (Labour Party, 1990; Liberal Democrats, 1992). The opposition parties also called for a national health strategy, with clear health targets, something that the Thatcher government had resisted. This was subsequently introduced by the Major government in the form of the *Health of the Nation* strategy (DH, 1992). These examples illustrate that the Major government was pragmatic enough to adopt policies advanced by its political opponents.

Party politics after 1997

New Labour

After 1979, the Labour Party shifted further to the left, reflected in its 1983 election manifesto, which called for further nationalisation, state control of industry, withdrawal from the European Community, nuclear disarmament and increased spending on welfare and public sector projects. With regard to health, it reiterated its commitments to phase out charges and to remove private practice from the NHS. These were accompanied by more radical aims, to take a major public stake in the drugs industry, and to take over parts of the private health sector and prevent its expansion.

Labour's defeat at the 1983 and 1987 General Elections forced a rethink. Under the leadership of Neil Kinnock (1983–92) and John Smith (1992–94), organisational changes were made to strengthen the Party leadership's control of the policy process, accompanied by policy reviews. Policy became less rooted in ideological considerations and more pragmatic, reflecting the Party's desperate desire to gain office (Jones, 1996). This process was continued by Tony Blair, following Smith's sudden death in 1994. Blair rebranded the Party as 'New Labour', and moderated its socialist principles. Notably, he secured revision of the symbolic Clause Four of the Labour Party constitution, which had committed it to state ownership, replacing it with a general statement about the importance of the community, equity and social justice. Blair also further strengthened the leadership grip on the Party's policy-making process (Webb, 2000).

In justifying these changes, Blair appealed primarily to the overriding imperative to gain office. But ideas also played a part. Blair drew on communitarian ideals, which emphasised the importance of balancing community values with individual responsibilities (see Etzioni, 1993; Tam, 1998). Communitarianism is a rather imprecise philosophy and well suited to those adopting a pragmatic approach. According to Driver and Martell (2002), there are different types of communitarianism. They argued that the approach adopted by New Labour promoted conservative values, was focused on individuals, was prescriptive and emphasised responsibilities as a condition for having rights.

A further key aspect of Blair's philosophy was the so-called 'Third Way' (Giddens, 1998; Driver and Martell, 2002). The essence of the Third Way was a set of governing principles that incorporated elements of both socialism and neoliberalism. The Third Way endorsed an inclusive and fair society with equality of opportunity, reflecting socialist principles. But it also incorporated neoliberal ideas by encouraging the use of markets and the private sector. It echoed neoliberal values by highlighting the importance of individualism and the entrepreneurial role of the modern state in resolving solutions to social and economic problems. The state was seen as requiring modernisation to make it fit for purpose, which included a pragmatic approach ('what counts is what works') and the break up of traditional state bureaucracies. The goal was to 'modernise' state institutions and to create new partnerships (with the private and voluntary sectors) that responded more effectively to the needs and preferences of the public. Blair supported public service reforms that increased choice, used market mechanisms, increased competition and promoted greater private sector involvement.

These changes in Party leadership, organisation and direction had ramifications for the Labour Party's policies on health. By 1987, it had already retreated from the most contentious statements contained in its previous manifesto. A new health strategy subsequently emerged (Labour Party, 1990, 1992). Labour pledged to abolish the Conservatives' internal market, proposing that the newly created NHS trusts would be brought back under local NHS control, and that the purchasing of services by 'fundholding' GPs would end. However, there were signs that Labour was beginning to accept some aspects of government policy. It proposed changes to the allocation of resources within the NHS to create incentives for providers that performed well. Labour was increasingly cautious about making spending commitments on the NHS, and earlier pledges to phase out health service charges were not repeated.

Another policy review in the mid-1990s reflected growing acceptance of the Conservatives' reforms. The Labour Party published further policy documents (Labour Party, 1994, 1995), which took a pragmatic approach. It accepted the division between purchasers and providers of healthcare, and said it would retain NHS trusts. However, it also proposed replacing GP fundholding with a system of commissioning covering all GPs. Hostility to the private sector also remained, as demonstrated by a commitment to abolishing tax relief on private health insurance.

Labour's victory, with a 179-seat majority in Parliament in the 1997 General Election (followed by a majority of 167 in 2001), gave it the legitimacy and ability to effect policy change. However, it was impossible to completely reverse 18 years of Conservative reform, even if Blair's government had wished to do so. During the period 1997–2000, New Labour set about implementing its manifesto commitments on health, including a key pledge to reduce waiting lists by 100,000 during the lifetime of the Parliament (DH, 1997). The internal market was reformed rather than totally dismantled. GP fundholding was replaced by local primary care commissioning groups, and the division between commissioners and providers remained. The Labour government fulfilled its commitment to get rid of health insurance tax breaks for the elderly. This contrasted with its decision to expand the role of the private sector in the financing, building and running of hospitals through private finance initiative (PFI) schemes (Shaw, 2004).

Labour adhered to the previous government's spending plans (Toynbee and Walker, 2001), which restricted health spending in the early years of the Blair government. However, financial pressures led to the allocation of further resources from contingency funds, and subsequently to a review of health spending, an unprecedented expansion of resources for the NHS (see Chapter Seven), and a new blueprint, in the form of *The NHS Plan* (DH, 2000).

In the period up to 2000, Labour policy closely reflected proposals developed in opposition. But with the advent of *The NHS Plan*, government policy began to depart from these principles (see Baggott, 2004; Greener,

2004a; Crinson, 2005). These developments reflected a desire by Blair and his allies to undertake a more radical reform programme for the NHS. Blair (2010) stated that he regretted not taking on NHS reform earlier in his term in office. In the early years of New Labour, radical reform was resisted by the Department of Health and its Secretary of State, Frank Dobson, a traditional 'old' Labour stalwart (Blair, 2010; Mandelson, 2011). His replacement by the 'Blairite' Alan Milburn signalled a more radical era. However, this was a 'gradual, pragmatic process rather than a one-off overarching "big bang" set of reforms' (Mays et al, 2011, p 6).

There were several strands. First, a greater role for the private sector in the NHS. PFI schemes were expanded, and a similar scheme for primary healthcare capital projects introduced. A concordat was agreed with the independent healthcare sector aimed at bringing about greater collaboration with the NHS (IHA and DH, 2000). The sector was offered opportunities to run 'failing' NHS services. A further opening was provided by the programme of independent sector treatment centres (ISTCs) run by private operators.

A second key area of policy change was the introduction of a new system of resource allocation in the NHS. Labour retained the division between purchaser and provider introduced by the Conservatives, but sought to replace existing contracts for healthcare with longer-term, comprehensive healthcare agreements. It later decided to introduce 'payment by results' (PBR), where health service providers would be paid on the basis of work done (see Chapter Seven). Although this differed in detail from the Conservatives' internal market, it nonetheless represented a shift back towards competition and the use of market forces. This policy was combined with policies to give NHS patients a choice of providers, including private sector suppliers. Another part of this new landscape were the new foundation trusts, created by New Labour to give providers more freedom to respond to market forces and patient choice. Labour also backtracked to a limited extent on its policy on GP fundholding, by piloting 'practice-based commissioning' (PBC) schemes (see Chapter Seven).

A third area of health policy that underwent considerable development after 2000 was health service quality and regulation. In opposition, the Labour Party had expressed a desire to improve the regulation and monitoring of care, proposing a Quality Commission. In office, Labour established a raft of new national bodies to set and monitor standards of health and social care (see Chapter Seven). In addition, new national service frameworks (NSFs) were introduced setting out standards and models of care for particular condition areas (for example, coronary heart disease, diabetes) or patient/user groups (children, older people). Labour also introduced a new quality assurance system – clinical governance – aimed at making NHS organisations more responsible for improving the quality of care provided. After 2000, regulation became much more 'top-down', in the form of performance targets, metrics and enforcement processes. New and more powerful central regulatory bodies were also established (see Chapter Seven).

Another area of policy activity for New Labour was public health. During the 1980s and 1990s, the Labour Party had been very critical of the Conservative government's record in this field. Once in office, the Blair government introduced a review of health inequalities (DH, 1998a), a new White Paper on public health (DH, 1999b), and appointed a minister for public health. It promised to ban tobacco advertisements (which, after delays and controversy over certain exemptions, was eventually introduced in 2003), and established an independent Food Standards Agency. The NHS was urged to give priority to public health and inequalities. Health Action Zones (HAZs) were established, to provide greater focus for efforts to improve health in areas of high need. The government was also prepared to use social and economic interventions to combat poverty. It set a long-term commitment to abolish child poverty, and introduced new programmes aimed at improving children's wellbeing (through Sure Start programmes). It also aimed to tackle unemployment and regenerate economically deprived areas (through the New Deal programmes).

The Brown government

For some, the departure of Blair in 2007 heralded a partial move back towards Old Labour. However, his replacement, Gordon Brown, Blair's Chancellor of the Exchequer and long-term rival for the leadership, was an active and willing participant in the New Labour project. Following his accession, he set out his future policy priorities, including health (Evans, 2008). This upheld the principles of an NHS free at point of use, available when needed and regardless of ability to pay. Brown stated that the NHS would be his immediate priority, but there was to be no reversal of the reform programme begun under Blair. Despite Brown's opposition to foundation trusts (see Chapter Three), he did not propose their abolition. Nor was there to be any retraction of the private sector's growing involvement in NHS provision. Instead, the new Prime Minister focused on initiatives to improve access to GPs, ensure patients were treated with dignity, improve basic care (for example, food and hygiene), and strengthen services for the elderly. Brown also stated his commitment to clarify accountability in the NHS, and put more power in the hands of local staff and patients. He signalled a move away from the top-down target culture with a greater emphasis on local targets and initiatives (see Chapter Seven).

Brown initiated a review by the eminent surgeon Lord Ara Darzi (whom he appointed as a health minister) to explore how NHS services could be improved. This was seen as an effort to depoliticise NHS reform. Even so, the Darzi Review (DH, 2008) and the government's response to his recommendations did not reverse the direction of policy set by New Labour.

The Darzi Review identified key principles for the NHS: that services should be fair, personal, effective and safe (DH, 2008). The Review's main recommendations were that the local NHS should devise plans to develop services, to be led by professionals and involving the public. It also called for closer working between the NHS and other bodies, such as the private sector, local authorities and the voluntary sector, to enable more integrated services. An NHS Constitution was recommended to clarify NHS core principles and values, as well as the rights and responsibilities of staff and service users. A new system of quality improvement was recommended, whereby health service providers published more information about the quality of their services, and demonstrated much stronger and more visible leadership. The Darzi Review called for greater patient input in the rating of quality, and that patients should be able to make informed choices in healthcare. This included a right to make choices and measures to enable patients to hold budgets for healthcare, which reflected a key principle behind the Review: that care should be more personalised. It also recommended that commissioning of health services should be more effective in generating improvements in quality, and that GPs should have a greater role in commissioning. The Review emphasised the importance of access and quality in primary care, greater choice of GPs for patients and new primary care centres. It also called for greater efforts by the NHS and its partners to prevent illness and to maintain good health.

The Conservatives and coalition government

Conservative policy after 1997

Following his defeat at the 1997 General Election, John Major resigned as leader of the Conservative Party and was replaced by William Hague. The new leadership began to revise its policies. The Party acknowledged that Labour had continued to dominate on health issues, and that this seriously affected Conservative electoral prospects (Bale, 2010). The initial response was to match Labour's spending commitments on the NHS, to maintain services free at the point of use, and to rule out privatisation (Conservative Party, 2001). Even so, the Conservatives endorsed policies likely to extend the independent sector, including a scheme that would oblige the NHS to meet maximum waiting times based on clinical need, if necessary by paying for treatment in a private hospital. A new partnership between the NHS and the independent sector was also proposed, alongside measures to grant tax relief on employers' private medical insurance.

Following the Conservative Party's defeat at the 2001 General Election, Hague resigned as leader. His replacement, Iain Duncan Smith, was an ineffectual leader, who resigned after only two years, following a loss of confidence among his backbenchers (Bale, 2010). Despite his short tenure, he did exert some influence on his Party's policies. Duncan Smith initiated several policy reviews that paved the way for Conservative policies at the 2005 General Election (Conservative Party, 2003; Evans and Williams, 2002; Williams, 2002; Clark and Kelly, 2004). After resigning from the leadership, he founded the Centre for Social Justice, and later served as Secretary of State for Work and Pensions in the coalition government between 2010–15, overseeing the controversial reform of welfare payments.

In 2003, Duncan Smith was replaced by the Thatcherite, Michael Howard (Bale, 2010). Subsequently, the Party's 2005 General Election manifesto covered a range of policies, many of which had been developed under Duncan Smith's leadership (Conservative Party, 2003, 2005). These included a 'patient passport' scheme, which would enable NHS patients to receive a subsidy from the taxpayer to pay for private healthcare. In addition, independent healthcare providers would be able to secure the right to supply services on behalf of the NHS. Patients would have access to treatment in independent hospitals that could perform operations at a standard and price acceptable to the NHS. Other policies focused on the following themes: decentralisation of commissioning and service provision, with an end to central targets; greater patient choice; a reduction of NHS bureaucracy, including the abolition of some NHS bodies and cuts to others; and more rigorous inspections and accountability. The Conservatives reiterated that they would at least match Labour's spending plans, and pledged to cut waiting lists. They also highlighted public health issues, which had become more prominent since the previous election, proposing action on hospital infections, cancer screening, alcohol misuse, drug abuse and sexual health.

Cameron's leadership

After the electorate returned the Blair government to a third term in office in 2005, Howard was replaced by David Cameron. Promising a fresh approach, Cameron began yet another round of policy reviews. As the next general election approached, health policy commitments were developed by the Party leadership, with the shadow Health Minister (Andrew Lansley) playing a crucial part. A Green Paper on the NHS was produced in June 2008 (Conservative Party, 2008), followed by a *Renewal plan for a better NHS* (Conservative Party, 2009). Cameron (2009) sharpened the focus of his Party's plans by setting out the top priorities for health and the NHS. This was followed in 2010 by the general election manifesto (Conservative Party, 2010b). In addition, the Conservatives produced policy documents on specific issues such as public health (Conservative Research Department, 2007; Conservative Party, 2010a) and patient choice and accountability (Conservative Party, 2007b). The main themes of these policies were as follows.

Funding and privatisation

The Conservatives abandoned the patient passport policy and subsidies for private medical insurance in 2006. They focused instead on public funding, making significant commitments to prioritise health expenditure. NHS spending was exempted from planned budget cuts. Moreover, the Conservatives were the only party at the 2010 General Election to pledge an increase in health spending year on year. The endorsement of a publicly funded healthcare system, coupled with a shift in emphasis away from private health spending, was a significant move, as it brought the Party much closer to Labour's position. However, the Conservatives made no secret of their plans to expose the NHS to competition from the independent sector. Their policy would allow patients to choose any provider meeting NHS standards, and at a price acceptable to the NHS, which was an extension of Labour's policy to extend choice and to increase competition. The Conservatives intended to continue Labour's policy of PBR, but with modifications, so that payments to providers could be more closely aligned with performance against health outcome measures.

Decentralisation

The Conservatives drew up an NHS Independence Bill (Conservative Party, 2007a). This enshrined the core principles, which included: a universal national health service for all based on clinical need, not ability to pay; the provision of comprehensive services; services based around the needs and preferences of patients, families and carers; and the need to promote health while trying to reduce health inequalities. Although the core principles identified by the Conservatives were similar to those set out by Labour, there were key differences in policy detail. The Conservative Party's proposals, for example, included an independent NHS board, appointed by the Secretary of State for Health, and reporting to Parliament. This board would be responsible for improving health, allocating resources and securing health services. The Secretary of State for Health would set the overall objectives and outcomes for the NHS as a whole. The Conservatives stated that political targets focusing on processes would be abolished, although health outcome targets would be retained.

The Conservatives remained committed to all NHS trusts becoming foundation trusts. They also reiterated previous promises to give GPs more powers over budgets and commissioning. The Party returned to its familiar pledge to reduce health bureaucracy by reducing public bodies and cutting NHS administrative costs, but although mergers between NHS bodies were welcomed, no reorganisation was proposed at this stage (Gainsbury, 2009).

Choice

The Conservatives outlined a vision of a patient-led NHS where patients would be in control of the care they received. This meant greater choice of secondary care provider, as indicated above. They also proposed greater choice of primary care provider. In addition, a manifesto commitment was made to introduce individual budgets for people with long-term conditions, a policy already adopted by New Labour. In addition, the Conservatives pledged to create a new statutory watchdog (Healthwatch) to act on behalf of patients and the public (Conservative Party, 2007b, 2010a).

Public health

The Conservative Party manifesto proposed that the Department of Health (DH) should become the Department for Public Health (Conservative Party, 2010a). This was an attempt to prioritise public health issues and to distance the Department from the NHS. The Conservatives had argued that public health budgets would be ring-fenced and over time transferred to a new structure, separate from healthcare resource allocation. The manifesto stated that separate public health funding would be provided to local communities (Conservative Party, 2010b), with a 'health premium' weighting public health funding towards the poorest areas with the worst health outcomes. There was also a commitment to expand the numbers of health visitors, who play a major role in preventing illness and health promotion, especially in deprived areas.

The Conservatives pledged to implement a range of measures to improve diet, levels of exercise, reduce smoking and alcohol abuse (Conservative Research Department, 2007; Conservative Party, 2010a). The emphasis was mainly on encouraging individual responsibility to improve lifestyles, but also included measures to strengthen corporate social responsibility. With regard to obesity, for example, the Party backed industry-led initiatives to reformulate food products and reduce portion sizes. It also endorsed 'proportionate' regulation of food advertising and health campaigns by government and industry to encourage healthy diets.

Explaining Conservative health policy

Conservative Party health policy developed significantly after 2005. Although policies were retained, some established commitments were dropped and new policies took their place. How can this be explained?

The impact of consecutive election defeats cannot be underestimated. As with Labour after 1987, this prompted a fundamental rethink of strategy and policy. It also led to the choice of a relative newcomer as leader. Cameron's election as Party leader represented a significant break with the past (Dorey, 2007). Although Eton-educated and affluent, Cameron was more open than his predecessors to consider alternative policies, and had more freedom to experiment.

In addition, there was a personal factor that many believe was significant. One of Cameron's children, Ivan, was born with a rare and severe medical condition that required around-the-clock care and treatment. Tragically, in February 2009, Ivan died at six years of age. Cameron put on record the impact of his family's experience on his views of the NHS: 'I believe that the creation of the NHS is one of the greatest achievements of the 20th century. When your family relies on the NHS all the time ... you really know how precious it is' (quoted in Elliot, 2009). For many people, this made Cameron a more genuine and credible steward of the NHS than many other Conservative politicians.

After taking up the Party leadership, Cameron launched several policy reviews, two of which were relevant to health policy (Dorey, 2007; Public Services Improvement Policy Group, 2007; Social Justice Policy Group, 2007). These reviews were chaired by senior Conservative figures (the former by Stephen Dorrell, a previous Health Minister, and the latter by Iain Duncan Smith). The review groups also included people with expertise from outside the Party. The reviews made many detailed recommendations. Not all became Party policy, but many were accepted. The function of the reviews was primarily to strengthen the legitimacy of the policy direction set by the new leadership (S. Lee, 2009).

The recommendations of these reviews were thrust into a mix that consisted of Party consultations on health policy and ideas put forward by Conservative or pro-market think tanks such as the Conservative Research Department, the Centre for Policy Studies and the Adam Smith Institute (Brown and Young, 2002; Mason and Maxwell, 2008), which have influenced Conservative health policy in the past. These were joined by newer centre-right think tanks such as Policy Exchange, Reform and the Social Market

Foundation (Bosanquet et al, 2007; Hamblin and Ganesh, 2007; Furness and Gough, 2009). There was a strong element of cherry picking by the leadership from such reports. For example, recommendations for devolving responsibility to local clinicians, reducing central regulation and targets, and increasing choice and competition were taken on board. However, calls for new charges and alternative ways of funding the NHS were rejected (Brown and Young, 2002; Charleson et al, 2007; Furness and Gough, 2009).

Notably, the leadership's position on health policy contrasted with that taken by many Conservative MPs. According to one survey, two-thirds of Conservative MPs supported tax relief on private medical insurance, a policy rejected by the Cameron leadership (Sky News, 2009). Moreover, right-wing elements within the Party disliked the NHS, and supported alternative models of healthcare. In 2009, these views were publicly aired by Conservative MEP Daniel Hannan, who described the NHS as a '60 year-old mistake' (Summers and Glendinning, 2009). His comments produced a swift defence of the NHS from Conservative leadership. Although rebuked by Cameron, the suspicion remained that Hannan was not a lone maverick. He was linked to senior figures on the Conservative frontbench, some of whom were believed to be sympathetic with his perspective (Helm and Syal, 2009).

Other factors may also have shaped the Conservatives' policies. For example, special interests, such as the private healthcare industry and the food, alcohol and tobacco industries, are traditionally close to the Party and enjoy close links with its MPs. In January 2010, it was revealed that senior Tory MPs in charge of health policy had accepted donations from private healthcare companies, while others had undertaken consultancy work or accepted benefits in kind (Kirby, 2010). Although these interests were declared, and no impropriety should be implied, such links potentially provided a useful channel for influencing policy debates (see Chapter Six).

Coalition politics

Following the 2010 General Election, no party had an overall majority in Parliament. After five days of negotiations, the Conservatives formed a coalition government with the Liberal Democrats (Adonis, 2013). The Coalition was led by David Cameron, with Nick Clegg, the 'Lib Dem' leader, as Deputy Prime Minister. In the past the health policies of the Liberal Democrats had often been at odds with the Conservatives. As Adonis (2013) observes, there were deep differences between the two party manifestos at the 2010 General Election. Even so, both parties were now under a centre-right leadership, and there was more common ground. There were also significant policy similarities. The Liberal Democrats, like the Conservatives, were sympathetic to greater devolution of decision-making in the NHS

(Liberal Democrats, 2008, 2010). However, they wanted to establish elected local health boards, not supported by the Conservatives. The Lib Dems also shared the Conservatives' desire for a reduction in both NHS bureaucracy and central targets. The two parties also agreed that there should be more choice in healthcare and more freedom for commissioning bodies to secure services from different types of provider. Both acknowledged the need to act on the key public health problems of smoking, alcohol and obesity, as well as tackling health inequalities. It was significant that the NHS barely featured in the coalition talks, and was not initially identified as a key area of disagreement (Timmins, 2012).

In an attempt to create a more coherent set of aims and priorities for the coalition, a programme was agreed (HM Government, 2010a). Fifty-four commitments in this programme were health-related (28 related to the NHS, 21 to public health and 5 to social care). Specific commitments included: to increase health spending in real terms year on year; to end 'top-down reorganisations'; to cut the costs of NHS administration by a third, alongside a significant reduction in health bodies; to strengthen the power of GPs in commissioning; to provide for directly elected members of primary care trusts (PCTs); to create an independent NHS board to allocate resources and provide commissioning guidelines; and to encourage greater involvement of independent and voluntary service providers in the NHS. With regard to public health, commitments included: to give local communities more control over public health budgets, linking payments to health outcomes; to give greater incentives to GPs to tackle public health problems; to explore ways of improving access to preventive healthcare for people living in disadvantaged areas; and to introduce policies to tackle alcohol and drug abuse.

Table 2.1: Coalition policies on health and social care

Manifesto source/	NHS	Social care	Public health	Total
Conservative	9	1	9	19
Liberal	5	2	2	9
Both	6	2	7	15
Compromise	4	0	2	6
Neither	4	0	1	5
Total	**28**	**5**	**21**	**54**

The White Papers and the NHS Bill

When the coalition government's NHS reforms for England were outlined in a White Paper, *Equity and excellence: Liberating the NHS* (DH, 2010a), there was much surprise at the radical nature of the reorganisation proposed. Although many elements were trailed in advance – especially in previous Conservative policy documents – the approach proposed did not sit easily with the coalition's earlier commitment to avoid top-down reorganisations (see Timmins, 2012). The path taken was seen as a political risk, potentially undermining the efforts made by Conservatives to 'detoxify' the NHS as a political issue (Bale, 2010; Timmins, 2012).

The White Paper proposed the abolition of PCTs and strategic health authorities (SHAs), and the transfer of their commissioning functions to local consortia of GP practices (later reformulated and renamed clinical commissioning groups, CCGs). At a national level, an NHS commissioning board (since renamed NHS England) would be created to allocate funding, issue guidelines, monitor the commissioning process and directly commission some services (see Chapter Seven). This body would implement priorities set by the Secretary of State for Health, who would set a policy framework in the form of a mandate, and allocate an overall budget for the NHS. It was declared that all NHS trusts would become foundation trusts, and there would be more competition between providers, including from independent suppliers. The new NHS market would be regulated by the current foundation trust regulator, Monitor. In addition, the Conservatives' earlier proposal for a new system of patient and public involvement (PPI) – Healthwatch – was endorsed (see Chapter Eight).

Although the key focus was on the NHS, *Equity and excellence* proposed important changes in the structure of public health – namely, the transfer of key public health responsibilities and functions to local authorities (those with social service responsibilities), and the creation of a national public health service (Public Health England) to integrate existing health improvement and health protection expertise. A further White Paper, *Healthy lives, healthy people* (DH, 2010b), clarified the details. A new, ring-fenced, public health budget would be established for the national public health service and local government public health functions. Areas with high health needs were promised additional funding in the form of a 'health premium', and there would be a focus on reducing health inequalities.

In addition, businesses, the public sector and voluntary organisations were to be given a key role in health improvement. Employers would be encouraged to support employees to stay healthy. Commercial interests in food, obesity and alcohol would be expected to work in partnership with government to establish a 'responsibility deal' setting out how businesses in these sectors could contribute to a healthy diet, increased physical activity and safe drinking. Change4Life, the Labour government's social marketing programme for health, would become a broader social movement with a bigger contribution from business, the voluntary sector and local government.

The coalition promised to increase the number of health visitors by 4,200, and to give them more responsibility for children's health and community development. Although there would be less emphasis on the 'nanny state' and more on 'nudging' people into adopting healthy lifestyles (through incentives to eat healthily and to take exercise), initiatives were promised on specific public health problems, such as alcohol, tobacco and obesity.

The coalition also proposed new bodies to improve health and to bring together NHS services and social care. Health and wellbeing boards would be established as statutory committees in local authorities (see Chapter Eight). They were created mainly to satisfy the Liberal Democrats, who were concerned about the negative impact of coalition reforms on the collaboration and integration of health and social care. They were also seen as compensation for dropping the Liberal Democrats' proposal (contained in the coalition agreement) to make PCTs partially directly elected (see Timmins, 2012).

The government's NHS and public health reforms were included in the Health and Social Care Bill introduced in January 2011. As the Bill moved through its early parliamentary stages, criticism intensified, most of this levelled at the NHS reorganisation (see Chapter Four). In the face of these pressures, the coalition government agreed to 'pause' the legislative process to consider possible amendments (see **Box 3.3**). Although the broad thrust of the legislation remained, many concessions were made.

It might appear that the Conservatives tried to railroad the Lib Dems with a more radical Bill than they had agreed to, but the story is more complex than this. The Liberal Democrat leadership was happy to sign up to the original Bill. Only when its activists began to rebel, following the introduction of the Bill into Parliament, did the leadership shift its position. The Bill was also poorly understood by the Conservative leadership. Both the Liberal Democrat and Conservative leaders later acknowledged that the reforms were not politically feasible, and this paved the way for substantial amendments, explored further in Chapter Four.

In the years following the enactment of the Health and Social Care Act in 2012, until the 2015 General Election, important changes in the coalition's health policy occurred. The architect of the reforms, Andrew Lansley, was replaced as Secretary of State for Health by Jeremy Hunt, who adopted a different policy style. He pursued a more pragmatic, less overtly ideological approach than his predecessor. Hunt was also more attuned to the problems of the new system. He was prepared to intervene where necessary to ensure that measures were being implemented in line with the government's policies and targets. There were also significant changes brought by events. Concerns about patient safety and service quality provided a major challenge for the coalition, especially following the report of the public inquiry into the Mid Staffordshire NHS Foundation Trust in 2013 (see Chapter Seven). This agenda demanded a more interventionist approach from the Department of Health, and sat ill with the 'choice, decentralisation and markets' philosophy of the Health and Social Care Act.

Conclusion

Parties are important vehicles of change in health policy. They play a crucial role in setting the terms of political debate and in shaping the policy agenda. Party ideologies can lead them to adopt certain policies, which can then become government policies if they gain office. In this sense they are important 'battering rams of change', as described by Crossman (see Chapter One).

However, the link between party ideology and government policy is not straightforward. Party ideologies have themselves been subject to wider influences over the years, notably with regard to the permeation of neoliberal ideas across all mainstream parties. Furthermore, party policies are influenced by a range of other considerations, primarily the need to win elections, which may override ideological principles. Ideological factors may be thwarted by political and technical constraints of implementation, for example. Policy learning may also be relevant, as governments discard ideological party policies that are ineffective or impractical, and choose more pragmatic approaches. There is also a certain amount of 'path-dependency' in health, with governments retaining elements of their predecessors' policies, which limits the impact of party ideology. Governing parties may find themselves adopting policies introduced by their predecessors, or may borrow policy ideas from their rivals in order to address a policy problem. This is consistent with the moving consensus model of Rose (see Chapter One), which suggests substantial policy continuity between governments irrespective of which party holds office.

Not only has there been 'remarkable continuity' (Crisp, 2011) between the parties in government, but there have also been substantial policy changes under governments of the same party. This does not seem to fit well with either Rose's or Crossman's model, and is perhaps better explained by changing political circumstances (that is, where new problems arise or existing ones become more significant), electoral competition (where the party in office has to modify its policy because it fears losing votes) or internal party conflict (on either ideological or pragmatic grounds).

The experience of the coalition government between 2010–15 adds to an already complex picture. Both the Liberal Democrats and the Conservatives had to compromise in the formulation of health policy. These compromises were initially quite clear, as set out, for example, in the coalition agreement. Then, with the legislative plans, the situation became rather messy, with the reforms being criticised within government by Conservative politicians as well as Lib Dems. The final outcome, which was the result of a complex array of external and internal pressures, was very unpredictable, and demonstrates the limited capacity of party competition models to explain policy outcomes.

Summary

- Health is an important issue in party politics.
- There are significant political and technical constraints facing parties when in office, which limit their influence.
- Although parties can act as 'battering rams of change', there is evidence of a moving consensus in health policy.
- There is substantial evidence of policy change under governments of the same party.
- It is particularly difficult to predict the policies of coalition governments.

Key questions

1. What are the key differences in health policy of the main political parties today?
2. Have these differences stayed the same, narrowed or widened in recent years?
3. Why has health been a prominent issue in general elections?
4. Can you give examples of where a political party has borrowed or adapted its opponents' policies?
5. How, and to what extent, did coalition politics affect party influence on health policy between 2010 and 2015?

three

Central government and health policy

Overview

This chapter examines the role of central government institutions in health policy. It begins by looking at the functions, organisation and culture of the Department of Health (DH), and then explores the specific roles of ministers, civil servants and advisers. It also considers health and health-related responsibilities across government, and examines how these are led and coordinated. In this context, the role of the Treasury and the Prime Minister's Office is explored. Finally, the chapter examines the interface between central government institutions and external organisations and experts in the formation and implementation of policy

Central government (or 'the executive') comprises government departments and agencies as well as the core institutions – the Treasury, the Cabinet Office and the Prime Minister's Office. Many of these organisations have an interest in health policy (see **Box 3.2**). Nonetheless, the best place to begin is with the department with overall responsibility for health and the NHS, the Department of Health.

Department of Health

History of the Department of Health

The Ministry of Health was created in 1919 (Gilbert, 1970; Honigsbaum, 1970). Its principal duty, vested in the Minister of Health, was 'to take all steps as may be desirable to secure the preparation, effective carrying out and coordination of measures conducive to the health of the people' (Ministry of Health Act 1919). Prior to the NHS, the Ministry did not have responsibilities for a comprehensive health service. However, it possessed important public health responsibilities, including environmental health, housing, water supply and sanitation, as well as oversight of local government.

After the Second World War, the Ministry of Health acquired responsibility for the NHS, but lost control of important public health responsibilities when local government was ceded to the Ministry of Housing and Local Government in 1951. This negatively affected morale in the Department, and focused the Ministry's attention on health services, in particular hospital services, to the detriment of public and community health (Webster, 1996). During the post-war period, the Ministry of Health was not a prestigious department. Its senior minister was not guaranteed Cabinet rank (and between 1945 and 1968 was more often outside rather than inside the Cabinet). This compounded the weakness of the Ministry in interdepartmental politics. In addition, it was regarded as a rather cautious, reactive and essentially non-interventionist department (Klein, 1995; Mohan, 1995; Webster, 1996), although it later adopted a more proactive stance, drawing up national plans for services and initiating NHS reorganisation (see Chapter Seven).

The creation of the Department of Health and Social Security (DHSS) in 1968, from a merger of the health and social security ministries, effectively guaranteed Cabinet status for its senior minister, the Secretary of State for Social Services. The DHSS was a big spending department, employing large numbers of civil servants, responsible for a range of politically sensitive social welfare issues, including the NHS. The Departments of Health and Social Security were subsequently demerged in 1988, but by this time the health portfolio had expanded and become more significant politically, in its own right. Ever since, the Secretary of State for Health has been a Cabinet-level appointment.

The current responsibilities of the DH can be summarised as follows. It is the principal government department for UK-wide health and care matters, and represents the UK government in international and European fora. It is responsible for coordinating policy and action on health and care matters affecting the UK as a whole, such as infectious diseases or biological threats. Otherwise, its remit is confined to England, where it supports ministers in fulfilment of their statutory duties (see **Box 3.1**). Elsewhere, the devolved governments are responsible for most health and healthcare matters (see Chapter Nine).

Box 3.1: Statutory responsibilities of the Secretary of State for Health

The NHS Act 1946 (Part 1, s 1(1)) imposed a duty on the Minister of Health (now the Secretary of State for Health) 'to promote the establishment in England and Wales of a comprehensive health service designed to secure improvement ... in the physical and mental health of the people of England and Wales and the prevention, diagnosis and treatment of illness and for that purpose to provide or secure the effective provision of services ...'. Some minor changes were made by the NHS Reorganisation Act 1973 (Part 1, s 2(2)), and by the NHS Act 1977 (Part 1, s 1(1)). Subsequently the consolidating NHS Act 2006 amended the duty to reflect the devolution of health service duties and responsibilities to Wales.

In contrast, the changes proposed by the Cameron government in 2010 were more far-reaching and highly controversial. The aim was to transfer significant duties and responsibilities to the NHS in order to give more autonomy to the NHS and less central direction from Whitehall. The original Health and Social Care Bill removed the Secretary of State's duty to provide or secure the provision of services, replacing this with a general duty to exercise functions in relation to other bodies to secure those services. This, along with a new ministerial duty to promote autonomy in the NHS, raised two concerns. First, that ministerial accountability to Parliament for the NHS would be reduced, and second, that the ministerial duty to promote a comprehensive health service would be severely weakened in practice by passing on the duty to provide services to other parties (for a detailed discussion, see House of Lords Select Committee on the Constitution, 2011a, 2011b). The government agreed to reiterate the Secretary of State's existing duty to promote a comprehensive health service by including this in the Bill (which became law when the Health and Social Care Act was passed in 2012). Furthermore, a new clause was added, clarifying the Secretary of State's responsibility to Parliament for the provision of the health service. Other amendments clarified that the Secretary of State must exercise functions 'to secure that services are provided in accordance with this Act'. And duties contained in the original Bill to promote autonomy in the NHS were subject to the overriding ministerial duty and responsibilities set out in section 1(1) (the duty to promote a comprehensive health service). NHS bodies – including NHS England and clinical commissioning groups (CCGs) – were also required to be consistent with this general duty. Some critics remained dissatisfied, and pressed for the Secretary of State's duties to be strengthened or clarified further, especially with regard to ensuring the provision of services (Kmietowicz, 2013). Notably, the Health and Social Care Act did clarify a number of other specific duties already placed on the Secretary of State for Health, for example, with regard to public health and health research. It also specified new duties with regard to service quality improvement, the NHS constitution, the reduction of health inequalities, and education and training.

Internal politics of the Department of Health

As Ham (2004) observed, the DH is not a monolith. It contains different types of personnel and cultures. Differences also arise from the internal structure of work within the Department. The Secretary of State for Health, as the most senior politician in the Department, is formally accountable to Parliament for the DH's activities (see **Box 3.1**). In theory, ministerial responsibility is extensive and reflects the principle, encapsulated in Bevan's phrase, that 'when a bedpan is dropped on a hospital floor its noise should resound in the Palace of Westminster' (cited in Nairne, 1984). In practice, however, such comprehensive responsibility has long been regarded as a constitutional fiction (Royal Commission on the NHS, 1979). Moreover, successive governments have attempted to devolve operational responsibility to NHS bodies (see **Box 3.1** and Chapter Seven). Nonetheless, ministers must answer Parliamentary Questions (PQs), carry legislation through Parliament, respond to debates and give evidence to select committees (see Chapter Four).

The Secretary of State issues strategic statements and guidance on health and social care policy (including the mandate, which formally sets out the key priorities for the NHS). As departmental policy must be consistent with the government's overall policies, the Secretary of State must engage in discussions with other ministers. S/he will also seek to ensure that the Department's view is reflected in wider public policy debates, while striving to secure the resources and powers needed to achieve health and care policy objectives. This involves being a member of formal Cabinet committees and informal policy working groups. It also requires effective working relationships with the Treasury, the Cabinet Office and the Prime Minister's Office as well as other departments. Despite attempts to shift responsibilities on to NHS organisations, the Secretary of State remains the public face of the DH, appearing in the media, promoting the Department's agenda and responding to issues of public concern. The DH's statutory powers are vested in the office of Secretary of State. In practice, however, there is considerable delegation, to junior ministers, policy advisers and civil servants. In addition, specific functions have been 'hived off' to special agencies, accountable to the Secretary of State, discussed further below.

At the time of writing, there are five junior ministers: four MPs and a member of the House of Lords (who acts as the Department's spokesperson in the Upper House). Each minister has specific responsibilities for areas of policy and services (such as public health, health services or social care).

In practice, much of the burden of everyday government business falls on their shoulders. Junior ministers are active in the policy process, negotiating with outside organisations, piloting legislation through Parliament, and implementing policy changes. In some cases, junior ministers remain in the Department for some time, building up considerable expertise and knowledge (Crisp, 2011). This provides a useful apprenticeship for future Secretaries of State (Ham, 2000). Since the 1980s, five Secretaries of State of Health (Kenneth Clarke, Virginia Bottomley and Stephen Dorrell [Conservative] and Alan Milburn and Andy Burnham [Labour]) previously served as junior ministers in the Department.

The particular style of the Secretary of State can make a crucial difference to the Department's approach to policy-making and to policy direction (see Ham, 2000; Edwards and Fall, 2005; Baggott, 2007, Storey et al, 2010). For example, Frank Dobson, Secretary of State in the Blair government between 1997–99, was said to be a collegial and consensual policy-maker who sought to establish a good working relationship with the health professional groups, and who listened carefully to advice from civil servants. According to Blair and other senior colleagues, he had little time for radical reform (Blair, 2010; Mandelson, 2011). Dobson's successor, Alan Milburn, was described as a more driven character, with a clear objective to radically reform the NHS, and a keen eye for policy detail (Crisp, 2011). It was said that he preferred to work with individual professionals who shared his vision rather than professional groups as a whole. John Reid, who followed Milburn, has been described as a tough and uncompromising policy implementer who demonstrated little enthusiasm for the health brief (he is reported as greeting news of his appointment with the words "Oh fuck, not health!"; Hammond, 2009). His successor, Patricia Hewitt, was described as a more emollient character, who tried to build bridges with the professional organisations while attempting to set a new agenda that emphasised primary care and community-based models of care, although she struggled to do so in the context of financial deficits and growing criticism of NHS privatisation. Hewitt's successor, Alan Johnson, was seen as having a becalming influence on health policy and as a force for stability (Jarman and Greer, 2010), much of his short term in office being taken up by the Darzi Review of the NHS and its early implementation. The final Labour Health Secretary in this period, Andy Burnham, was in post for less than a year, and it is therefore difficult to shape a judgement about his particular policy style.

The Cameron government had only two Secretaries of State between 2010–15. The first, Andrew Lansley, developed a reputation for having a somewhat single-minded approach (Timmins, 2012; D'Ancona, 2013). Only after his proposed NHS reforms attracted overwhelming opposition (from within government itself, from Parliament, and among professional and other stakeholders) did he backtrack significantly on some of the most controversial elements. Lansley was replaced by Jeremy Hunt who demonstrated a greater willingness to work with professional groups, but was also willing to intervene when politically necessary. Following the Conservatives' victory at the 2015 General Election, Hunt was reappointed as Secretary of State for Health.

Civil servants

Traditionally, senior civil servants (such as the Permanent Secretary and other senior grades) influenced policy by providing advice to ministers. Even middle-ranking civil servants contributed to policy formation – by briefing their superiors on specific issues, liaising with outside interests and garnering expert advice (see, for example, Baggott et al, 2005). Furthermore, civil servants' role in implementing decisions involved considerable discretion, enabling them to shape the detailed application of policies.

However, civil service influence over policy appears to have diminished in recent decades. Former DH civil servants and senior NHS managers have detected a decline in the traditional channels of influence, a trend accentuated under the Blair government (Baggott, 2007). Some observed a distrust of the traditional civil service based on suspicion of its principles of 'neutrality'. This was reflected in ministers seeking policy advice from elsewhere – such as individual experts and special advisers (see also Dorey, 2005; Edwards and Fall, 2005, p 201; Sheard and Donaldson, 2006). In addition, the performance of civil servants has been more closely monitored, reducing their discretion in the implementation process. Linked to this, a new breed of 'managerialist' civil servant has emerged, the implications of which are discussed later.

It appears that the influence of civil servants with a health professional background has diminished even more dramatically. The DH and its predecessor bodies have always employed civil servants drawn from the health professions and other experts. The distinction between these specialists and the other, generalist, civil servants is long-standing. At one time this was clearly reflected in the structure of the Department. Until the mid-1990s, the Department had separate medical divisions that were managerially as well as professionally accountable to the Chief Medical Officer (CMO). This was superseded by an integrated management structure, although the specialist civil servants remained 'professionally' accountable to their respective professional leader.

Some observers believe that professional power, and in particular medical power, was diminished as a result. This and other factors weakened the role of the CMO. The CMO (who is the medical adviser for the government as a whole, and not just the DH) was regarded as a check on the power of Secretaries of State for Health, and as a key influence on policy (Edwards and Fall, 2005; Sheard and Donaldson, 2006). CMOs have also acted as a channel for influence, and were regarded key 'go-betweens' in the relationship between government and the medical profession (Ham, 2000). However, the removal of management responsibilities, cuts in medical staffing levels in the Department, and declining morale appear to have undermined the CMO's role and influence (The BSE Inquiry, 2000; Sheard and Donaldson, 2006; Sheard, 2010).

Under Sir Liam Donaldson (CMO, 1998–2010), this decline was arrested to some extent. Donaldson took on managerial responsibility for medical standards and quality (Sheard, 2010). Even so, the appointment of a medical director of the NHS in 2007 led to the transfer of responsibilities for clinical quality and patient safety. Bruce Keogh, a leading cardiac surgeon, was appointed to this new post (which is now based within NHS England). He has since been active in tackling key issues around quality and safety, for example, with regard to faulty breast implants, and investigating problems at hospitals with high death rates in the aftermath of the Mid Staffordshire scandal. Even so, there has been concern that the establishment of the medical director role not only displaced existing modes of liaising with the medical profession, but also imposed a more managerial and top-down model of interaction with the profession (see Jarman and Greer, 2010).

Liam Donaldson was an effective campaigner within the DH and across government on public health issues such as smoking, obesity and alcohol abuse. His successor, Dame Sally Davies, was initially appointed on an interim basis, which some believe weakened her position. It was also pointed out that Dame Sally is not a public health specialist, but a haematologist and medical researcher by background. There were fears that her background would make it less likely that she would focus on controversial public health lifestyle issues (Scally, 2013). However, she has commented on issues such as alcohol, smoking, obesity and drug abuse, and has raised controversial policy issues, including sugar taxes to combat obesity.

Although professional power within the Department may have decreased, other developments suggest that professionals retain considerable influence over policy. Under the Blair government, senior clinicians were brought in as national clinical directors (also known as 'czars') for priority areas such as cancer, heart disease, mental health, diabetes, older people, children, emergency services and primary care (Cox, 2001; Burns, 2004; Sheard, 2010). They were appointed on a part-time and temporary basis (although some have held posts for longer periods). This incorporation of senior clinicians created new opportunities for professional influence over policy (see also Chapter Six). They have had access to health ministers, and in some cases, to the Prime Minister. Their influence is difficult to judge and has been variable (Storey et al, 2010). Even so, there is some evidence that they can be important players in the policy process (Burns, 2004; Edwards and Fall, 2005; Baggott, 2007; Crisp, 2011).

The national clinical directors have been regarded as an important channel for medical influence (and are a target for other lobby groups, such as the drug industry and patients' groups). It is possible that they have narrowed the channels of clinical influence, bypassing traditional forms of lobbying and expert advice (Baggott, 2007). But they may also be manipulated by government, providing a useful scapegoat if policies prove unsuccessful. There have been fears that national clinical directors could be drawn into defending government policy on political grounds (Burns, 2004), but the high professional standing of post-holders has alleviated these concerns.

In recent years, there has been disquiet about the use of czars and other advisers across government, particularly with regard to a lack of transparency about processes of appointment and the lack of clearly defined roles (PASC, 2010), although this criticism perhaps applies less to the appointment of national clinical directors than other posts. Nonetheless, as czars fell out of fashion, rumours of a likely cull of the health czars spread. In 2012, five DH czars left their posts, while the others were given only temporary contracts (Calkin, 2012), suggesting that they may be being phased out. Nonetheless, at the time of writing, there are 23 national clinical directors in post (now based within NHS England, rather than the Department of Health).

The appointment of a leading surgeon, Ara Darzi, as a health minister in the Brown government is a further illustration that doctors retained significant policy influence. Darzi led a major review of the NHS, and set out a framework for reform (see Chapter Two). Notably, previous governments have appointed doctors to health ministerial posts in the past. Indeed, the first Minister for Health, Christopher Addison, was a doctor.

Another key feature of the DH, already mentioned, has been the rise of 'managerialist' civil servants. Within the Department, the traditional civil servant has, to a large extent, been replaced by those with a background in NHS management (Baggott, 2007; Jarman and Greer, 2010). Day and Klein (1997) found that this led to important cultural changes. The traditional civil service approach – which emphasised risk avoidance and written communication, was process-oriented, collegial and minister-centred – was challenged by the managerialist approach, which emphasised risk-taking, was NHS-centred, outcome-oriented, individual rather than collegial, and emphasised verbal communication. The result was a hybrid culture. Civil servants became more focused on performance management and delivery. However, elements of the traditional civil service ethos – in particular, the overriding goal of protecting ministers from criticism – remained strong.

Jarman and Greer (2010) acknowledged that the Department is culturally split between public servants and managers, and that the latter are in the ascendant. They note that this has been born out by the implementation of political preferences consistent with managerialism but inconsistent with the traditional civil service ethos. Their research also found that only a minority of senior civil servants (one in ten) within the Department had a traditional civil service background. Around half had an NHS background, the remainder coming from the private sector, local government or from other professional backgrounds.

Special advisers

All government departments, including the Prime Minister, have special advisers. In November 2014, there were over a hundred ministerial advisers (Cabinet Office, 2014). One of their key roles is to provide and develop policy ideas for ministers. They have been described as providing 'brain power for ministers' (cited in Baggott, 2007). Unlike civil servants, they are not expected to be politically impartial. They can influence policy (Edwards and Fall, 2005; Baggott, 2007; Jarman and Greer, 2010), and have been used to counteract the power of the traditional civil service. Political advisers also play an important part in defending government policy. They act as a counterweight to ideas and arguments hostile to government coming from the media and Parliament. Some advisers act as 'spin doctors', influencing the media and the public perception of issues (see also Chapter Five). Special advisers are central to the process of monitoring the implementation of policies within the Department and in the NHS. They act as the eyes and ears of ministers, and feed back problems of implementation.

Special advisers are used by the core institutions of the executive, the Prime Minister's Office and the Treasury, to coordinate departments. From a departmental perspective, however, they can help fight battles with other departments, especially with the Treasury (Crisp, 2011). Special advisers also mediate between departments and external organisations, such as pressure groups. In turn, they are seen as valuable political contacts by lobbying organisations (Sheard and Donaldson, 2006).

It is difficult to generalise about special advisers. It appears that they vary significantly in quality. Lord Crisp (2011, p 156) stated that some special advisers 'were very able and added value' while others were 'completely useless and just got in the way'. It is also hard to judge their influence. Much depends on who is employing them. DH advisers are generally seen as less influential than those advising the Prime Minister (Baggott, 2007).

There has been a degree of public concern about special advisers (see PASC, 2012), in particular, about a lack of transparency and accountability in their work, the dangers of them exceeding their brief, and potential conflicts of interest. In an attempt to address some of these concerns, there have been attempts to limit the number of advisers (although these have been relatively unsuccessful). There is now a code of conduct for special advisers, whereby they must declare conflicts of interest, gifts and hospitality. They are vetted when taking up roles with external organisations after serving in government. Guidance has also been issued on the conduct of special advisers on quasi-judicial issues.

The DH, like other departments, also employs management consultants to provide various services including policy advice and evaluation – the Department spent £5.4 million on consultants in 2013/14 (DH, 2013b). One of the main firms is McKinsey & Company (Davies, 2012). McKinsey has been involved in many health policy reviews and initiatives. It is often said that there is a revolving door, with key personnel moving between government and the firm. Examples include David Bennett, who worked for McKinsey before becoming a policy adviser to Tony Blair, and later became the chief executive of Monitor. Another is Penny Dash, who currently works for McKinsey, and was formerly Head of Strategy at the DH. However, there is little direct evidence about how much influence McKinsey has over policy or how this compares with other management consultancy firms.

Structure of the Department of Health

During the 1980s, structural changes were undertaken within the DH to separate health policy from management (see Edwards and Fall, 2005). In 1989, this culminated in the creation of a new body, the NHS Management Executive, which was based at Leeds. This physical separation of policy and management is now widely regarded as a mistake (Edwards and Fall, 2005; Crisp, 2011; Greer et al 2014a). Government acknowledged this when the NHS Executive (NHSE, 'Management' having been dropped from its title) acquired policy-making functions in the mid-1990s. Under the Blair government, NHSE was marginalised, particularly after the appointment of Alan Milburn as Secretary of State (Edwards and Fall, 2005). The arrangement was inefficient as senior NHSE staff, though based in Leeds, spent most of their time in London supporting ministers (Crisp, 2011). In 2000, the posts of DH Permanent Secretary and Chief Executive of the NHS were combined (only to be separated again in 2006), and the NHSE's functions repatriated to the main body of the DH.

The NHS reforms introduced by the coalition government reprised previous efforts to divide policy from management. However, there are important differences, chiefly, that there is now a legislative basis to this arrangement. NHS England (see Chapter Seven), the body responsible for delivering NHS objectives, and overseeing commissioning and the allocation of resources in England, is a statutory body, and its relationship with the Secretary of State for Health is defined in legislation. Nonetheless, given the political significance of health policy and the NHS, it is likely that similar problems of demarcation between policy and management will be repeated. Notably, stakeholders have already expressed confusion about the interface between NHS England and the DH (Ipsos MORI, 2013).

Agencies

A significant amount of health policy activity is undertaken by arm's-length agencies. These are not ministerial departments, but are nonetheless part of government. They fall within the overall responsibilities of the Secretary of State, are appointed under his or her powers, and are allocated resources to carry out their specific functions. These bodies vary enormously in size and in their freedom from ministerial and departmental influence. The four main types of health agency are as follows. *Special health authorities* are appointed by the Secretary of State to manage specific areas of activity, such as litigation or blood transfusion. *Executive agencies* undertake specialised areas of work on behalf of the Department, and include the Medicines and Healthcare Products Regulatory Agency and Public Health England. *Non-departmental executive public bodies*, such as the Care Quality Commission (CQC), Monitor, the National Institute for Health and Care Excellence (NICE), and NHS England (see Chapter Seven), govern or regulate important aspects of health services. Meanwhile, *non-departmental advisory public bodies* bring together expert advice on particular issues, such as professional remuneration (for example, the Review Body on Doctors' and Dentists' Remuneration) and medicines (the Commission on Human Medicines).

The special health authorities have the least independence. They operate under a strictly defined policy and resources framework set by the DH. Executive agencies can exercise considerable operational freedom, but are more subject to departmental influence than non–departmental public bodies. In the case of the latter, a greater degree of independence is acknowledged in legislation (their powers and duties are specified in statute). Even so, they are subject to departmental influence on key strategic matters (and indeed, can be 'leaned on' by ministers and the Department on operational matters too). Advisory bodies can be highly independent, and may be able to resist departmental influence when making reports and recommendations. But no body is entirely autonomous. Government can exercise influence through policy and resources, and by appointments to these bodies. It should also be noted that there are variations in degrees of autonomy within the above categories. For example, NICE enjoyed considerable freedom as a special health authority (before becoming a non-departmental body). Monitor has been given much more freedom than CQC (although the latter has recently been given more autonomy). Much depends on the specification of independence in statute and agreements, the political nature of the issues under consideration, and the relationship between the leadership of the agencies and the Department (and particularly between ministers and the chairs of these bodies).

During the latter half of the 2000s, as part of a broader programme across government to cut bureaucracy, a process of rationalisation was undertaken that reduced the number of health bodies, their staffing and budgets. In 2010, the number of bodies had fallen by more than half, to 18. They employed 18,000 (4,000 less than in 2004), and annual spending was cut from £2.5 billion to £1.6 billion (DH, 2010c). Subsequently, the coalition further aimed to reduce the number and costs of arm's-length bodies, as part of a broader policy of reducing the size of the state and public expenditure. The overall number of health bodies, however, increased. Many of the new bodies were created as a direct result of policies to rationalise functions and to move functions out of the DH.

A shrinking department

DH staffing levels have fallen over the past two decades due to hiving off functions to arm's-length bodies, a broader attack on the size of central government, and the shifting of responsibilities to local NHS bodies (discussed further in Chapter Seven), There has also been a greater use of secondments from outside bodies (including the private sector). In 2013/14 there were around 2,300 (whole-time equivalent) staff in the Department, about half the number from the early 1990s; around a fifth of staff do not hold permanent contracts.

The DH has been frequently restructured over the years. At the time of writing, it is organised under seven directorates: the Chief Medical Officer; finance and the NHS; social care (and local government and partnerships); public health; innovation, growth and strategy; strategy and external relations; and chief operating officer. The Department is overseen by a strategic board chaired by the Secretary of State for Health which includes the department's ministers, the Permanent Secretary and the heads of each directorate, as well as five non-executive directors.

Performance of the Department of Health

The DH's status grew under the Blair government. It was credited with embracing Blair's modernisation agenda (Baggott, 2007; Crisp, 2011). Its reputation was subsequently tarnished, however, by a mounting financial crisis in the NHS, which led to the resignation of the Permanent Secretary, Sir Nigel (now Lord) Crisp, in 2006. A review of the Department undertaken by the Cabinet Office (2007) was then highly critical. Although the Department was credited for achieving the majority of its targets, several weaknesses were identified. These included concerns about strategic management and leadership, weaknesses in communication, insufficient focus on policy outcomes and the use of evidence, and problems working with other departments and external stakeholders. A follow-up review was more positive, noting improvements in leadership, analytical capabilities and strategic capacity (Cabinet Office, 2009). Staff morale, identified as poor in the 2007 report, had also improved. A further review (DH/Cabinet Office, 2012) picked up problems identified in the previous reports. It highlighted three key areas for improvement: the need to build a common purpose and strong sense of ownership of the change agenda; the imperative to work differently to achieve more, notably in light of the loss of key levers with which to direct performance (see below and Chapter Seven); and to get the right people in the right place with the right skills.

One of the long-standing criticisms of the DH (and its predecessor departments) has been its failure to give sufficient attention to public health and to collaboration across government to promote health and prevent illness. It has often been seen as the Department for the NHS rather than a Department for Health. In the past there have been regular calls for the Department to focus more on these issues and less on the NHS. During the late 2000s, the Conservative Party endorsed greater independence for the NHS, and that the DH should focus on public health (Conservative Party, 2007a, 2010a). The Conservative manifesto of 2010 stated that it should be renamed the Department of Public Health (Conservative Party, 2010b), but this did not make it into the coalition agreement (see Chapter Two). Although the Department's name has not changed, however, its formal duties and responsibilities have altered. Following the coalition reforms it ceded important functions to NHS England, and many DH staff moved across to this new organisation. Meanwhile, public health reforms led to other staff moving to another new agency, Public Health England.

The DH began to use a different language to clarify its new role. There is much talk of its role as the 'steward' of the health and social care system, rather than as the headquarters of the NHS. In reality, however, the Department has intervened in the NHS, on quality and safety issues for example (see Chapter

Seven). The political importance of health makes it very difficult to let go of the NHS. Furthermore, the reiteration of ministerial accountability (see **Box 3.1**) reinforced this. Ironically, the Department is in a much weaker position to exert leverage. As Greer et al (2014a) observed, the DH has lost key powers as a result of the Health and Social Care Act 2012. Moreover, as some of these powers have accrued to other central government bodies (such as Monitor and NHS England), this is a recipe for instability, incoherence and turf wars (see also Ham et al, 2015).

Other departments and the core executive

Although most health policy activity takes place within the DH, it has long been acknowledged that key decisions affecting health and care are made by other central government departments and agencies (see **Box 3.2**). However, it has often proved difficult to get these bodies to work together, as they have different priorities.

> **Box 3.2:** Departmental responsibilities and health-related issues
>
> *Cabinet Office:* voluntary and community sector; coordination of government policies; efficiency and reform; civil service reform.
>
> *Department for Business, Innovation and Skills (BIS):* universities, science and technology, research and innovation; employment and skills, workplace training; further education and lifelong learning; employment relations; consumer affairs; trade and competition; corporate governance; regulation and deregulation.
>
> *Department for Communities and Local Government (DCLG):* fire, resilience and emergencies; climate change and sustainable development; housing and homelessness; neighbourhoods and communities; community empowerment and the big society; diversity and equality; faith, community cohesion and minorities; regeneration and economic growth; planning; troubled families; regional bodies and local government; decentralisation and localism.
>
> *Department for Culture, Media and Sport (DCMS):* culture and heritage; the media and creative industries; National Lottery and the Big Lottery Fund; promotion of arts and sport; tourism; gambling; equality and human issues; women and LGBT issues.
>
> *Department for Education (DfE):* education of children and young people (from 'early years' to 19 years of age); school-based health and personal education,

school sport; childcare; care, support and protection of children; apprenticeships and further education.

Department of Energy and Climate Change (DECC): energy policies; climate change; fuel poverty; nuclear safety.

Department for Environment, Food and Rural Affairs (Defra): the environment; climate change and sustainable development; agriculture; food and drink; rural affairs; natural environment, water supplies and biodiversity.

Department for International Development (DfID): international development including preventing illness and deaths in developing countries.

Department for Transport (DfT): transport policy and planning; transport safety and accidents; sustainable travel (including walking and cycling).

Department for Work and Pensions (DWP): Income Support for people in financial need and poverty, unemployed people, people with disabilities and their informal carers; child poverty; pensions; maternity benefits; family policies including parental leave and child maintenance; rights and opportunities for disabled people; ageing society; employers' issues; labour market issues; job centres and employment programmes; health and safety.

Home Office: security and terrorism; border control and immigration; police, criminal justice and public order; violent crime; antisocial behaviour; civil contingencies; drugs and alcohol abuse.

Ministry of Defence (MoD): health and welfare of armed forces personnel; Defence Medical Services for service personnel and their families including health service provision and commissioning of services from the NHS.

Ministry of Justice (MoJ): judicial and criminal justice system; prisons and probation services; human rights; victims of crime; legal aid.

The Treasury: public expenditure allocation; efficiency and value for money; taxation; tax credits.

Note: Some functions are exercised through government agencies such as the Food Standards Agency, the Health and Safety Commission and Sport England. Some functions are shared by departments (for example, training and employment skills, and criminal justice).

In the past, departmental relationships on health matters have varied considerably. At one end of the spectrum there has been outright distrust and overt hostility, evident in the relationship between the DH and the former Ministry of Agriculture, Fisheries and Food (MAFF) on issues of food safety, especially during the 1980s and 1990s (The BSE Inquiry, 2000). Some areas are marked by multilateral disputes. For example, alcohol policy, where the departments concerned with the consequences of alcohol misuse (such as violence and disorder, ill health and accidents) – which include DH, DfT and the Home Office – have often battled with other departments, such as those representing business, trade and industry (Baggott, 1990, 2010b).

Coordinating policy and joined-up government

The lack of coherence of central government has often been acknowledged, and successive governments have tried to promote 'joined-up approaches'. One suggestion, which resurfaced from time to time, was for a 'super department' to coordinate social policy, including health (Webster, 1996). A merger between the Ministries of Health and Social Security in the late 1960s, as noted earlier, was regarded as unsuccessful. In the 1970s, further attempts to join up government took the form of the Joint Approach to Social Policy (JASP), based on cross-departmental policy analyses by the Central Policy Review Staff, a think tank located in the Cabinet Office (Blackstone and Plowden, 1988; Challis et al, 1988), and other initiatives to get departments to consider the wider impact of their spending programmes (see Deakin and Parry, 2000). This was also regarded as ineffective. Another approach was to establish a cross-government ministerial post to coordinate policy. For example, the creation of a Minister for the Disabled in the 1970s was regarded as a moderate success in raising disability issues across government (Ashley, 1992). In 1997, the Blair government appointed a Minister for Public Health to coordinate policy across government. After a promising start, the post was effectively downgraded when its incumbent was replaced by a less senior minister (Baggott, 2010a).

Core executive

The Cabinet itself is not a forum for extensive policy debate, except in times of crisis (Smith, 1999). Nonetheless, its subcommittees, Cabinet committees, have an important role in agenda setting and decision-making. These consist of ministers drawn from several departments with a stake in the policy area, as well as others who have a coordinating or strategic role. The Home Affairs Cabinet Committee is the main forum for discussing health policy business. Its membership includes the Secretary of State for Health, the

Home Secretary, and the Secretaries of State for Defence, Work and Pensions, Communities and Local Government, Education, Transport, Environment, Food and Rural Affairs, Energy and Climate Change, and Culture, Media and Sport. The Lord Chancellor (and Secretary of State for Justice), Attorney General, Secretaries of State for Scotland, Wales and Northern Ireland and Secretary of State for Business, Innovation and Skills are also members of the committee, as are Cabinet Office and Treasury ministers. It is currently chaired by a minister without departmental responsibilities. Health ministers are represented on other Cabinet committees (such those on social justice, public expenditure efficiency, and the National Security Council subcommittee on threats, hazards, resilience and contingencies). They also sit on interdepartmental ministerial task forces that monitor and promote implementation of key priorities across departments, for example the integration of health and social care.

Coordination of policies also falls within the remit of the most powerful central government institutions. These include the Prime Minister's Office ('Number 10'), the Cabinet Office (which supports the Prime Minister and has a coordinating role across government) and the Treasury (which holds the government's 'purse strings'). Although these institutions are all involved in strategic direction and coordination, there are significant tensions between them (Burch and Holliday, 2004). Under New Labour this was given a further twist by the fraught political relationship between Prime Minister Tony Blair and Chancellor Gordon Brown (Campbell, 2008; Blair, 2010; Rawnsley, 2010; Mandelson, 2011). In the health arena, there were major disputes, over NHS spending and on foundation trusts, for example (Campbell, 2008; Rawnsley, 2010; Mandelson, 2011). In 2002, Alan Milburn, Secretary of State for Health, with Blair's support, argued that NHS providers should have greater freedom to make their own decisions, including more financial autonomy. Gordon Brown strongly opposed this, partly because it undercut Treasury financial controls, and partly because of his growing hostility to Blair and his allies (including Milburn). Blair backed down in the face of this 'endless, rancorous and destabilising' debate (Blair, 2010, p 491). Milburn felt betrayed at the dilution of his reform package, and subsequently resigned (Mandelson, 2011).

Between 2010 and 2015, the usual departmental, ideological and interpersonal conflicts that have characterised most governments were compounded by party political conflicts within the coalition (see **Box 3.3**).

Box 3.3: Conflict within the coalition government

The formulation of the coalition's NHS reforms revealed a great deal of conflict and confusion within central government (see Timmins, 2012). In particular, there was a lack of oversight by the core executive of the plans of Secretary of State for Health, Andrew Lansley. According to Timmins, the Coalition Agreement was a political exercise within Number 10. There was no input by DH civil servants, and little opportunity for Lansley to say much about his plans. He apparently attempted to challenge the pledge not to undertake top-down reorganisation, and other aspects of the agreement that were at odds with his policy. He was not a lone critic. Timmins' sources were scathing about the NHS commitments in the Coalition Agreement (their comments included: "a fudge", a "cut and shut job" and "a spatchcocked mess"). The DH supported Lansley's radical plans to reorganise the NHS, in spite of the Coalition Agreement. The White Paper on NHS reform was published in July 2010 (DH, 2010a). According to Timmins, at this stage concern was expressed in the Coalition Committee (which oversaw key decisions) particularly by Chancellor of the Exchequer, George Osborne. Nonetheless, the reforms went ahead. At this point the Lib Dems supported the reforms. Indeed, Nick Clegg, the Lib Dem leader and Deputy Prime Minister, and chair of the Home Affairs Cabinet Committee, signed off the White Paper (with a warm letter, according to Timmins). Later, under pressure from Party activists, senior Lib Dems changed their position and demanded changes to the legislation as it passed through Parliament (**Box 4.3**).

The White Paper and the Health and Social Care Bill were also criticised by some within the Conservative Party. After spending several years trying to build public confidence in their policies on the NHS, there was frustration among Conservative ranks that Labour had been handed a golden opportunity to attack them (BBC, 2012). As the Bill passed through its parliamentary stages, Lansley was increasingly attacked by his own side. *The Times* reported that 'a number ten insider' had said that Lansley 'should be taken out and shot' (Sylvester, 2012). Following the intervention of Cameron and Osborne, the DH was instructed to reach a compromise with the Bill's critics. The legislation was paused, and a short 'listening exercise' with stakeholders conducted.

This was a chaotic way of making key decisions. It was as much an indictment of the coalition's poor decision-making and consultation processes as of the much-maligned Secretary of State for Health. A key factor was that Number 10 lacked policy expertise in health policy at a vital time, when the reforms were being formulated. The Prime Minister did not initially have a specialist health adviser. Moreover, the Delivery Unit and Strategy Unit, created under New Labour, had been discontinued. The coalition responded by bolstering policy-making capacity (for example, the Prime Minister appointed a special adviser on health) and strengthening the Prime Minister's Policy Unit in 2011 (renamed the Policy and Implementation Unit). The Prime Minister also appointed more 'political' special advisers, with connections to the Conservative Party and right-of-centre think tanks. The Policy and Implementation Unit continued to attract criticism in some quarters for not being political enough, and was mostly staffed by civil servants (PASC, 2012). However, subsequent appointments gave it a more political and radical complexion (see West, 2013).

Number 10 and the Cabinet Office

The intervention of the Prime Minister in health policy is not new. In the 1970s, Harold Wilson intervened in the dispute over pay beds (see Chapter Two), and later established a Royal Commission on the NHS. In the late 1980s, Margaret Thatcher initiated a review of the NHS that led to the internal market reforms. Under Blair, however, prime ministerial intervention in health policy became more sustained and systematic (Baggott, 2007). There were several reasons for this. First, health and the NHS was a key government priority. Second, this policy area was a 'test bed' for New Labour's public service modernisation programme. Third, Blair's style of government was 'presidential', allowing much more direct intervention in departmental affairs than hitherto (Driver and Martell, 2002). Finally, prime ministerial intervention was facilitated by changes in central government processes.

Many of the key policies of this period – greater choice, competition, more use of the private sector and greater autonomy for NHS service providers – were attributed to Number 10. Furthermore, Number 10 took a closer interest in the details of policy. For example, the national service frameworks (NSFs) (see Chapter Two), which set out plans and service models for condition areas and population groups, were closely scrutinised and influenced by the Prime Minister's Office (see Hogg, 2002; Baggott et al, 2005) and by the Treasury. *The NHS Plan* of 2000 was also strongly influenced by Number 10 and the Treasury (see below). More routinely, Blair and his advisers regularly held meetings with the chief executive of the NHS, almost every fortnight (Crisp, 2011), which focused on progress with reform and targets.

The increased influence of Number 10 in the Blair era was linked to the activities of the Prime Minister's special advisers (Dorey, 2005; Short, 2005). Previous Prime Ministers retained health policy advisers. Margaret Thatcher, for example, appointed a businessman, Sir Roy Griffiths, as a health adviser. He exerted considerable influence over health policy in the 1980s, including NHS management changes and community care reforms (Wistow and Harrison, 1998). Blair's health policy advisers were regarded as highly influential over policy (*Society Guardian*, 2000; Baggott et al, 2005; Baggott, 2007; Jarman and Greer, 2010). Simon Stevens, the current chief executive of the NHS, was Blair's policy adviser between 2001 and 2004, having earlier advised the Secretary of State for Health. He was regarded as very influential (Seldon, 2004, p 633), and closely associated with many health policies introduced after 2000, including patient choice, NHS market reforms, foundation trusts and the increased use of the private sector.

In contrast, the Cameron government lacked a special adviser on health in the early stages. This was partly blamed for the mishandling of NHS reform (see **Box 3.3**). Subsequently, special health advisers were appointed, and this may have played a part in steadying the ship thereafter.

The intervention of Number 10 in policy matters was reflected in the reorganisation of institutions at the heart of government. Under Blair, the Prime Minister's Office was restructured, with the creation of a policy directorate to monitor the implementation of policies across government. There were also changes in the Cabinet Office, which coordinates policy across government (Kavanagh and Seldon, 2000; Burch and Holliday, 2004), placing greater emphasis on supporting the Prime Minister and 'government-wide' initiatives. These included a Prime Minister's Strategy Unit (PMSU) (to examine longer-term strategies and cross-departmental issues), a Delivery Unit (to oversee implementation) and an Office of Public Service Reform (which was fairly unsuccessful and short-lived). Meanwhile, the Prime Minister's Policy Unit (created back in the 1970s) continued.

In the 2000s, the PMSU was heavily involved in policy development (Baggott, 2007) in areas such as alcohol policy, global health and GM food, for example. Meanwhile the Delivery Unit monitored the implementation of policies and reforms, particularly with regard to the government's public services modernisation programme (HM Government, 1999b). Its activities included bi-monthly 'stocktakes', meetings attended by the Prime Minister, where departments would be held to account for their performance (Barber, 2008). Periodically, the Unit produced delivery reports, analysing departmental performance, and a league table to compare departments' performance. The Delivery Unit subsequently introduced capability reviews that analysed departments' ability to meet their objectives. It also had a role in spending reviews and the formulation of public service agreement (PSA) targets (discussed further below).

The Delivery Unit saw the DH as a key department. Its relationship with the department seems to have been cordial, largely because it delivered the government's objectives (at least until 2005/06, when financial problems were revealed). In general, it was seen as an effective institution in driving performance improvement while strengthening the Prime Minister's power (Seldon, 2004; Rawnsley, 2010). Its work was later subsumed into the Cabinet Office.

The coalition, despite its opposition to the performance management regime of New Labour, created its own systems of accountability and oversight in Whitehall. Instead of PSA targets, departments set out strategic priorities with structural reform plans and business plans. Monthly progress reports were produced. Performance was monitored by a number of bodies including the Treasury's Performance and Reform Unit and the Efficiency and Reform Group of the Cabinet Office. There was also oversight from the Prime Minister's Policy and Implementation Unit, and from a new Implementation Unit set up in 2012 within the Cabinet Office to coordinate the delivery of policy by departments.

It is acknowledged that despite the Prime Minister's power and resources, he cannot control all policy, all of the time (Smith et al, 2000). Indeed, departmental ministers have their own political resources, and the Prime Minister's approach is generally one of alliance-building rather than dictatorship (Richards and Smith, 2002). Prime Ministers have adopted an informal approach when dealing with policy issues. Informal bilateral discussions with senior ministers and other advisers were a key feature of the Blair era (Seldon, 2004), a technique also used extensively by Margaret Thatcher (Kavanagh and Seldon, 2000), but less so by John Major, who had a more collegial style (Seldon, 1994). The 'bilateral axis' between Number 10 and the DH has been remarked on (Baggott, 2007), with insiders arguing that although the former often drove the latter in a particular direction, the Department was able to exercise much influence over policy details.

The political perspective of health ministers and the closeness of their relationship with the Prime Minister has often been an important factor shaping the relationship between Number 10 and the DH. For example, the appointment of 'Blairite' ministers after 1999 helped to ensure a consensual dialogue with Number 10, as health ministers were keen to implement the Prime Minister's policies. This contrasted with the period 1997–99, when Frank Dobson was at the helm. But affinity does not always make for a good bilateral relationship. Despite being close to Cameron, Andrew Lansley's tenure at the DH was tempestuous to say the least (see **Box 3.3**).

The Treasury

The Treasury has provided a counterweight to the policies driven by Number 10. It is a small but powerful department that derives its influence from its control of the budget. It negotiates with the major spending departments on the overall size of their budget, and monitors their expenditure. Designated Treasury civil servants 'shadow' spending departments, meet with departmental civil servants, and also observe how services operate and what they achieve. Over the past few decades, the Treasury has moved beyond the control of public spending towards matters of policy and management (Deakin and Parry, 2000; Richards and Smith,

2002). Its concern with value for money has led to a greater focus on policy objectives and outcomes.

The Treasury's influence over departmental policies was strengthened by the introduction of comprehensive spending reviews (CSRs) and PSAs in the late 1990s. CSRs set out overall public expenditure, efficiency targets and departmental budgets, in the context of the government's priorities over the coming years (currently five years ahead). PSAs identified key priorities and targets for each department (and in some cases, such as obesity and health inequalities, some cross-departmental priorities and targets). The performance of each department was monitored against these objectives. In 2007 there was a significant change to PSAs. They were reduced in number and more closely aligned with key thematic priorities. In addition, strategic priorities were set for each department. Although the system was changed by the coalition – which discontinued PSAs – departments must still set out their strategic aims and are expected to meet key objectives (some of which still have targets associated with them).

Policy actors from the health arena have acknowledged the Treasury's substantial influence over health policy (Baggott, 2007). Its control of expenditure sets important parameters for policy development. Its role in promoting efficiency has had an effect on the DH directly by forcing it to cut staff numbers, which has affected capacity (Greer et al, 2014a). The Treasury has helped to shape DH priorities, objectives and targets. However, there is much agreement that, although providing an important counterweight to Number 10, the Treasury has usually played a secondary role in policy development (see Baggott, 2007).

Relationships between central government and outside organisations

Central government is bound to the outside world by many relationships. It has links with voluntary organisations, local authorities, the NHS, professional bodies, pressure groups, trade unions, business organisations, think tanks, research institutions and individual experts, among others. These policy stakeholders are examined further in Chapter Six. Relationships with these organisations and individuals are important in the formulation and implementation of policy. They supply expertise and information that is useful in the policy-making process. They also provide political support for policies, and can help implementation through their cooperation. Together, government and non-governmental bodies and individuals form policy networks that shape and implement policies (see Chapter One).

Government consults outside interests and experts in a variety of ways. It may issue proposals (in the form of a Green Paper, or a consultative document) for comment. Or it may establish an inquiry – such as a Royal Commission, a committee of inquiry or a public inquiry – to take evidence from interested parties. It also consults through a system of advisory committees. Representatives of outside organisations and individual experts are co-opted onto these bodies, which make policy recommendations. Organisations and individuals also meet directly with ministers, civil servants and special advisers to put their case on a particular issue.

Post-war governments adopted a consultative style, and engaged closely with groups and individual experts (Stewart, 1958). This approach began to break down during the 1970s, a time of growing social conflict marked by a decline in consensus on key social and economic issues (Baggott, 1995). During the 1980s the Thatcher government adopted a hostile approach to some producer groups that had formerly enjoyed a close relationship with government, such as the BMA, for example. Important reforms were introduced with little or no prior consultation. This was illustrated by the NHS internal market reforms of the late 1980s, which emerged out of a small working group appointed by the Prime Minister to formulate policy ideas (Butler, 1992; Timmins, 1995; Ham, 2000). This 'top-down' approach led to a failure to acknowledge political and practical barriers to implementation. Government subsequently had to rebuild relationships with producer groups in order to secure their cooperation in implementing policy (Baggott, 1995).

The Major government was portrayed as more consensual, and heralded a re-emphasis on consultation and building effective working relationships with outside organisations (Baggott, 1995; Baggott and McGregor-Riley, 1999). This led to some improvement in relationships with stakeholders, although prior consultation remained patchy and inadequate on some key policy issues. The Major government was not afraid to confront organised interests, although with less overt hostility than its predecessor. Because the Major government lacked the political resources of Thatcher's – having a smaller parliamentary majority coupled with an increasingly hostile media and a resurgent Labour opposition – it was forced to compromise on policy issues, particularly at the implementation stage.

On taking office, the Blair government called for an inclusive approach to policy-making. The government argued that by consulting outside experts, those who implement policy and those affected by it, early in the policy-making process, it would be possible to develop policies that were deliverable (HM Government, 1999b). In this period the government's inclusive style was reflected in a host of task forces appointed to explore a range of policy issues, including health (Platt, 1998). The formulation of *The NHS Plan* in 2000 was an example of this style of policy-making. It was formulated with the help of modernisation action teams (MATs) involving people drawn from NHS management, the professions, the voluntary sector, and health consumer and patients' groups, social services, trade unions and local government. Most MATs were chaired by a minister, with the prevention and inequalities team chaired by the CMO. In addition, civil servants from the DH, the Treasury and the Prime Minister's Office (including the Prime Minister's adviser on health) were involved in the MATs. Research has shown that MAT discussions were inclusive and wide-ranging (Baggott et al, 2005; Baggott, 2007).

Despite the goodwill built by *The NHS Plan* process, the Blair government attracted criticism for its autocratic style and for failing to consult adequately. Relationships with producer groups, notably the BMA, deteriorated. After 2000, reform ideas tended to emanate from special advisers, business organisations and think tanks, rather than from organisations representing professionals, health workers, patients and the public (see Chapter Six).

As Alvarez-Rosete and Mays (2008) noted, important changes did take place in the health policy process from the late 1990s. There was sign of a shift to a more open and inclusive style of governance, marked by greater pluralism and the involvement of more policy actors. However, they also observed that the extent of the change was modest. Government continued to adopt a centralised approach, as most initiatives came from government sources, and it sought to maintain control over policy processes and policies.

It is difficult to detect differences in policy style between the Blair and Brown governments, as the latter's tenure was comparatively short. The Darzi reforms, initiated by Brown, were relatively uncontroversial and based on extensive consultation. However, the momentum of the earlier reforms – choice, competition and foundation trusts – continued.

The coalition's policy style was more chaotic, due to the interaction of party politics and central government institutions (see Chapter Two and **Box 3.3**). After initially charging ahead with radical reform, with little consultation, the government was forced to pause the legislation to allow for consultation with stakeholders. The NHS Future Forum (an independent advisory panel including members drawn from the professions, local government, NHS management, service providers and the voluntary sector, as well as patients' representatives) was established as a vehicle for this. It made a series of recommendations to government, and most of the controversial issues in the Bill were addressed – although not necessarily to the satisfaction of all critics (see Chapter Four).

Surveys of stakeholders have revealed that although they are broadly positive about how the DH engages with them, certain shortcomings have persisted (Ipsos MORI, 2012, 2013). The key problems are that consultations are often too short; that engagement needs to be more consistent; that different parts of the DH need to work with them in a more joined-up way; and that engagement needs to be more open and more of a two-way process (with more feedback on consultations, for example). Stakeholders also pointed out that the Health and Social Care Act 2012 had a negative impact on many stakeholder relationships with the department, but that this did not appear to have a lasting effect on relationships with officials.

Conclusion

This chapter has explored the institutions at the heart of health policy-making. It has shown that health policy is not the sole preserve of the DH, but involves other central government institutions. The important roles of core executive institutions such as Number 10 and the Treasury have been identified. Although there appears to have been a centralisation of health policy in recent years, such intervention is not unprecedented. Prime Ministers have previously intervened in health policy and the NHS, but under the Blair administration, these centralising tendencies became more systematic. Centralisation appears to have been part of an attempt to impose a more rational policy-making style within central government. The clarification of goals, centralisation, target setting, PSAs, monitoring and the joining up of central government activities all reflect this. The shift in the balance of power between ministers and their special advisers relative to departmental civil servants was also an indicator of this approach.

The coalition initially adopted a rather hands–off approach to health policy that proved politically disastrous. This was replaced with a more interventionist approach. However, during the implementation phase of the NHS reforms, the DH once again seems to be have been given freedom to manage the process (although with central oversight and scrutiny). Even so, this occurred in the context of a policy to allow the NHS more autonomy from the centre (see Greer et al, 2014a). If such a policy is carried through fully, central policies will carry less weight. Whether or not this is likely to happen is discussed further in Chapter Seven.

Summary

- Although the DH is the main focus for health policy, other government departments have health-related responsibilities.
- Health is a key policy area for the Prime Minister, the Cabinet Office and the Treasury.
- There was an increase in the intervention of the core institutions of central government in health policy, particularly under the New Labour governments.
- Special advisers have become very influential over health policy, particularly those working for the Prime Minister. Civil servants appear to have become less influential over policy formation but retain an important role in relation to implementation

Key questions

1. Why does Number 10 intervene in health policy?
2. Many believe that the influence of civil servants within the DH has been weakened in recent years. Is this the case, and if so, why has this occurred?
3. What are the main functions of special advisers?
4. How is health policy coordinated across government departments?

four

Parliament and health policy

Overview

This chapter looks at the impact of Parliament on health policy. It begins with a discussion of the health interests of MPs, and then moves on to analyse the role and function of the House of Commons in relation to health policy. This is followed by an examination of the role of the House of Lords.

Over 30 years ago, Ingle and Tether (1981) argued that Parliament had minimal influence over health policy. They argued that Parliament was largely powerless when faced with a majority government, and that the House of Commons did not scrutinise health policy and administration effectively. The ability and commitment of MPs to raise issues of concern to their constituents was acknowledged, but the tools of the trade (debates and questions) were found wanting. Scrutiny by the House of Lords was rated as high quality, although the Chamber lacked 'clout' (Ingle and Tether, 1981, p 47). This chapter examines whether or not Ingle and Tether's findings are still relevant today.

Health policy interests of MPs

Individual background and personal factors

MPs' interests are shaped by a range of background and personal factors (Richards, 1972). Some MPs have worked in healthcare, including, for example, Dr Richard Taylor, the former independent MP for Wyre Forest (2001–10), who was an NHS consultant. Medically qualified MPs in the 2010–15 Parliament included Dr Sarah Wollaston, who chaired the Health

Select Committee (see below), and Dr Dan Poulter, who served as a DH minister. Other MPs have previously worked in the NHS as nurses, dentists or in other health occupations. Some MPs have an interest in health arising from personal or family experience of illness. Examples from the 2010–15 Parliament include Laura Sandys and Paul Maynard, both of whom have epilepsy and have been active in Parliament in raising awareness of the issues facing people with this condition. Others have health policy interests as a result of working with health charities, while some sit on NHS boards as non-executive directors.

Constituency interests

MPs' interests are shaped by constituency factors. Local NHS staff and patients may approach them to raise issues of concern. Sometimes this will relate to an individual matter, such as problems accessing services. MPs undertake a 'welfare officer' role, where they take on cases raised by individual constituents. But there are also broader issues of local interest, such as the closure of a hospital facility. Involvement in local health matters is driven by civic duty, and to some extent, by political calculation. MPs are keenly aware of the importance of health issues to their constituents. Moreover, local press, radio and television take a close interest in health issues, and this offers opportunities for MPs to maintain and raise their profile with voters.

Economic interests and other affiliations

MPs have a range of health-related economic interests and other affiliations, which they are required to declare in the interests of openness and transparency. This does not necessarily mean that they will be controlled by these interests and contacts, but it is important to acknowledge them as potential factors for influencing MPs' judgements and decisions. Some MPs have a stake in healthcare businesses, such as shareholdings in pharmaceutical companies, for example (see House of Commons, 2014). Some are paid to advise organisations in the health sector, some of which have a commercial interest in NHS contracts. A small number of MPs are company directors in the health and care sector or in businesses with health implications (such as food and drink companies). Some MPs have links with trade unions in the health sector (such as Unite), and receive donations to their constituency parties from these sources.

Collective interests

MPs and Peers (members of the House of Lords) may develop health policy interests by participating in various parliamentary events and activities. They often attend parliamentary receptions, hosted by outside organisations, where they receive information from business interests, professional organisations, charities and pressure groups. This might involve highlighting new research, raising awareness about particular conditions, identifying problems and possible solutions (Baggott et al, 2005).

All-Party Parliamentary Groups (APPGs) are also useful in enabling MPs and Peers to develop health interests. They are mainly fora for backbench MPs, although ministers attend them, usually to respond to an issue of concern. Although not official committees, APPGs are acknowledged by Parliament. In 2015, 618 APPGs were registered. Of these, 143 were 'country groups' (focusing on issues relating to a specific nation state). Of the remaining 475, known as 'subject groups', 96 directly covered health topics (although others, for example, climate change, considered issues relevant to health). Health subject groups included: specific diseases (for example, diabetes, breast cancer and osteoporosis); public health issues (obesity, drug policy reform, smoking and health); certain groups (older people and ageing, and children); and health service providers, services and treatments (emergency services, maternity services and the drugs industry).

APPGs are seen as a useful way of informing MPs and Peers, and as a means of persuading them to raise issues. They are regarded as a useful channel of communication between outside groups and Parliament, and as a means of building cross-party support (as they are open to members of all parties) (Baggott et al, 2005; Baggott, 2007). They provide a useful forum where MPs and Peers can discuss issues and put their views to ministers, and where the latter can explain their policies. However, their shortcomings include duplication and overlap between committees, and limited resources. Health APPGs appear to be most effective when they have a clear focus to their work and assistance from external organisations, which includes administrative and financial support. For example, the British Heart Foundation provides the secretariat for the APPG on heart disease, and the APPG on cancer receives administrative support from Macmillan Cancer Support. Any support must, however, be declared (see Register of All Party Groups, 2015).

In addition, each parliamentary party contains health subject committees, which consider policy issues. While there is uncertainty about their exact role, and their policy influence is generally regarded as low (see Jones, 1990), they are primarily a means by which party leaders can manage dissent among backbench MPs or as a means of communication between frontbenchers (government ministers or opposition shadow ministers) and backbenchers. Nonetheless, the health subject committee of the governing party can occasionally be influential (Baggott, 2007). For example, when Labour was in office between 1997–2010, the Parliamentary Labour Party Health Committee chair had access to ministers. Ministers appeared before the Committee to explain their policies. On controversial issues the Committee was used to secure concessions (for example, on the issue of foundation trusts where opinion on the Labour backbenches was hostile). Ministers also used the Committee to gauge party backbench opinion and to 'firefight' backbench discontent.

Scrutiny, accountability and policy influence

Parliamentary questions, debates and early day motions

Parliamentarians have several instruments with which to question government, obtain information or put a case or argument (see Silk and Walters, 1998; Rush, 2005). MPs and Peers can table questions, initiate or contribute to debates, and initiate or support early day motions (EDMs). What follows relates to the House of Commons, but similar procedures exist in the House of Lords.

Parliamentary Questions (PQs) are directed at ministers (including the Prime Minister, in the House of Commons only) and receive a written or oral response. Each department faces 'oral questions' around once a month (the Prime Minister, once a week), providing an opportunity for MPs to challenge ministers in the House. MPs can also ask Urgent Questions on issues where the Speaker agrees that an immediate answer is required. Both oral and written responses appear in the parliamentary record (see www.parliament.uk/business/publications/hansard/). For example, on 10 October 2013, 12 Questions were answered by the DH on topics including school milk, complementary medicine and mental health services. Today more than one in ten PQs in the Commons is answered by the DH.

The number and proportion of health questions has risen substantially since the 1960s (see Baggott, 2007). In the 1960–61 session of Parliament, 971 health questions were asked, representing 7 per cent of the total. By 1980–81, the number of health questions had risen to 2,169, but this represented the same proportion as 20 years earlier. The number and proportion of questions has since risen, and in 2002–03, almost 14 per cent of Questions in the Commons were answered by the DH. In 2012–13, 5,739 MPs' Questions were answered in the Commons by the DH, representing 12.2 per cent of the total on all topics (46,902) in that session.

MPs and outside organisations have commented that PQs are useful to obtain information about health issues not in the public domain and to raise concerns (Baggott, 2007), although ministers can refuse to answer questions if the cost is too high, the information is unavailable centrally, the matter is commercially sensitive, or it is not in the public interest to divulge it (see Select Committee on Public Administration, 2002).

In the health domain, as in other policy areas, ministers have been able to limit the impact of PQs. The establishment of arm's-length institutions (see Chapter Three) has enabled ministers to refuse to answer questions about operational matters. Following the creation of foundation trusts in 2003, the DH informed MPs that such questions should be directed to these new institutions. Furthermore, ministers have used commercial confidentiality to deter MPs probing the involvement of private contractors in running NHS services and projects.

Parliamentary debates provide another opportunity to scrutinise government policy. Although the government effectively controls the parliamentary agenda, there are opportunities for the opposition parties and backbench MPs to initiate debates. Those launched by opposition parties can put real pressure on government. Such 'set-piece' debates are usually reserved for high-profile issues. In the days allocated for opposition debates in 2010–12 (an unusually long parliamentary session), six focused on the subject of the NHS (plus an emergency debate on the Health and Social Care Bill).

Backbenchers can also initiate debates. In 2010, the Backbench Business Committee was set up to organise these debates. Some take place on the floor of the House, others in a room near Westminster Hall (in the Palace of Westminster). A number of sessions are allocated to debate particular issues of importance. In the session 2010–12, eight were on a health or social care topic (including contaminated blood products, drugs policy, the care of older people and assisted suicide). In addition, short adjournment debates are held on specific topics, often local issues, on most days when the House is sitting. Although adjournment debates are poorly attended and attract little media coverage, they do guarantee a response from the minister responsible (Baggott et al, 2005). As **Box 4.1** indicates, health is a popular topic for adjournment debates in the House of Commons.

Box 4.1: Adjournment debates: health and social care topics

7–31 January 2013

7 January   Newark Hospital

8 January   Female genital mutilation*

8 January   Liverpool Care Pathway*

9 January   Diabetes*

9 January   Antibiotics (intensive farms)*

10 January   Education support for children with cancer

14 January   Vascular services, Wycombe Hospital

16 January   Personal Health and Social Education*

21 January   East Midlands Ambulance Service

22 January   Hospital services, South London*

22 January   Dementia services, Gloucester*

23 January   Terminal illness; access to medicines*

23 January   Progressive supranuclear palsy*

29 January   Epilepsy

30 January   Horsemeat*

30 January   Children's services*

There was also a backbench debate on dementia on 10 January.

 * Westminster Hall debate.

Source: House of Commons Debates, 2012–13

MPs also present petitions from the public. There is a long-standing practice whereby citizens can make a written appeal to an MP entailing a request for action. The MP who receives the petition can either give a short statement on the petition, or place it behind the Speaker's chair. The text of the petition is published in *Hansard* and a copy sent to the relevant government department.

More recently, government has introduced an e-petitions process. In 2011 a central website was created to allow petitions to be created online by citizens for others to endorse. Since September 2012, e-petitions that receive substantial support are expected to receive a response from the relevant government department; some are also debated in Parliament. A petition receiving 100,000 signatures can be considered for debate in Parliament, but for this to happen, it must be supported by an MP who agrees to initiate a debate. In addition, the Backbench Business Committee must also agree that a debate can take place, and schedule it accordingly.

On 11 October 2013, 571 e-petitions were open on health topics, while a further 1,336 were closed (each is open for one year). In total, the DH has had a total of 1,907 e-petitions (open and closed) since the process began. This is the fourth largest across government departments (the Treasury received the most, with 3,292). Some health e-petitions have received large support. The 'Drop the Health Bill' e-petition (closed 16.5.12) attracted 179,464 supporters, and was debated on 13 March 2012. The debate was not secured via the Backbench Business Committee, however, but due to a motion moved by the opposition.

E-petitions are a channel for expressing public sentiment, and can lead to parliamentary debates. However, there is some concern that they may raise public expectations that are subsequently not met. As there is no guarantee of a response from government or Parliament, this could increase public cynicism. Also, there is confusion because the e-petition process – which is a government initiative – is distinct from the traditional petitioning of Parliament procedure (Procedure Committee, 2012, 2013a; Hansard Society 2012).

Another instrument is the EDM. EDMs are formal motions submitted for debate (although they are rarely debated). Instead, they serve as statements about an issue, institution or policy, which MPs (excluding ministers, government whips and other MPs serving in an official capacity) may initiate, support and amend. They are used to express opinions on issues of general interest, to promote political debate, to give prominence to a campaign or event or to the work of an outside organisation, or to highlight local issues (Procedure Committee, 2013b). A minority of EDMs (around 2 per cent) are used to oppose statutory instruments (see below), while some are used to criticise individuals or organisations. EDMs can provide a useful barometer of opinion. When supported by a large number of MPs, particularly backbenchers of the governing party, they can capture the attention of government. According to the late Lord Ashley (1992, p 193), a seasoned campaigner on health and disability issues, 'over 100 signatures on a motion is usually regarded as significant.' Health issues are popular subjects for EDMs, being the subject of over 10 per cent of the total number tabled (Baggott, 2007). In the 2012–13 session of Parliament there were over 1,300 EDMs, attracting an average of around 25 signatures each. Two of the 'top 10' EDMs (that is, those receiving the most support) were on the NHS (securing 214 – the highest for any EDM that session – and 155 signatures respectively).

The various parliamentary instruments are relatively weak when used in isolation. However, they can be effective when deployed in a coordinated manner and coupled with external pressure from the media and pressure groups (see Chapter Six) (Baggott, 2007). They can be used by outside organisations to mobilise MPs and get them to raise the profile of an issue. For example, between 2010-13 the Joint Epilepsy Council (JEC, a coalition of epilepsy groups) worked with MPs on the APPG on epilepsy (for which the JEC provides a secretariat) to promote three Commons debates on this issue. Members of the APPG also raised PQs and initiated EDMs during this period. The value of PQs, debates and EDMs is that they indicate parliamentary opinion. If this opinion is strong, the government will be more likely to give concessions. Parliamentary opinion expressed in this way (and through other channels such as party committees, APPGs and select committees; see below) can attract the attention of health ministers and civil servants to an issue that is currently low on the political agenda, or conversely, may indicate opposition to a policy currently being pursued.

Select committees

Select committees are official committees of the House of Commons that inquire into policy, administration and expenditure (Dorey, 2005; Russell and Benton, 2011; Benton and Russell, 2013). They take written and oral evidence from individuals and organisations (including ministers and civil servants), and publish reports with recommendations. Some have a wide-ranging brief across government, such as the Public Accounts Committee (PAC) (which examines the use of taxpayers' money by government departments and agencies) and the Environmental Audit Committee (which examines cross-departmental action on environmental issues), and cover health issues as part of their remit. Others examine the work of particular departments and related agencies, such as the Health Committee, which focuses on the DH and health policy, national health agencies and public bodies including the NHS, and public health issues such as obesity (see **Box 4.2**).

Select committees consist of backbench MPs (numbering between 11 and 14). Their composition reflects the balance of seats held by the parties. However, they are expected to act in a non-partisan way. To reflect this, some are chaired by MPs from opposition parties. For example, in the 2010–15 Parliament, Labour chaired 11 out of the 28 select committees (Conservatives chaired 15 and Lib Dems 2).

There have been several concerns about the weakness of select committees, in particular that they lack resources, independence and powers to challenge the government. However, as research has shown, they can have considerable influence. Between 1997–2010, 40 per cent of their recommendations were accepted by government in part or in full (Russell and Benton, 2011). A slightly higher proportion of measurable recommendations (44 per cent) was actually implemented to some extent. The same study found that there were other, more subtle, ways in which they could exert influence, including contributing to debates, influencing agendas, drawing together evidence, exposing failings, improving the quality of government decision-making and brokering between government actors. In addition, committees can be influential where government fears criticism and seeks to pre-empt this. The influence of select committees and their ability to hold government to account has been due to several factors (PCRC, 2013a; Liaison Committee, 2012). First are efforts to reduce the influence of the government (and the opposition) parties over the selection of committee members and chairs. Following a number of cases where appointments to chair select committees were blocked by party whips, reforms were eventually implemented in 2010, making most of these appointments subject to secret ballot by all MPs. Members of the committees are also elected by secret ballot (although this is organised by each party). Second, the lack of resources of select committees was addressed by increasing their staffing resources, including the appointment of assistants and advisers to support their work, and it was also agreed that chairs would be remunerated for their additional responsibilities. Third, committees have received additional powers, to conduct pre-appointment hearings for senior posts, and to conduct pre-legislative scrutiny (see below). Fourth, committees have done more to publicise and raise the profile of their work in the media. Even so, there is still room for improvement (Russell and Benton, 2011; Liaison Committee, 2012; Benton and Russell, 2013; PCRC, 2013a). Shortcomings have been found in following up recommendations; an inability to commission appropriate research; evidence of poor attendance and lack of attention to detail from some committee members; and a continuing failure by some in government to take select committees seriously.

Box 4.2: The Health Committee

The Health Committee has been perceived as a useful scrutiny body by observers and policy actors (Baggott, 2007). However, it has operated within the constraints facing all such committees. These include limited resources to conduct inquiries; a lack of publicity for reports; insufficient time for debating reports; and limited opportunities to follow up recommendations in a systematic way. Things have improved somewhat with greater independence from the party whips, more resources and a more proactive approach to publicising their work.

The Health Committee, like all select committees, has the potential to influence policy. Policy actors cited by Baggott (2007) noted that the Committee could be influential, particularly in highlighting neglected issues and helping to get 'less fashionable' issues (such as mental health and sexual health) on to the agenda. They noted that pressure groups are keen to have their recommendations endorsed by the Health Committee as they believe it adds weight and credibility to their case (see also Baggott et al, 2005). However, they also pointed out that the Committee's influence over policy was limited when it went against the grain of current government policy.

A major study found that between 1997–2010 the Health Committee published 59 specific scrutiny reports (plus one monitoring report and two reports on appointments), making 1,820 recommendations (Russell and Benton, 2011). Of the 59 reports, 7 per cent were deemed to be agenda setting, 27 per cent examined proposals, 19 per cent reviewed progress, 44 per cent responded to failures and 3 per cent were 'follow-up' inquiries. Compared with the average for all departmental committees, the Health Committee undertook proportionately much more inquiries that were 'responding to failure' (the average for all committees was 15 per cent) and much less on 'reviewing progress' (average 42 per cent). The Health Committee's success in having recommendations fully or partly accepted was 35 per cent, slightly lower than the average for all committees (40 per cent). Similarly, the proportion of measurable recommendations partially or fully implemented (37 per cent) was less for health than the average for all committees (44 per cent).

In practice, it is difficult to evaluate the influence of any select committee, as they are only one of several potential channels of influence (alongside party politics, the activities of pressure groups, media and public opinion, and other parliamentary processes). Moreover, much depends on forces within government that may make the committee's recommendations more acceptable or not. Select committees also operate in quite subtle ways. There are many of examples of where they have facilitated policy shifts and changes and specific decisions, although they cannot claim to have been the sole or main initiator of these developments.

Two inquiries shed light on the role of the Health Committee in relation to policy. The inquiry into smoking in public places (Health Committee, 2005a) strengthened the resolve of some within government for tougher action on smoking. The government initially opted for a partial ban on smoking in licensed premises, but the Committee was instrumental in pressing for a comprehensive ban, backed by health groups and some business interests. The Health Committee's (2011a) report on public health provided a sharp analysis of the weaknesses of the government's policy to transfer NHS public health functions to local authorities and to restructure national public health expertise and oversight to a new executive body. Most of the Committee's recommendations were eventually accepted and implemented by the government in its Health and Social Care Act 2012 (see **Box 4.3**).

Other departmental committees also have an interest in health-related matters, and have covered such issues in their inquiries. Examples include the Transport Committee (road safety), the Environment, Food and Rural Affairs Committee (environmental health and food safety) and Home Affairs (alcohol and drugs). As mentioned, cross-departmental committees, such as PAC, are also important as they consider health and the NHS as part of their remit. PAC, much-feared in Whitehall, is conventionally chaired by an opposition MP. In the period between 2010–15 it produced critical reports on issues such as out-of-hours primary care services, managing NHS consultants, NHS efficiency savings and the NHS IT programme.

Legislation

Primary legislation takes the form of Acts of Parliament, which result from Bills approved by both the Commons and the Lords and given Royal Assent. The House of Commons is the most powerful legislative body and can enforce its will on the Lords (discussed further below). Secondary legislation is made by governments under powers already granted to them by previous Acts.

If a governing party (or parties) has a majority in the House of Commons (that is, has more MPs than the other parties put together), it is able to control the legislative process. The bigger the majority, the greater the degree of control. This is because on most legislation, MPs do not have a free vote, but are subject to party discipline. Party discipline is a process (enforced by special MPs called party whips) that seeks to ensure that MPs vote in line with their party leaders, although MPs occasionally rebel against the party line. In 2003, for example, 62 Labour MPs voted against (and a further 50 abstained) the Health and Social Care Bill, which introduced the controversial policy of foundation trusts. The government's majority was only 35. During the final stages of the Bill its majority fell further, to only 17. Although the Bill became law, the government had to make concessions to appease the rebels. The coalition government also faced opposition to its health legislation from its own MPs, and was forced to make significant changes to its Health and Social Care Bill (see **Box 4.3**).

Nonetheless, it is very rare for a government with a substantial majority to be defeated on a vote in the Commons. In reality, Parliament's main function is to scrutinise the government's legislation and to raise concerns, which can lead the government to rethink its proposals. MPs (and Peers) can propose their own amendments to legislation. These can be successful if they get sufficient support from Parliament, although this is unlikely without government consent.

Some issues cut across party lines, including matters of conscience such as embryo research, abortion and genetic testing. On such matters, MPs are usually permitted to debate and vote in a non-partisan way. MPs may also bring forward Private Member's Bills (PMBs) on these or other issues. However, the government's control of the parliamentary timetable means that its consent is necessary in order to have any chance of success. The success rate for PMBs is very low. In the last 30 years, around 10 per cent of PMBs introduced in the Commons or Lords have become Acts of Parliament (and less than 5 per cent did so in the period 2000–01 to 2009–10; see HCIO, 2010). This compares with an almost 100 per cent success rate for government Bills. An example of a successful PMB was the Human Fertilisation and Embryology (Deceased Fathers) Bill, which became law in 2003. This clarified the law on the registration of deceased fathers on birth certificates where the child is conceived through fertility treatment. The government was prepared to amend the law, but did not have sufficient space in its legislative programme. Indeed, government departments often use MPs and Peers to introduce legislation that is important, but not a major priority for government. In 2012–13, nine of the ten PMBs that became law were generated in this way.

Parliament can influence policy indirectly by using legislative procedures to raise issues and concerns. MPs can intervene in debates on government bills to plant ideas for future legislation. PMBs are also useful in raising issues, even if they have no chance of becoming law. They can be used to test parliamentary opinion, in an effort to persuade the government to introduce its own legislation. For example, government legislation to ban tobacco advertising in 2002 followed many PMBs on the subject over previous decades. In recent years MPs have introduced Bills on a range of health issues including alcohol marketing, the regulation of soft drinks, and support for carers, to name just a few.

MPs get opportunities to debate, propose amendments and vote on various stages of a Bill as it passes through Parliament. A key point in the process is the committee stage. Public bill committees (known as standing committees until 2007), appointed in proportion to the party strengths in the House of Commons, undertake scrutiny of the Bill. The government's in-built majority on these committees (when it has a majority in the House as a whole), coupled with the system of party discipline, enables government to exert considerable control over the committees. Research has shown that although these committees are undertaking more scrutiny, discussing more amendments and proposing more changes than 30 years ago, the government is less likely to accept amendments from backbench MPs and the opposition parties (Thompson, 2013). Also, government amendments represent an increasing proportion of the amendments moved or tabled in these committees (from 21 per cent in 1967–71 to 30 per cent in 2000–10). This is not to say that the committees are simply a rubber stamp for government Bills, however. Governments do accept amendments from backbench and opposition MPs, and in the modern era are more likely than in previous times to adopt amendments from these sources (that is, by introducing them as government amendments). And amendments are sometimes accepted in whole or in part at post-committee stages of the Bill, following further consideration by government and consultation with MPs and external organisations (such as pressure groups, charities, business organisations, trade unions and professional groups). In particular, the report stage (where the relevant public bill committee reports back to the whole House) is often the most appropriate point for the government to table an amendment that reflects these deliberations.

Concern has been expressed about the quality of legislative scrutiny, and in particular, the role of public bill committees. The influence of whips over appointments and amendments has been highlighted, and measures proposed to limit their power, for example, by making appointments subject to similar procedures as select committees (PCRC, 2013a; Russell et al 2013). It has also been pointed out that public bill committees do not have a permanent membership, so are unable to build up expertise and a culture of cross-party working (PCRC, 2013a; Russell et al, 2013). Indeed, they often exclude those with expertise, especially if they are likely to be critics of the legislation. For example, in 2011, Conservative MP Dr Sarah Wollaston, a former GP, was unable to secure a seat on the committee considering the Health and Social Care Bill (Russell et al, 2013).

A number of changes have been introduced to improve the quality of legislative scrutiny. Pre-legislative scrutiny is undertaken (by Commons' select committees or by joint committees of both Houses) prior to their formal introduction to Parliament. The committee responsible examines the Bill in draft form and considers evidence from government, outside organisations and individuals. An example is the Draft Care and Support Bill, considered by a joint committee in 2012–13. The committee took oral and written evidence and also undertook an online consultation exercise with carers. The committee reported that the Bill needed to focus more on prevention and the integration of health, social care and other relevant services (such as housing), calling for more powers to mandate joint budgets (House of Lords and House of Commons, 2013).

Although recent governments have endorsed the pre-legislative procedure, only a minority of Bills are subject to such scrutiny. A number of bodies recommended that this process should be extended to more Bills, and that committees are given sufficient time to scrutinise them properly (Modernisation of the House of Commons, 2006; PCRC, 2013a, 2013b). There have also been calls to make available more information about forthcoming Bills, and to make it easier for outside groups and the public to influence legislation. A public reading stage for Bills, enabling comments on proposed legislation, was piloted. In addition, public bill committees now hold evidence-gathering sessions, usually prior to considering amendments to Bills. Although seen as a positive step, there is often insufficient time between the evidence-gathering sessions and committee discussions of amendments. This reflects broader criticism that more notice is needed to consider evidence and amendments to Bills, to enable meaningful debate (Modernisation of the House of Commons, 2006; PCRC, 2013b).

Over the years the increasing volume of legislation (in terms of primary legislation as well as secondary legislation) has been blamed for a decline in its quality (PCRC, 2013b). Key changes have been proposed. PCRC (2013b) called for quality standards for legislation. These would set out good practice, including the provision of information on the objectives of the legislation, clarification of the relationship between new and existing legislation, details of the costs and impact of the legislation, and the use of processes of consultation to take the views of outside organisations and individuals.

Health policy actors and observers are sceptical about the impact of Parliament on legislation (Baggott, 2007), especially when governments have a large majority, as has been the case for most of the period since 1979 (with the exception of the Major government between 1992 and 1997). However, the situation under the coalition government was different. Although the Conservative and Liberal Democrats had a good working majority, they were not able to steamroll legislation through quite as easily as the Thatcher and New Labour governments. **Box 4.3** examines the case of the Health and Social Care Act 2012, which was passed only after a large number of amendments.

Box 4.3: Health and Social Care Bill, 2011–12

The Health and Social Care Bill was introduced into the House of Commons in January 2011 to provide statutory underpinning for the coalition government's NHS reforms. The measures were enacted in 2012 in the face of great hostility from organisations representing health professions and the NHS workforce (including the BMA, Royal College of GPs and Royal College of Nursing) and other pressure groups (such as 38 Degrees, Keep Our NHS Public and UK Uncut). It was attacked by the Labour Party, a substantial section of the Liberal Democrat Party and also by elements of the Conservative Party.

As the Bill passed through its parliamentary stages, it was criticised by select committees, notably the Commons Health Committee (2011a, 2011b, 2011c) and the House of Lords Select Committee on the Constitution (2011a, 2011b). It was also criticised by senior figures, including former ministers from across party lines such as Lord Owen, Alan Milburn, Dame Shirley Williams, Lord Mackay and Lord Tebbit. Former NHS chief executive, Lord Crisp, described the reforms as 'a mess'. Specific concerns included: the speed and scale of the reforms; the increased scope for competition and privatisation; barriers to providing integrated care services; a lack of accountability relating to shifts in responsibility from the Secretary of State to the NHS Commissioning Board and local clinical commissioning bodies (see **Box 3.1**); and problems with governance of local commissioners. In addition, there were criticisms of the clauses on patient and public involvement (PPI), and on public health.

Initially, the government decided to tough it out. The Secretary of State for Health, Andrew Lansley, bolstered by support from the Prime Minister, David Cameron, and Deputy Prime Minister, Nick Clegg, gave few concessions. However, things began to unravel in March 2011 (Timmins, 2012) when the Liberal Democrats' Spring Conference voted against their leadership's motion of support for the NHS reforms. Under pressure from Liberal Democrat members and parliamentarians, the Lib Dem leader Nick Clegg called for changes to the Bill. Conservative MPs also became concerned, although most still supported Lansley. In response, Cameron instructed Lansley and the DH to undertake a consultation on the Bill, in effect, 'pausing' the legislation. This was a highly unusual step. To facilitate this listening exercise, the DH set up the NHS Future Forum to report back within weeks. The Forum was headed by a doctor, and its membership included clinicians, health service managers and service users. Local authority social services and voluntary organisations were also represented.

The government responded positively to the Future Forum's recommendations (NHS Future Forum, 2011) and introduced many changes to the Bill. In addition, further debates in Parliament brought other amendments. In all, over 2,000 amendments were proposed, and 375 substantive changes were made (Timmins, 2012). The government was defeated on two votes (both in the Lords): the first (which was eventually accepted by the government) gave mental health equal priority with physical health. The second concerned a review of the tax treatment of voluntary organisations supplying health services (this was accepted by government in a modified form; it agreed to review all providers of NHS services, including the voluntary sector, with regard to taxation as well as other relevant issues that might affect their ability to provide health services on behalf of the NHS).

It is impossible to list all the amendments made to the Health and Social Care Bill during its stormy passage through Parliament, but the most significant, perhaps, are as follows:

- Clarification of the Secretary of State's responsibilities for health services (see **Box 3.1**).
- GP commissioning consortia renamed as clinical commissioning groups (CCGs).
- CCGs to have responsibilities for local residents not registered with local GPs.
- Changes to CCG governance (for example, composition extended to include other clinicians and lay people; requirements to declare and manage conflicts of interest).
- Research, education and training enshrined as core responsibilities of the NHS (with clear duties placed on the Secretary of State for Health, the NHS Commissioning Board [now NHS England] and CCGs).
- Restrictions on foundation trusts' ability to earn income from non-NHS sources. In addition to a limit introduced by the government, that foundation trusts must not earn more from non-NHS sources than from the NHS, they would have to report on the impact of non-NHS income generation on NHS services. Also, any trust wishing to increase the percentage of its income derived from non-NHS sources by 5 per cent or more would have to secure the support from a majority of its board of governors.
- The duties and powers of Monitor, the regulator of the NHS market, were amended to place greater emphasis on promoting integration of services to improve quality and reduce inequalities while preventing anti-competitive behaviour that operates against the interests of service users.
- The clause on setting maximum prices for NHS services was amended in an effort to discourage price competition (and the 'cherry picking' of NHS services by the private sector).
- With regard to PPI, the Bill was amended to strengthen the individual patient's voice in how services are commissioned for them. In addition, CCGs were required to report on their PPI activities. Another change was to give the new

national Healthwatch body greater independence from its host (the CQC) by requiring that a majority of its board members must not be members of the CQC.

- There were many amendments to the public health provisions of the Bill, which transferred important functions to local government and to a new national body, Public Health England. These included statutory protection for directors of public health, provision for statutory guidance on their appointment, termination, employment terms and conditions, and greater involvement of the new health and wellbeing boards (see Chapter Eight) in NHS commissioning plans. In addition, the government promised to amend other relevant legislation, for example, to establish the legal status of the director of public health as a chief officer in local authorities where they are based.

Secondary legislation

The ability of MPs to scrutinise legislation has been adversely affected by the rise in secondary legislation, also known as 'delegated legislation' (see Silk and Walters, 1998, pp 146-151; Rush, 2005). Primary legislation grants powers that enable ministers to make further legal provisions. Most secondary legislation takes the form of statutory instruments (of which there are various types, including regulations, orders and rules). The number of statutory instruments has increased over the last 30 years – in 2014, there were 3,494 (see www.legislation.gov.uk/uksi). Although an efficient way of dealing with routine and uncontroversial matters, they enable government to avoid scrutiny on some important matters. There are few opportunities to debate secondary legislation, and most become law without a debate or vote. Even when debated, they cannot be amended and are rarely rejected. There is a special committee (established jointly between the Commons and the Lords) that scrutinises secondary legislation, but it is overworked, confines itself to technical matters (that is, consistency with the relevant primary legislation), and has no powers to amend secondary legislation or to prevent it from coming into force. However, government does withdraw a small number of statutory instruments each year that have attracted intense criticism from the committee. Other parliamentary bodies also examine powers and processes relating to statutory instruments (including the House of Lords' Secondary Legislation Scrutiny Committee, the Lords' Delegated Powers and Regulatory Reform Committee, and the Commons Regulatory Reform Committee).

A large amount of secondary legislation is produced on health matters (an example was the somewhat tortuously-titled 'NHS Bodies and Local

Authorities Partnership Arrangements, Care Trusts, Public Health and Local Healthwatch Regulations 2012' [SI No 3094]). Although statutory instruments are mainly technical, they do affect the implementation of health policy. In the main the instruments are developed quietly, usually in consultation with affected interests. However, they occasionally become the subject of public controversy. For example, when in 2013 the government brought forward regulations under the previous year's Health and Social Care Act, opponents believed that it was seeking to stimulate competition in health services above and beyond the provisions in the Act (and thereby reneging on previous assurances). As a result of protests from doctors and other health pressure groups, the government had to revise the regulations.

Finance

Parliament has little influence over government's public spending decisions (see Hansard Society Commission on Parliamentary Scrutiny, 2001; Parliament First, 2003). However, it does have a role in reviewing expenditure plans, and examines how money has been spent. For example, departmental select committees, including the Health Committee, scrutinise public expenditure and make recommendations in their reports.

A number of specialist offices and committees also monitor expenditure. The National Audit Office (NAO), headed by the Comptroller and Auditor General (CAG), audits the government's accounts and issues reports on specific topics, including health and NHS programmes and services. The CAG/NAO undertakes an initial investigation and produces a report. PAC (see above) follows up these reports and can revisit issues if necessary.

A non-parliamentary body, the Audit Commission, performed an important role in the auditing of local public bodies and the assessment of value for money in government policies and programmes. It produced reports on a range of health policy issues such as partnership working, financial management in the NHS, care in the community, children's health and health service targets. These reports often highlighted inefficiencies as well as variations and gaps in policy implementation, prompting changes in policy and practice. In 2010 the coalition government announced the abolition of the Audit Commission. It was eventually closed down in March 2015.

Redress of grievances

As noted earlier, MPs have a 'welfare officer' role (Richards, 1972, p 164), which involves helping constituents who are facing problems with government and public bodies, including maladministration, delay, unfair decisions and incompetence. MPs engage in many activities for their constituents. This includes contacting authorities on their behalf, and raising PQs, EDMs or debates to gain attention for their plight.

In addition, patients and their families can take up administrative and clinical complaints with the health ombudsman, appointed by Parliament. There is a health ombudsman for each country of the UK. In practice, these posts are combined with other posts – for example, in England the health ombudsman also serves as the parliamentary ombudsman and investigates complaints against other government bodies. In Wales, Northern Ireland and Scotland the health ombudsmen also undertake parliamentary and local ombudsmen roles).

Although health ombudsmen can shine a light on harmful and unfair practices, their role is restricted. Complainants are expected to take up the matter initially with the relevant health service body or clinician. Private health service providers are covered by the ombudsman's powers, but only when providing services funded by the NHS. The health ombudsman cannot look at policy matters, investigate issues that are not identified through specific complaints, nor enforce compliance with recommendations (which can include financial redress). However, an additional power was granted to produce special thematic reports, based on earlier investigations. This has been used to highlight areas where many complaints have been upheld, notably with regard to long-term care and NHS complaints procedures.

In recent years there has been criticism of the English health ombudsman for not fully investigating systematic failings in health services raised by multiple individual complaints. There have also been shortcomings in communication and working with other regulators. These have led to pressures to reform the health ombudsman's powers and practices.

House of Lords

The House of Lords has a significant scrutiny role, and can make matters uncomfortable for government. In some situations, it may persuade government to amend legislative proposals. However, its power to delay and block legislation is severely limited by statute. The will of the House of the Commons (and by implication, the will of the government) tends to prevail. Unlike MPs, Peers are not elected by public constituencies. Amid concerns about its lack of democratic legitimacy, many attempts have been made to change the composition of the Lords. The Blair government removed most of the hereditary Peers (who sit in the House by virtue of birth), but was unable to abolish them completely. Attempts by New Labour, and subsequently the coalition, to introduce democratic elections for peers, have failed.

Interests

Although Peers are not elected by the public, they are not isolated from public concerns, or from special interests. Individuals and organisations frequently bring matters to the attention of Peers, who raise these issues on their behalf. Peers have a wide range of health interests. Some have commercial and financial interests, as directors or shareholders of companies in the health field, or whose business affects health. Others have an interest arising out of a career in the health service, have led trade unions in this field, or been involved in professional bodies at a senior level. Examples include Lords Winston, Turnberg and Walton, who are all prominent members of the medical profession. Others have served as non-executive directors or in some other lay capacity on NHS bodies (for example, Lord Chan and Lord Harris of Haringey).

A large number of Peers are ex-MPs, many of who have taken an interest in health matters while in the House of Commons (an example was the late Lord Ashley, who campaigned in both Houses on behalf of disabled people). Some are former health ministers, and maintain an active interest in health issues. For example, Baroness Cumberlege, a minister in the Major government, who has a long-standing interest in health issues, particularly with regard to maternity and childbirth issues, has served on NHS bodies and has been involved with several health organisations – as a patron of the National Childbirth Trust, a trustee of Cancer Research UK and vice-president of both the Royal College of Nursing and the Royal College of Midwives.

In addition, other Peers take a keen interest in health policy as a result of their former or current roles in academia, the civil service, science and the voluntary sector. Examples include Baroness Pitkeathley (former director and now vice-president of Carers' National Association); Lord Allen (member, Mencap), Baroness Greengross (former director, Age Concern), Lord Bragg (President, Mind), Baroness Gould (President, British Epilepsy Association), Lord Smith of Clifton (trustee and director of the Stroke Association) and Baroness Morgan of Drefelin (chief executive, Breakthrough Breast Cancer).

Scrutiny, legislation and influence

The House of Lords uses similar instruments to the House of Commons when scrutinising government. Peers can table questions to ministers (each department, including the DH, has a minister in the House of Lords) and raise debates. The House of Lords also has select committees, although they are not focused on specific departments. Health matters fall within the remit of several committees – including the Science and Technology Committee, the European Union (EU) subcommittee on social policy and consumer affairs, and committees dealing with delegated legislation (mentioned above). Health issues are also covered by ad hoc committees, established for a particular purpose (for example, the Mental Capacity Act Committee, which reported in 2014). Peers use committees to hold government to account, to highlight problems with policies and services, and to propose changes to policy. For example, the Science and Technology Committee has explored several important health issues such as stem cell research, infection control and antibiotic resistance.

One of the key functions of the House of Lords is legislative scrutiny (Russell, 2013). The government and Commons rely on the Lords to undertake the routine but important task of examining proposed legislation. This helps to identify loopholes and inconsistencies in proposed laws, and gives the House of Lords a certain amount of leverage. Failure to secure its cooperation can delay important legislation. Because of the relative weakness of party discipline in the House of Lords, it can defeat the government on votes more easily than can the Commons, thereby forcing government to reconsider its proposals (Baggott, 2007). It is often argued that debates in the House of Lords can be more persuasive because they are not conducted in such an adversarial atmosphere as in the Commons. Peers can be persuasive because of their expertise, understanding and knowledge of health policy and the NHS. They can be particularly influential on issues that cut across party lines, such as stem cell research, alternative therapies and euthanasia.

Between 1979 and 1997 the Conservative government was defeated in the Lords on an average of 14 times each parliamentary session. Between 1997 and 2010, the Labour government was defeated on 528 occasions in the Lords (almost 40 defeats per session). Between May 2010 and February 2015, the coalition suffered 99 defeats (around 20 per year) (see www.parliament.uk). Although the Commons is the most powerful Chamber, it has been estimated that around four in ten government defeats in the Lords are not reversed (Hazell, quoted in Timmins, 2012). The government often offers a compromise to avoid delaying the legislation or to prevent rebellion among backbenchers in the Commons. It should also be noted that in many cases the matter will not be put to a vote, following informal agreement between the government and its opponents in the House of Lords, enabling the government to move its own amendment. Notably, the Lords was very influential in the debates on the Health and Social Care Bill in 2011 and 2012 (**see Box 4.3**).

In summary, the House of Lords can influence the details of legislation, help to get issues on the agenda, and can contribute to important debates, particularly those cutting across party lines. Its effectiveness is, to some extent, undermined by its currently undemocratic composition. But this is counterbalanced by the greater independence of peers from the system of party discipline and their repository of knowledge and experience. It is vitally important that any reforms to democratise the House of Lords do not remove these important attributes.

Conclusion

Health remains an issue of considerable importance to MPs and Peers, and, if anything, is higher on their agenda than it was 30 years ago when Ingle and Tether wrote their book. But parliamentary scrutiny, of public policy generally and health in particular, remains limited, and influence over policy is marginal. Parliamentary accountability has been described by David Hinchliffe, former chair of the Health Select Committee, as 'a nonsense' and 'largely mythical' (Edwards and Fall, 2005, p 189). Reforms such as the introduction of departmental select committees (for example, the Health Committee) appear to have little direct impact, although their influence is probably greater than commonly thought. For many years people have argued for a comprehensive programme aimed at strengthening the powers of Parliament, enabling MPs and Peers to hold government more closely to account and exert greater influence over policy (Commission to Strengthen Parliament, 2000; Hansard Society Commission on Parliamentary Scrutiny, 2001; Parliament First, 2003). There have been some positive changes (for example, with regard to backbench business, pre-legislative scrutiny and evidence gathering for public bill committees). It also appears that MPs are becoming more rebellious. But longer-term factors associated with the decline of Parliament, such as 'strong government', the 'presidential style' of recent Prime Ministers, and the growth of secondary legislation have outweighed any positive effects of reform (Riddell, 2000).

Nonetheless, Parliament is not irrelevant. In certain circumstances it can have greater influence over policy, notably with regard to conscience issues. Parliament can also be influential when government has a small majority, is in a minority, or it faces serious divisions within its ranks. When they combine with other political actors, such as pressure groups and the media, MPs and peers can provide a counterbalance to government, and may help to shape agendas and contribute to policy changes, particularly in the longer term. Parliament is still an important arena where outside individuals and organisations can advocate or oppose policy ideas. Moreover, its scrutiny powers can be used to shed light on government policy and administration, and thus generate wider pressures for change.

Summary

- Health is an important issue for MPs and Peers.
- A variety of factors shape MPs' interests including background and personal factors, constituency interests, membership of groups or committees in Parliament, economic interests and affiliations.
- MPs have a variety of activities in which they may engage to raise issues and scrutinise government in the health policy arena, although these are relatively weak in promoting policy and ensuring effective scrutiny of government.
- Select committees have an important potential role in health policy and in strengthening accountability. However, they have only a limited impact on policy, and face obstacles in holding government to account.
- Government dominates the process of legislation. Parliament can exert some influence over primary legislation, in particular circumstances, yet as long as government has a large parliamentary majority and party discipline remains strong, there are few opportunities to change government policy.
- Parliament's powers over finance are weak. However, by highlighting waste and inefficiency, it can cause the government considerable embarrassment.
- Parliament helps to secure redress for those who have faced problems at the hands of government and the NHS. There is scope for increasing the powers of ombudsmen in this field.
- The House of Lords has played a useful role in scrutinising health policy. It can influence the details of legislation in some circumstances.
- Only a comprehensive programme of reform will strengthen Parliament and enable it to exercise influence over health policy and hold government more closely to account.

Key questions

1. What factors shape MPs' and Peers' interests in health policy?
2. What are the main parliamentary activities used by MPs and Peers to raise issues and scrutinise the government's health policies?
3. How effective are select committees in influencing health policy and scrutinising government in this field?
4. Has Parliament become stronger in its ability to influence and scrutinise health policy in recent years?

five

The media and health policy

Overview

This chapter examines the role of the media in the health policy arena, as it has an important role in the policy process (see Chapter One). The media shapes the perception of problems and policies, and can be manipulated by other policy actors, such as government and pressure groups. But it is also a policy actor in its own right that can influence policy outcomes as well as perceptions.

What is the media?

The media is not easy to define (Torfing, 1999; Devereux, 2007). It is a catch-all term for the many ways in which communication takes place between people. The term 'mass media' covers means of communication with large groups of people, with traditional forms of mass media including television, radio and the print media. Much attention has been paid to these forms of media as they involve communication from one entity to many, giving rise to opportunities to manipulate public opinion. Traditional media are now accompanied by new media technologies that enable person-to-person as well as mass communication (such as the internet and mobile phone technology).

The mass media doesn't just communicate news, views and information; it also has enormous political, cultural and economic significance (McQuail, 2005), conveying values, ideas and meanings. It is important in shaping shared identities and cultural environments (hence film and music are considered part of the mass media). And it has a crucial political dimension, as a channel of debate and as a means of exercising political influence.

The media has experienced substantial changes over the past few decades (Dean, 2013; Richards, 2013), with the key developments as follows:

- *Technological changes:* these include the rise of the internet, mobile phone technologies and the means of communication linked to these new media (websites, blogs, email, messaging, Twitter and social networking sites). Technological changes have reduced the cost of traditional media and enabled their expansion into other formats (for example, print media and multi-channel TV becoming available through computers and mobile phones). These changes have resulted in a proliferation of mass media forms, which are increasingly interlinked, and have led to significant changes in the way news is made. Users can now create and disseminate content and become news makers. We also now have 24-hour rolling news in a variety of forms (notably through the internet and satellite TV channels), creating a constant demand for new stories.
- *Concentration of media corporations:* media corporations have become larger and fewer in number. There has been a growth in cross-media ownership and cross-national ownership (for example, NewsCorp). This gives these firms, and the individuals who control them, a great deal of power, despite the fragmentation of the media industry.
- *Regulation and accountability:* fears of the power and lack of accountability and practices of media corporations (notably the phone hacking scandal in the UK) has created pressures to strengthen media regulation. The Leveson Inquiry, set up in response to these concerns, produced recommendations to provide statutory underpinning for press regulation and complaints, to safeguard personal information and privacy, and to establish greater transparency in relationships between the press and politicians (and also between the press and the police).
- *Quality of media coverage:* it is argued that while there is now more mass media, the quality of news and information provided has declined. Perversely, the media tend to chase the same 'big' story, in effect, narrowing the news agenda. Associated with a perceived decline in quality is a decline in specialist and investigative journalism.

Media coverage of health and illness

According to Callaghan and Schnell (2011, cited in Boero, 2013) there are three ways in which the media can shape public policy: by deciding which issues to cover; by elevating some issues over others; and by the framing of issues (see also Dean, 2013; Richards, 2013). This section explores key aspects of media coverage of health and illness, focusing particularly on the potential for bias in the selection and reporting of issues.

Selection bias

Media coverage of health issues expanded in the second half of the 20th century (Entwhistle and Beaulieu-Hancock, 1992; Ali et al, 2001), partly because of their increasing 'newsworthiness' (see **Box 5.1**). Although health and illness is extensively covered, some issues do receive more attention than others, and several biases have been identified (see Karpf, 1988; Seale, 2002), including:

- an overwhelming concern with hospital-based medicine and technology at the expense of primary and community-based services;
- a preoccupation with 'health scares' at the expense of long-term chronic illness and more serious underlying threats to health;
- a focus on 'newsworthy' diseases and medical conditions, which do not reflect the actual burden of mortality and morbidity in society;
- a focus on 'bad news' at the expense of 'good news'.

Stories about healthcare services have been identified as the largest single category in both TV and newspaper health news (Harrabin et al, 2003; Millward Brown, 2004). Hospital news predominates, although increasingly coverage is given to GP and community-based services, public health and alternative therapies (Seale, 2002).

The media tends to concentrate on dramatic health threats, irrespective of the level of risk they pose. To demonstrate this, Harrabin et al (2003) compared the number of deaths in the UK from various health threats with the number of news stories on each topic. They found that for every story on smoking reported on BBC News there were 8,571 deaths from smoking-related illness, but for every news item on HIV/AIDS, there were only 20 deaths. New infectious diseases are extremely attractive to journalists, as indicated by media coverage of SARS (Washer, 2004) and the 'flesh-eating bug', necrotising fasciitis (Gwyn, 1999).

Some medical conditions consistently receive more media attention than others (Henderson and Kitzinger, 1999). Bartlett and colleagues (2002) found that cancer and reproductive health issues were more likely to be reported in newspapers than heart disease, diabetes and mental health. Robinson et al (2013) suggested that there was under-reporting of mental health, respiratory and musculo-skeletal conditions in the press, compared with illness rates for these conditions, although cardiovascular disease, the condition associated with the highest mortality and morbidity, was the most frequently covered topic. Other researchers found that breast cancer attracted more attention than other cancers (Saywell et al, 2000; Clarke and Everest, 2006).

The health of some population groups attracts more media interest than others. The plight of sick children, for example, is very appealing to the media (Seale, 2002; Baggott et al, 2005). In contrast, illness in older people has attracted less interest, and women's health issues tend to be covered more often than men's health (Bartlett et al, 2002).

Box 5.1: Factors that indicate 'newsworthiness'

- Availability of 'visuals' or 'images' that clearly illustrate a problem or attract attention.
- A human interest aspect, if possible, portraying actual individuals or families.
- Affects children.
- Potentially wide implications – could affect a large proportion of the population.
- Novelty of the story, or at least a new angle on something familiar.
- Unusual, rare occurrence, an out-of-the-ordinary event.
- Likely to provoke a strong emotional reaction from most people.
- Raises ethical, moral or other controversial issues.
- Can be related to the current news agenda, perhaps continuing a current story but in a different way.
- Fits in with underlying public preconceptions.
- Relates to a minority or maverick view against the establishment.
- Concerns greed or venality.
- Involves sex/sexuality.
- Involves violence or serious harm, especially against the innocent or vulnerable.
- Involves celebrities.
- Implies a significant future threat to the public.
- Relates to an unpredictable pattern of events that lie ahead.
- Involves an invisible or powerful threat or scare.
- Has dramatic consequences, in particular, death.
- Involves conflict, crisis or scandal.
- Involves fault or blame, or criticism of people in high places.
- Involves new technology or a scientific breakthrough.

Sources: See Karpf (1988); Bell (1991); Negrine (1994); Entwhistle (1995); Entwhistle and Sheldon (1999); Franklin (1999); Gwyn (1999); Jennings (1999); Doyle (2000); Harrabin et al (2003); Dean (2013)

However, it is wrong to see selection bias as fixed – notably, breast cancer was once a taboo subject for the media. Public health issues such as smoking, alcohol abuse and obesity now receive much more coverage than before

(Gard and Wright, 2005). Meanwhile, some formerly 'low-profile' illnesses, such as prostate cancer, bowel disease, stroke and arthritis, have received much more media attention in recent years, as have traditionally unfashionable topics such as mental health and the care of elderly people (Millward Brown, 2004). The media's desire for new angles and stories can lead to 'neglected' topics being covered, as exemplified by recent media interest in the neglect of elderly people in hospital and care homes. Increased media coverage may also result from successful campaigns on behalf of those with certain conditions and illnesses, and reflect new and more favourable circumstances (for example, greater openness about 'taboo' illnesses, or acknowledgement of the consequences of an ageing population).

The selection of news stories is perhaps influenced by the media's 'negativity' (Dean, 2013). Bartlett et al's (2002) research found that while good news and bad medical research news stories were equally likely to be issued as press releases, bad news was more likely to be reported by newspapers.

Bias in media reporting

The language used in the media shapes perceptions and assumptions about health and illness. This is perhaps most apparent in relation to impending health threats, invariably portrayed in apocalyptic terms. Obviously, the public must be alerted to possible risks to health and how to prevent or mitigate them. Even so, the portrayal of health threats can be counterproductive, creating fear and panic. It can also promote policy decisions that unnecessarily reduce people's autonomy and strengthen the power of governments and professionals.

The exaggeration of health threats involves metaphors of impending doom. Media messages about infectious disease or chemical/biological contamination frequently deploy military metaphors of a population under attack from a powerful enemy. However, in their study of the impending avian flu epidemic, Nerlich and Halliday (2007) found that 'disaster metaphors' (flood, earthquake, tsunami), rather than military metaphors or personification, were the most salient in media reports. Animal and bioterrorism metaphors were also deployed, as were historical frames, linking the impending threat to past events. This research also found that scientists contributed to the rhetoric of fear associated with the use of such metaphors by actively initiating them.

The reporting of health issues can reinforce stereotypes and existing assumptions about illness, inhibiting public understanding. For example, breast cancer, which predominantly affects older women, is usually portrayed as a bigger threat to younger women. Charities and patients' groups in this field are concerned about the media's obsession with breast cancer and young women (Saywell et al, 2000; Baggott et al, 2005). More generally, it appears that the media are preoccupied with breast, ovarian and cervical cancer in women, and prostate/testicular cancer in men. This could distort the public perceptions of health risks. A study of Canadian/US English-language magazines undertaken in the late 1980s (Clarke, 2004) found that breast cancer and prostate/testicular cancers were closely associated with stereotypes of femininity and masculinity, exacerbating fear of these diseases and diminishing awareness of other important causes of death.

Cancer has been portrayed in a way that does not match patients' actual experiences. Sontag (1991) argued that the dominant 'military' metaphors ('fighting cancer') were unhelpful and demoralised patients, justified brutal interventions, and stigmatised those diagnosed with the disease. While such metaphors are still widely used (Lupton, 1994; Clarke, 1999; Clarke and Everest, 2006), more positive coverage by the media can now be found. Seale (2001) found that 'sporting' metaphors (that is, winning/losing) were more common, and that cancer stories had become more positive, emphasising a personal struggle, but with chances of success.

Media reporting of mental health has been criticised for reinforcing negative stereotypes (Lawrie, 2000; Millward Brown, 2004). In particular, the portrayal of mental illness highlights rare psychotic behaviour far more often than the more common mental health problems such as anxiety and depression (Philo, 1996, 1999). This reinforces the stigma of mental illness and possibly discourages people from seeking help. Such coverage may have an impact on mental health policy, in ways discussed later.

Another example is childhood illness, which tends to be covered in a particular way. The vulnerability and helplessness of the child, the heroism of the parents and medical staff, the disruption of 'normal' childhood, are all emphasised. Perhaps most serious of all, the chances of successful intervention are exaggerated (Seale, 2005). This can produce an unhelpful distortion of reality for sick children and their families, raising expectations, preventing children from participating in their own care, and possibly restricting their activities more than clinically necessary. Some of these features were evident in the Child B case, which involved a health authority's refusal to sanction cancer treatment (Entwhistle et al, 1996).

Stereotyping also happens to health professionals and producers of healthcare products and services. There are 'villains' (Seale, 2002), such as the drugs industry and the tobacco companies, and more recently, the food and alcoholic drinks industries. NHS health authorities, managers and administrators are often depicted as heartless bureaucrats denying services to those in need (see Seale, 2005). While managers are depicted as a drain on the NHS, diverting resources from the 'front line', doctors and nurses are the 'heroes' (Karpf, 1988; Seale, 2005). However, this is not always the case. Allegations of poor or harmful practice against individual practitioners can lead to trial by media. Such cases are usually depicted as 'bad apples', leaving the reputation of professionals as a whole untarnished. Even so, there are signs that the media has become more critical (Ali et al, 2001; Seale, 2002).

Factual inaccuracy and irresponsible reporting

Goldacre (2008) gives an excellent account of the ways in which the media mis-report medical science. Researchers in the US found that health news stories consistently under-reported the costs, harms, benefits, existence of alternative options, and the quality of evidence, when covering healthcare products and services (Schwitzer, 2008; Brainard, 2011). In the UK, Bartlett et al (2002) revealed that studies that provided the highest quality of evidence (randomised controlled trials) were relatively under-reported compared with others (observational studies). Researchers subsequently found that half of news items reporting medical research trials were subject to 'spin' (that is, the presentation of information to create a positive or favourable impression; see Yavchitz et al, 2012). Meanwhile, Robinson et al (2013) concluded that there were significant differences in the quality of health reporting in the press, with the highest quality articles found in *The Times* and *The Independent* (quality broadsheet newspapers) and the poorest in *The Sun* (a tabloid newspaper).

Journalists must, of course, simplify research findings and present them in a way that the public can digest. Even allowing for this, there is often a failure to acknowledge the subtleties of research studies. There is too much reliance on press releases, public relations briefings and Press Association copy as a basis for articles. Journalists must be far more critical when using these sources (Dean, 2013; Robinson et al, 2013). Some media organisations employ specialist reporters, who can produce better quality articles on topics such as health (Science Media Centre, 2011; Dean, 2013). But their work is sub-edited, which can lead to inaccuracy and distortion. Further problems, pertaining particularly to the press and print media, include the use of misleading headlines, and poor quality pieces written by columnists renowned for writing strong opinionated articles (Science Media Centre, 2011; Dean, 2013).

Regulators have acknowledged the problems of inaccurate and irresponsible reporting. Lord Leveson's (2012) report on press regulation concluded that although science reporting was on the whole accurate and responsible, there were problems associated with unbalanced and irresponsible reporting. He was particularly concerned about the impact of 'sensational headlines of breakthroughs and scares' (Leveson, 2012, para 693), and very critical of the media's role in the MMR controversy (see **Box 5.2**). Leveson backed the use of media guidelines on science and communication (Science Media Centre, 2012). The Press Complaints Commission (the body then responsible for press self-regulation) adopted these guidelines and adjudicated complaints, which led some newspapers to acknowledge their errors (see Robbins, 2012).

Box 5.2: The MMR controversy

The media has often been criticised for giving too much attention to maverick viewpoints. One of the most notorious examples was media coverage of research suggesting a link between the MMR vaccine, autism and chronic inflammatory bowel disease, which misled the public about the balance of scientific evidence (Leveson, 2012). Dean (2013, p 327) called this 'one of worst cases of over-hyped journalism.' The media focused on Dr Andrew Wakefield's now discredited research, depicting him as a crusader against the medical establishment. The media also centred on the emotive accounts of parents who blamed MMR for their children's illnesses. This fuelled public fears about the safety of the vaccine, and prompted a fall in MMR immunisations (see Begg et al, 1998; Horton, 2004; Speers and Lewis, 2004). However, it should be acknowledged that the investigation that led to Wakefield's research being discredited was triggered by investigative journalism (Deer, 2011).

There have been calls for better training for journalists (including editors) in health and science matters (Science Media Centre, 2011; Association of Medical Research Charities et al, 2012), which have led to more resources in this field. In addition, health stories have been subjected to more scrutiny. An example is 'Behind the Headlines', available on the NHS Choices website, which examines the research evidence relating to media stories (www.nhs.uk). However, it would be wrong to blame poor reporting standards entirely on journalists, editors and their employers. Research has found health researchers are partly to blame for putting a positive spin on their work. Yavchitz et al (2012) found 'spin' in 41 per cent of abstracts describing research and 46 per cent of press releases. Similarly, Sumner et al (2014) found that 40 per cent of press releases contained exaggerated advice, 33 per cent overstated causal claims, and 36 per cent exaggerated inference to humans from animal research. In addition, they also discovered that exaggeration in news stories was strongly linked to overstatement in press releases.

What influences media coverage?

Although initiatives to improve the quality of health reporting are welcome, they do not address key factors shaping media coverage. To understand these, one has to explore the motivations, values and practices of media organisations and journalists as well as the constraints within which they operate. Media organisations contain many different interests and operate in a complex business environment (Keane, 1991; Newton, 2001), but none can ignore 'newsworthiness' (see the factors listed in **Box 5.1**). Stories do not require all these ingredients in order to be newsworthy. Moreover, some parts of the media emphasise some factors over others. The tabloids are more likely to respond to 'sex', 'celebrity' and sensationalism (although the traditional distinctions between the tabloids and quality press are somewhat blurred these days; see Sampson, 2004; Dean, 2013).

Journalists must entertain as well as inform (Miller and Reilly, 1994; Seale, 2003). Indeed, journalists reject the idea that health reporting must be purely factual, or that coverage must be commensurate with actual health risks (Harrabin et al, 2003). Ultimately, media organisations (including public service broadcasters) must sell their product, and the audience's desire to be entertained cannot be ignored.

Additional technical pressures and constraints lead to stories being 'packaged' in a way that oversimplifies them (Cottle, 2001). News is packaged in particular formats, often with a strong influence on visuals, which simplifies messages and can prevent critical and non-mainstream views from being heard. Similarly, Kitzinger (2000) discusses how media templates are used to portray issues in particular, stylised ways to reinforce interpretations, meanings and values. Although these can be reversed for dramatic effect (the classic 'man bites dog' story), that may prompt reinterpretation of an issue, stories are still subject to simplification. The result of packaging and stylisation may be that, as Franklin (1999) has argued, complex issues, and also more complicated *treatment* of issues, are excluded from the media agenda. There is much evidence of this in the health field, where stories on mental health (Philo, 1996, 1999), new infectious diseases and food safety threats (Miller and Reilly, 1994; Gwyn, 1999; Doyle, 2000; Washer, 2004; King and Street, 2005), sick children (Seale, 2005) and rationing (Entwhistle et al, 1996) have tended to follow a particular style of presentation.

The competitive pressure to entertain, along with technical constraints, impels the media towards simplification, exaggeration, stereotyping and the selection of particular issues over others. However, as Harrabin and colleagues (2003) observed, journalists maintain that they act in the overall public interest when reporting health. They point to examples of where they have acted in the public interest by highlighting NHS scandals and risks to health, and by campaigning on 'neglected' issues. There is also a belief that the need to simplify and entertain is counterbalanced by specialist correspondents who are better informed about health issues, and perhaps more likely to avoid sensationalism (Harrabin et al, 2003).

Over the years, investigative and campaigning journalism in the health field has challenged dominant and mainstream views, and has highlighted neglected groups, sometimes in the face of strong commercial opposition. An example is the work of *The Times* journalist Marjorie Wallace on schizophrenia in the 1980s that put this particular issue on the political agenda. However, it is believed that investigative reporting is in decline (Dean, 2013), and that this further undermines the ability of the media to hold government to account.

The journalist David Brindle (1999) has argued that the production of news is more chaotic than is realised, and journalists have considerable freedom to select issues and to report on them. To see them as mere puppets of media organisations in their quest for profit is too simplistic. Even so, proprietors do seek to influence content, although this is rarely done explicitly. As Dean (2013) notes, editors and journalists are well aware of the views of owners, and factor this in to their reporting and editorial decisions.

Health and the new media

There has been growing interest in the new media and health. In his book on the coalition's NHS reforms, Timmins (2012) noted the important role of social media (email, Facebook and Twitter) in raising issues and orchestrating opposition to the Health and Social Care Bill. Further analysis by King et al (2013) identified 120,000 tweets on the topic. Some users were more influential than others. They included a mix of professionals, politicians, activists, and mainstream commentators and journalists. The involvement of traditional media illustrates a general point made by Dean (2013) that old and new media increasingly interact with each other. King et al (2013) found that Twitter followed rather than led debate, and was more a means of sharing and reinforcing views than genuine debate. It acted as a focus for opposition, and importantly, enabled conversations across traditional hierarchical and professional barriers. The research was unable to pinpoint the precise effect of Twitter on policy, but acknowledged the role of celebrities, who have large numbers of followers, in generating interest in the issue through 'retweets'.

Drama

Drama and fictional accounts shape how health issues are perceived by the public, and can have implications for policy (Philo, 1999; Davis, 2005). They can also affect health behaviour. When a character in the popular television soap *Coronation Street* was diagnosed with cervical cancer, the charity

Cancerbackup experienced a large increase in calls to its helpline, and the number of smear tests rose by a fifth in Manchester alone (Wright, 2003).

The principal function of drama is to entertain. Representations of health issues are therefore tailored to fit the requirements of entertaining storylines and characters in a way that tends to simplify, exaggerate and reinforce stereotypes (Henderson, 1999). Particular attention has been paid to television soaps, regular mass-audience dramas based on the lives of a fictional community. As Seale (2002) has observed, soaps focus on acute illness and on young or middle-aged people. Deaths among soap characters are higher than in the population at large, and tend to be disproportionately violent (Crayford et al, 1997). There is stereotyping of certain types of illness (mental illness), population groups (elderly people) and gender roles (doctors/ nurses), reinforcing biases in news media described earlier (Seale, 2002). Even soaps that claim social realism contain inaccuracies that can distort public perceptions of illness (Henderson, 1999; Philo, 1999). However, drama can challenge stereotypes – as in the *EastEnders* storyline on schizophrenia in the late 1990s (Baggott et al, 2005) – or cover issues that have previously attracted little media attention, such as depression (recently covered by both *Coronation Street* and *EastEnders*). Indeed, research has shown that drama now portrays mental health issues more sympathetically and positively (Time to Change, 2015).

While health issues often appear in drama programmes, they are obviously central to medical dramas, such as BBC TV's *Casualty*. Such programmes are popular, and there is evidence that the public both trust and use information received from these sources (Kingsley, 1993; Davis, 2005). The need to be credible, and to avoid providing misleading information, is particularly important to these programme makers, who retain clinical advisers to ensure accuracy. Other programme makers also consult outside experts when portraying health issues, particularly those of a sensitive or controversial nature. In some cases, notably with regard to HIV/AIDS and mental illness, health consumer and patients' groups and professional experts have been consulted on scripts (Baggott et al, 2005; Goodchild, 2015).

Celebrities and illness

The modern celebrity culture has transformed the media (Sampson, 2004). Although celebrities are not political figures, like ministers or MPs, their actions can have a political impact (see **Box 5.3**). In the health field, celebrities can highlight specific conditions by lending explicit support to a particular health cause or charity. A prominent example was the public support given by the late Princess Diana to HIV/AIDS charities. Celebrity support can, however, be a double-edged weapon. Charities are often worried about celebrities portraying an inappropriate image (Batty, 2001). Also, celebrity support is often unequal, being less evident for stigmatised conditions such as mental illness (Cope, 2002). Even so, some celebrities have endorsed campaigns to challenge stigma and discrimination (for example, Time to Change in mental health, see below).

Celebrity illness is doubly compelling, as both 'celebrity' and 'illness' are newsworthy in their own right (see **Box 5.1**). When a famous person suffers from a condition, especially a high-profile condition such as breast cancer, media interest is intense, particularly when this person is youthful and vibrant. Hence the media frenzy that followed news of singer Kylie Minogue's breast cancer diagnosis in 2005. The impact of media coverage of celebrity illness can be enormous – the coverage of Kylie Minogue's illness was followed by an increase in rates of breast cancer screening (Chapman et al, 2005). However, this included young women, who are at lower risk and benefit less from screening than older women and for whom the harms of screening are likely to exceed the benefits (Kelaher et al, 2008). Indeed, it has been suggested more generally that by focusing on the experience of younger female celebrities with breast cancer, the media has misled women about the age-related risks of the disease (Cancer Research UK, 2006).

Sometimes celebrities galvanise public perceptions of a disease or condition. They may also campaign to improve research and treatment, as in the case of actor Michael J. Fox, who was diagnosed with young-onset Parkinson's Disease (see Fox, 2002). An American study found that celebrities who talked about their experience of cancer screening persuaded individuals to have tests (Larson et al, 2005). Another found that although celebrity illness can improve public awareness of a condition, it may mislead the public about how to prevent it (Hopkins, 2000).

Celebrities, even if not ill themselves, can become actively involved in health campaigns, expressing their support for a particular cause or issue, although there are mixed views on whether this should be actively encouraged. The positives (see Chapman, 2012) are that celebrities have a large following, increasingly in the new media such as Twitter. They are newsworthy, which attracts media attention. By speaking out on an issue, they can give it a profile and (if they have suffered from a particular illness) can bring an authenticity to an issue. They are seen as role models and can influence health behaviours. Negatively, celebrity involvement may be superficial and provide a weak foundation on which to promote health messages and issues (Rayner, 2012). This critique attacks the celebrity culture as being intrinsically harmful to health, by contributing to social trends such as the weakening of social bonds, inequality and consumerism.

The media and the policy process

Public opinion

The media can foster a climate of public opinion that encourages particular policy initiatives. For example, some sections of the media helped establish an atmosphere of consensus for policies on HIV/AIDS (Day and Klein 1989; Berridge, 1996; Miller et al, 1998; Williams, 1999; Seale, 2002). Furthermore, the media portrayal of the NHS as permanently in crisis has created a climate for reforms introduced by successive governments (Harrabin et al, 2003). The media can also demonstrate wider public concern about an issue and shape policies, as exemplified by the Jamie Oliver school meals campaign (see **Box 5.3**).

The media can promote public resistance to policies, as in mental health, for example (Rose, 1998; Philo, 1999). It is argued that the media has reinforced an extremely negative view among the public, promoting an exaggerated fear of people with mental illness. This, coupled with criticism of community-based care, makes it difficult for politicians to pursue a balanced policy in this field, and they are impelled by public safety rather than therapeutic concerns.

Even so, as Seale has commented, 'audiences may be treated like dupes, but they do not necessarily behave like them' (2002, p 43). People can resist media messages. The media may put forward different and contradictory views, which may reduce their impact, and people may have personal experiences that contradict media messages. Alternatively, the messages might conflict with their cultural attributes or value systems (Philo, 1999). However, media influence is often subtle and operates not by telling people what to think, but by shaping fundamental assumptions about issues and the way in which they are comprehended (Eldridge et al, 1999). These assumptions and interpretative frameworks are powerful and may outweigh those factors that promote resistance to media messages.

Policy-makers, and especially elected politicians, regard the media not only as an important barometer of public opinion, but as a source of policy influence (Harrabin et al, 2003). The media can generate debate on issues, which can lead to public pressure for or against policies. It can also shape public judgements about the effectiveness of governments and the competence of individual politicians.

The media can shape policy debates by using particular language and symbolism. These policy discourses define problems and possible solutions (Miller et al, 1998; King and Street, 2005). For example, with regard to obesity, it has been argued that an 'epidemic/universal threat/crisis/ timebomb' terminology is deployed in the media to exaggerate the problem and promote a response from government (Gard and Wright, 2005). At the same time, powerful imagery (in particular, the 'fat child/couch potato') is used to stigmatise people and to prioritise certain problems (obese and overweight children) and solutions (ban junk food, increase consumption of fresh fruit, increase exercise and sport), while ignoring other key issues, such as under-nutrition and deprivation among the poor. Further work on obesity, reviewed by Boero (2013), reveals a more complex picture. The framing of obesity is complex, contradictory and dynamic. Obesity is often depicted as a medical, genetic, moral or environmental problem beyond individual control, but at other times as a problem of individual willpower and self-control. Shugart (2011, cited in Boero, 2013) saw a shift towards the former, more fatalistic approach, but observed that this neither reduced the stigma of obesity or promoted debates about the role of social determinants. Further insights into the complexity of the framing of obesity were revealed by Ries et al (2011, also cited in Boero, 2013) in their study of newspaper coverage of obesity in the US, Canada and the UK. While obesity was principally reported as a lifestyle problem in all three jurisdictions, media coverage regarding the appropriate balance of responsibilities for tackling the problem (that is, between individuals, government and industry) varied between these countries.

Another example concerns healthcare-acquired infections. Media coverage of this issue increased during the 1990s (Childs, 2006). Reporting tended towards sensationalism, with much distortion about the causes of the problem (Childs, 2006; Koteyko et al, 2008; Chan et al, 2010). The media focused on cleanliness and hygiene, especially within a hospital context. Other important factors, such as the over-use of antibiotics, received much less coverage (as it was regarded by journalists as a relatively unexciting explanation! see Chan et al, 2010). Furthermore, healthcare infection was seen as primarily a hospital problem, despite the problems of infection in the community health and care settings. The media also focused on two main infections – MRSA and Clostridium difficile. Although undoubtedly serious and life-threatening, these represented a minority of healthcare-acquired infections. The media undoubtedly fuelled public concern and shaped the government's response, which was to target the two infections highlighted most in the media. Policies on antibiotic resistance were also endorsed by government, but overshadowed by its higher profile programme of hospital cleaning. It appears that this policy was pursued because the media would favourably portray it as a robust response (Chan et al, 2010).

Policy actors interviewed by Baggott (2007) supported the view that the media can influence both public opinion and government agendas. Only a minority of respondents thought that the media could drive the policy agenda, but most believed it strongly influenced the way in which the public thought about health issues and had the ability to push issues up the agenda (see also Doyle, 2000). Most saw the media as a negative rather than a positive force, in effect, blocking policies. Mental health policy was seen as an example of where this had occurred (see above). The tabloids were seen as a particularly negative force, especially in areas such as public health, where government policy had been dominated by a fear of being labelled a 'nanny state'. Even so, examples can be found of where the media has positively shaped policies and forced the government to take steps (see **Box 5.3**).

Box 5.3: The 'Feed Me Better' campaign

Amid public concern about rising obesity levels in children, the Labour government reintroduced minimum standards for school meals in 2001. However, problems remained, largely due to the lack of investment in the school meal service, low level of funding for ingredients, a system of competitive contracting that emphasised low-cost provision, and that many children – influenced by large-scale advertising and peer pressure – were choosing junk food.

Little more was done until a media campaign in 2005, headed by the celebrity chef, Jamie Oliver, forced the government to improve school meals in England (other parts of the UK having already adopted new policies following devolution). The trigger was Oliver's Channel 4 TV series *Jamie's School Dinners*. In the show, Oliver set himself the challenge of providing low-cost but nutritious school meals. The series was compelling viewing, illustrating the appalling state of school meals and the magnitude of the task of improving the diets of schoolchildren.

Public reaction to the series sustained the 'Feed Me Better' campaign, which called for higher nutritional standards and more investment in school meals. A website generated 5 million hits, and over 270,000 people signed a petition in support of the campaign. The campaign was picked up by TV news and the national press. Other celebrities endorsed the campaign (including sporting figures such as footballer Frank Lampard and the yachtswoman Ellen MacArthur). The issue was raised in Parliament and an EDM (see Chapter Four) attracted 159 supporters.

The government, which faced a general election later in the year, was caught off-guard. The Secretary of State for Education, Ruth Kelly, claimed that she was already looking at ways of improving school meals. Tony Blair publicly acknowledged the strength of the campaign and paid tribute to Oliver's efforts. Despite the political clout of private sector contractors, and the junk food industry, the campaign was difficult to oppose. The government responded with a three-year funding package for school meals (£280 million, partly subsidised by National Lottery funds) and new mandatory nutritional standards aimed at cutting salt, sugar and fats and increasing fruit and vegetables. It extended school inspections to cover food standards, and established an independent school food trust to encourage higher standards in school meals. Subsequently, in response to a follow-up programme on the campaign in 2006, the Prime Minister pledged that he would consider further recommendations from Oliver on how to improve school meals.

Although the new funding could have been more generous (it raised ingredient costs to only 50p per meal in primary schools and 60p in secondary schools), the campaign influenced public opinion and secured a positive response from government. The main factors behind this success were as follows:

- the campaign was led by a well-known celebrity, genuinely committed to doing something about a problem; the involvement of other celebrities added further strength to the campaign;
- the scale of the problem and the response required was clearly demonstrated;
- the issue related to one already on the political agenda – child obesity;
- the campaign used electronic media to engage the public and enlist support;
- the campaign was effectively cascaded to other media outlets, both broadcast and non-broadcast;
- government faced a general election, and, as the issue concerned many voters, it had to be seen to be doing something about the problem;
- the issue was taken up in Parliament; and
- the campaign was widely supported by pressure groups and public health organisations.

Subsequently Oliver and other school food campaigners were highly critical of the coalition government's policies on obesity and school nutrition (McSmith, 2010; Oliver, 2011). There was particular concern that new academies and free schools were exempt from the school food rules. The removal of ring-fenced funding for school meals was also criticised. However, the issue of school food and child obesity remained on the agenda. The coalition insisted that it remained a priority, backing a new a School Food plan (Dimbleby and Vincent, 2013), extending new school food regulations to new academies and free schools, and announcing universal free school meals for younger pupils in England.

The media works in complex ways, and this has become even more evident with the advent of new media. Government health policies do not automatically change according to the whim of the BBC, *The Sun* or the *Daily Mail*. Rather, it is the way in which stories cascade through the media and how policy–makers respond (Richards, 2013) that lead to such changes. As Harrabin et al (2003, p 25) commented, 'opinions really start to shift when a story breaks in the newspapers, is taken up by television and radio programmes and carried over to the next day's papers.' However, these dynamics are not well understood. Rather than being informed by one newspaper or programme, people's experience of the media is fragmentary (Seale, 2003), and they pick up information and meanings in different ways and in various settings (see also Eldridge et al, 1999). On some issues, but perhaps not on others, current media coverage may be able to stimulate public interest on the basis of accumulated understandings and information built up over time. Hence, media coverage of the same breadth and intensity may well have a different impact on public opinion and policy because of different contexts and circumstances.

Influencing the media

Government influence over the media

Health policy has been a very sensitive area for governments, which is not surprising given its attractiveness to the media. As Entwhistle and Sheldon (1999, p 125) commented, 'media reports of events in the health service are of key importance to politicians as one of the main currencies of success or failure.' Although not the first government, nor the last, to seek to manage the news agenda, the Blair government pursued a particularly robust and systematic approach to media management and spin (see Brindle, 1999; Newton, 2001; Jones, 2002; Harrabin et al, 2003; Oborne and Walters, 2004; Price 2011; Dean, 2013). However, particular concern was raised about practices in the New Labour era, such as the burying of bad news and attempts to smear opposition politicians and their families (Dean, 2013; McBride, 2013). Under New Labour, government public relations functions were highly centralised, with Number 10 exerting greater control over government communications. Press and information officers were subject to stronger pressure from their political masters (special advisers as well as ministers) (Dean, 2013). A strong emphasis on 'rapid rebuttal' was evident. Criticisms of government policies in the media were closely monitored and immediately countered, often in an aggressive manner (Jones, 2002). A closer integration of policy and presentation was observed, with the need to ensure a positive media response to policy becoming a key consideration (Fairclough, 2000; Newton, 2001). The head of DH communications once complained that Number 10 asked for policy announcements before the Department had actually devised the policies (cited in Dean, 2013, p 20). In addition, government often sought to describe policies in increasingly imprecise and simplistic terms (Fairclough, 2000; Newton, 2001). Indeed, policy documents – notably Green and White Papers – became more like sales brochures: glossy in appearance, using images and pictures, placing less emphasis on explaining policy options and decisions and thin on policy context and evidence. New Labour also publicised performance targets to counter allegations of service failures and shortcomings. The achievement of targets, although crude and sometimes counterproductive, can be used as evidence that reforms are working, and that cases suggesting the opposite are merely anecdotal.

News management continued under the coalition. However, it was initially less successful, as the debates surrounding the Health and Social Care Act perhaps indicated. Although the government managed to achieve its legislative objectives, thanks to many concessions, it lost the media battle. However, news management of health improved considerably in the last two years of the government. In particular, the coalition was able to portray itself in a much more positive light, especially with regard to its response to the Mid Staffs report (see Chapter Seven) and the quality and safety agenda.

Pressure groups and corporate interests

Professions, health consumer and patients' groups, voluntary organisations, single-issue groups and corporate interests are all keen to shape the way in which issues are portrayed. According to Karpf (1988), the media discourse of health matters was dominated by medical definitions and perceptions. Since she wrote in 1988, media coverage of medicine has become more critical (Bury and Gabe, 1994; Seale, 2002). There is greater scope for expressing alternative views, including lay perspectives (Entwhistle and Sheldon, 1999).

Although medical concepts and perspectives are more open to challenge today, professional organisations – such as the BMA and the Royal Colleges – remain active in seeking to influence the media. These organisations are well resourced and skilled in media relations. They are proactive, and do not simply respond to stories already in the media (Doyle, 2000). According to policy actors interviewed by Baggott (2007), journalists often turn to the BMA for potential stories and for scientific advice on medical issues. Other NHS 'producer' groups also place great importance on influencing the media, including trade unions (such as UNISON) and groups representing NHS organisations (for example, the NHS Confederation). Professional and producer organisations highlight the importance of good relations with the media (Baggott, 2007). It is perceived as an important forum for advancing policy ideas, a means of opposing policies, and as a vehicle for portraying their organisations in a positive light.

Patients and their representatives have a stronger presence in the media nowadays, and can exert greater influence than previously. Seale (2002), for example, has observed that the media identifies lay 'heroes' and highlights 'victims' of medical mistakes and 'survivors' of serious illness. The consumer and patient voice is heard more strongly, and this is, to some extent, down to greater responsiveness in the media to alternative and lay perspectives on health (Entwhistle and Sheldon, 1999) and a more critical approach to medicine and producer groups. It is also partly due to the 'halo effect' of the voluntary sector and charities (Deacon, 1999), which increasingly claim to represent patient and carer interests (Baggott and Jones, 2014).

Stronger advocacy by organisations representing patients and consumers, including charities and voluntary organisations, has had an impact. These groups have correctly perceived the importance of the media in raising awareness about medical conditions, their role in portraying health and illness, and as a means of influencing government policy (Baggott et al, 2005). Groups representing patients, users and carers have extensive contact with the media (Baggott and Jones, 2014).

Groups representing patients, users and carers try to change media images of illness. For example, Mind and other mental health groups and professional organisations have been extremely critical of media coverage (Philo, 1996). They have made great efforts to challenge stereotypes, most recently through the Time to Change programme (www.time-to-change.org.uk). However, as Baggott et al (2005) found in their study, many groups struggle to counteract media stereotypes. Often the media have a particular agenda or angle on a story that is not negotiable. As noted earlier, health consumer and patients' groups complain about the media's reinforcement of the inaccurate image that young women are disproportionately at risk from breast cancer. But if groups do not comply with media demands and requirements, they may forfeit opportunities to raise awareness about the condition.

Commercial interests also strive to influence the media. The pharmaceutical and medical technology industries have a clear motive to shape the perception of health issues and policies (Collier, 1989; Moynihan, 1998; Moran, 1999; Ferner, 2005). Their profitability depends heavily on funding for research and development, and ultimately on the funding of healthcare services. Their interests are suited by the media adopting an uncritical approach to medical technologies and drugs.

The Health Committee (2005b) concluded that a climate has been fostered where drug therapies are the intervention of choice. Medicines take up a large and increasing slice of the NHS budget. In the management of depression, for example, drug therapies have often been adopted in preference to other interventions (such as counselling) despite concerns about their relative efficacy, efficiency and safety. Drugs companies have been able to control the flow of information about their products, and have suppressed adverse research findings (Health Committee, 2005b). In addition, they have very large promotional budgets to shape the preferences of clinicians, and can promote public awareness of diseases and drug treatments (Moynihan et al, 2002; O'Donovan and Glavanis-Grantham, 2003). Moreover, as the Health Committee (2005b) noted, a major part of the industry's promotional activities involves working with journalists and patients' groups.

A similar situation is found in relation to medical technology, where equipment such as scanners and screening techniques are promoted without much consideration for alternative approaches. In many cases, the adoption of new techniques is not simply due to lobbying by manufacturers, but an alliance with professionals who want to get their hands on the latest equipment. In addition, health consumer and patients' groups, charities and journalists can be useful allies in the fight for approval of techniques and resources to fund them. The media tends to portray medical technology in a positive light, and to emphasise the benefits rather than the costs of these technologies (Karpf, 1988; Moynihan, 1998; Entwhistle and Sheldon, 1999; Moynihan et al, 2008). Nonetheless, it is unable to resist negative stories about drugs and other technologies, even when faced with the possibility of legal action and other threats from large corporations. It is doubtful that any of the major drugs scandals would have seen the light of day had it not been for the efforts of journalists and the courage of their editors. Despite its huge economic and political power, the drugs industry has a persistently bad image, uncorrected by the large amount of money spent on promotion, marketing and public relations.

Other industries have an interest in shaping the perception of health and health policy. The food, alcoholic drink and tobacco companies have been identified as major culprits in some of today's main public health problems, including obesity, food poisoning, chronic alcohol-related disease, alcohol-related accidents and injuries, lung cancer and heart disease. These are profitable industries, and have an incentive to oppose policies that reduce their commercial freedoms (for example, bans on promoting their products). These industries are highly politicised. They fund PR campaigns to combat adverse media coverage and to promote a more positive image. In addition, product promotion builds customer loyalty and shapes wider public perceptions about the legitimacy of products and their benefits and harms. Furthermore, as large advertisers, these industries can exert leverage over media outlets that rely on advertising revenue, shaping coverage of health issues related to their products.

Although the interests that shape media portrayal of health are distinct, they rarely operate in isolation. Health issues are usually propelled into the media by the combined activity of professional, consumer and business interests (Moynihan, 1998; Baggott et al, 2005; Health Committee, 2005b). For example, campaigns to raise the profile of prostate cancer have involved a range of organisations including the British Association of Urological

Surgeons, Macmillan Cancer Support, Cancer Research UK, Prostate Cancer UK, the Men's Health Forum and the Prostate Research Campaign. At the same time, medical technology companies and drugs companies in this field have lobbied for more resources to be allocated to the prevention and treatment of the disease. Various groups and organisations also come together to influence the portrayal of issues already on the agenda. Hence, as noted earlier, mental health user groups and clinicians have united to campaign against the negative images prevalent in this area.

Conclusion

It is clear from this analysis that in health policy, as in other areas of public policy, the media cannot be ignored. However, its role in health policy is complex. As Eldridge and colleagues (1999) have noted, the media is not a single ideological conspiracy, nor does its power exist in a social vacuum. The media is both a means of describing and making sense of policy issues, and a force for shaping policy (Terkildsen et al, 1998; King and Street, 2005). It has its own interests, but is also used by other interests, including government, to portray issues in particular ways and to support or oppose policies. The influence of the media tends to be indirect and involves other policy actors such as pressure groups, government agencies and Parliament.

In health policy, there is much evidence that the media is more effective as a negative force or veto power. This reflects the situation in other areas of public policy (Newton, 2001). Although instances can be found where the media has exerted direct and positive influence on decision-making, as in the case of the Jamie Oliver school meals campaign, such examples are fairly rare. Usually, the media operates at a more subtle level, helping to define and reinforce particular meanings and values, constructing issues and shaping agendas.

Summary

- Media coverage of health issues is extensive, and health issues are particularly newsworthy.
- The coverage of health issues in the media contains significant biases. Some diseases and conditions receive more (and more positive) coverage than others.
- Drama, not just news, can shape public perceptions of health and illness. Celebrities can also have an impact on public perceptions.
- The media can influence public opinion, which can affect both health behaviour and policy.

- The media is regarded mainly as a negative force, blocking policies, rather than a driver of the policy agenda. However, it can prompt government intervention by highlighting problems.
- Government seeks to influence media coverage of health policy issues, and these efforts have increased in recent years.
- Pressure groups also seek to influence the media, including professional and producer groups, commercial organisations, charities, and health consumer and patients' groups.

Key questions

1. What factors make a health issue 'newsworthy'?
2. Why do some health issues get more favourable coverage in the media than others?
3. How does the media influence the public perception of health issues?
4. How, and to what extent, does the media influence health policy?
5. Why does (a) government and (b) external interests and pressure groups seek to influence health issues in the media?

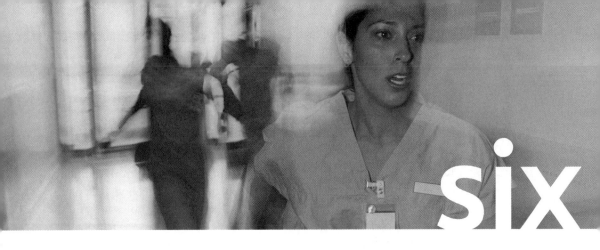

Policy networks and
health policy

Overview

The health policy arena is host to a range of representative organisations (such as professional groups and trade unions), campaigning organisations, think tanks, research bodies, commercial organisations, voluntary groups and charities. It also includes individual experts, researchers and campaigners. This chapter examines their interaction with governing institutions within health policy networks, their strategies and tactics, and discusses those factors that enable them to exert influence over health policy.

As noted in Chapter One, health policy can be seen as a developing within policy networks, which include various organisations and individuals from outside government. The rationale for such networks is that government lacks the capacity to govern alone. It needs external people and organisations to provide expertise, knowledge, research and ideas about policy. They are also useful as partners in the implementation of policy. They can inform sections of the community and the wider public about policy changes, and can even mobilise their resources to make policies work. External individuals and organisations are also needed as a means of strengthening the legitimacy of a policy. Their support can help convince public opinion and the media of the merits of government policy.

The roles of organisations and individuals are now examined in this chapter, along with the various lobbying tactics they use, and the resources that help them to exert influence over policy.

Interest groups: professional and labour groups

The medical profession

Over the past century, the medical profession has exerted strong influence over health policy. Its influence increased during the second half of the 20th century, due in part to the 'concordat' between the profession and the state on the NHS (Klein, 1995; Salter, 1998). Healthcare was nationalised, and the medical profession given both autonomy to practice and strong influence within the decision-making process. Doctors secured this position due to their political resources, including specialist expertise and knowledge, high social status, excellent political contacts and strong representative institutions. Indeed, with regard to the latter, the doctors' 'trade union', the BMA, gained a reputation as one of the most effective pressure groups in the country, while the prestigious Royal Colleges of Medicine, which represent specialists, could rely on the 'old boy network' to gain access to the highest levels of government. Meanwhile, the General Medical Council (GMC), responsible for medical regulation, standards of practice, education and training, continued to guard the privileges of professional autonomy.

Medical influence took a number of forms. The representative bodies of the profession – in particular the BMA – were enmeshed in the policy process and consulted extensively (see Eckstein, 1960). The relationship between the BMA and the government was close and consensual. Open conflict occasionally occurred, but was managed through an 'engineered consensus' (Klein, 1990). The medical profession exerted influence through advisory mechanisms and bodies established by government, and through medical divisions of the health department and the CMO (see Chapter Three).

During the 1970s, the consensual approach began to unravel, evident in the dispute over pay beds under the Labour government (see Chapter Two). Conflicts intensified under the Thatcher governments. Hostility to the public sector brought confrontation with doctors on issues such as NHS spending, reorganisation, GP contracts and the prescribing of medicines. In the late 1980s, the relationship with the BMA degenerated into open hostility (Ham, 2000). Even so, routine contact between the DH and the medical profession continued (McGregor-Riley, 1997).

During the 1990s, the Major government adopted a more conciliatory approach towards the BMA, and the traditional approach of 'mutual accommodation' was, to some extent, restored (Day and Klein, 1992). Nonetheless, DH-initiated contacts with the BMA declined in the early 1990s, as did the number of formal meetings between the two (Baggott and McGregor-Riley, 1999).

The election of the Blair government was heralded as a fresh start (Webster, 1998). New reforms were introduced in an atmosphere of consensus. Dialogue between the government and doctors' representative organisations were mostly cordial at the outset. However, there were tensions over the government's intentions to strengthen medical regulation, particularly in its relations with the GMC (see Irvine, 2003). The BMA also became disillusioned with the Blair government. It complained about doctors' workloads and the pace of the government's modernisation agenda. The BMA was furious when Blair identified it as part of the 'forces of conservatism' blocking public services reform. It became even more hostile when New Labour began to adopt market-style policies on the NHS (see Chapter Two).

Policy participants argued that the BMA had become weaker and lost influence in the latter years of the Blair government (see Baggott, 2007). However, others believed that it remained a big player and retained influence. The Royal Colleges consolidated their position, with the Royal College of Physicians regarded as particularly influential by some commentators (Sheard and Donaldson, 2006; Baggott, 2007). This was attributed to the effective leadership of these organisations and their willingness to work constructively behind closed doors – unlike the BMA, they rarely challenge the government in public.

Doctors were able to influence policy in other ways. National service frameworks (NSFs), introduced by the Blair government, were formulated by committees dominated by doctors (Hogg, 1999; Baggott et al, 2005). Meanwhile the czars (mostly drawn from the medical profession) were a channel for medical influence. To some extent, these offset the declining influence of medical civil servants within the department (see Chapter Three).

Gordon Brown's government sought to mend fences with the profession. As noted in Chapters Two and Three, Brown appointed a senior clinician (Lord Darzi) as Health Minister. Darzi was charged with undertaking a review of the NHS based on wide consultation, working closely with the medical profession.

The coalition government subsequently continued to take advice from senior doctors, emphasising the importance of clinical involvement and leadership in reform. However, it was not afraid to upset the medical profession's representative bodies (as the controversy over the Health and Social Care Act showed; see Chapters Three and Four). Although individual surgeons and GPs were courted by government, and as a result exerted some influence over policy, the profession as a collective force was initially weakened. But along with other external organisations, the professional bodies campaigned successfully for amendments to the legislation.

As the health policy arena has become more crowded (see Chapter Three), medical organisations have not found it as easy to dominate the policy process. Nonetheless, they retain considerable influence over policy. They increasingly work alongside other professional groups such as nurses and managers, organisations representing patients, carers, and users, other voluntary organisations, single-issue campaigners and also occasionally commercial interests.

Most observers believe that the medical profession retains considerable influence. One reason is that doctors and their organisations are smart political operators, and are well connected within the political system. And the medical profession continues to exert much influence over the public. Despite occasional NHS scandals and rising patient assertiveness, trust in the profession remains high. Medical organisations are well organised in how they deal with media. Furthermore, the profession influences how we think about healthcare, and its power remains entrenched in healthcare institutions, and in the values of the healthcare system. Notably, according to Alford's model, mentioned in Chapter One, the dominant professional monopoly interest can maintain its supremacy through its ability to define the values of the healthcare system, its professional status and knowledge, and control over the supply of professional services. This has been challenged in recent years by the corporate rationalisers – the bureaucratic, corporate and managerial interests that seek greater accountability and efficiency in health services – and, to an extent, by community interests, but nonetheless, medicine retains its position as a powerful structural interest (see also Harrison, 2001).

Nurses

When the NHS was created, nurses were excluded from policy formation and the decision-making machinery (Hart, 2004). In the intervening years, nurses became more vociferous. They have campaigned on pay and conditions, and have also sought to improve their professional status (Sibbald et al, 2004; McKee et al, 2006). There have been significant achievements as a result – the creation of a nurses' pay review body in the 1980s, and the Project 2000 reforms, which raised the status of nurse education and training. Nurses have extended the role of nursing (for example, triage services in urgent, accident and emergency care, and nurse prescribing). Furthermore, senior posts have been established for highly qualified nurses (nurse consultants, nurse practitioners, clinical nurse specialists and matrons). Some, however, argue that these developments have divided and fragmented the profession, by creating a nursing elite (Salter, 1998). In addition, it is believed that government policies have posed a direct threat to nursing interests, including the introduction of internal markets in healthcare, privatisation and the growth of managerialism in the NHS (Salter, 1998; Hart, 2004).

Nurses do possess a number of resources within the policy process. They are the largest section of the workforce, and have much public support. Acknowledgement of the extended role of nurses has placed a premium on their knowledge and expertise, and they are now consulted extensively on policy issues. Government has realised that many reform initiatives depend on political and practical cooperation from nurses' organisations, but while nurses' representatives are now more involved in policy discussions, their influence remains weak relative to the medical profession (Hart, 2004).

The Royal College of Nurses (RCN) – the largest nursing trade union, with around 370,000 members – is regarded by other policy actors as having leaders who are 'good operators' in relation to government and the media (Baggott, 2007). The trade unions, UNISON and Unite (discussed further below), which represent a broader range of public service and NHS workers, also organise nurses. However, as Hart (2004, p 201) has written, 'the division and lasting enmity between nursing's trade unions and professional associations is almost unique in British labour history'. More recently, the RCN and other trade unions have sought greater cooperation, but often take a different perspective on key issues (Hart, 2004).

In summary, nursing organisations participate in the networks that shape policy, but lack the same quality of access as doctors on the most important issues. Nurses are popular with the public, despite scandals that have revealed poor nursing care (as at Mid Staffs; see **Box 7.3**), and government does not welcome an open fight with them. But they have gained comparatively little, and what has been achieved is somewhat 'double-edged' in that it may undermine the unity, and ultimately the leverage, of the profession within the policy process.

Managers

In the eyes of government, the growth in managerialism within the NHS since the 1980s strengthened managers' status. However, they lack public support, partly because of a poor media image, which persists today (see Chapter Five). While senior NHS managers exert individual influence over policy (see Edwards and Fall, 2005), they have lacked a powerful collective voice. The Institute of Health Service Management (IHSM), which had quite a high policy profile in the 1980s and 1990s, became less prominent (and was rebadged as the Institute of Healthcare Management, focusing more on professional standards). In contrast, the NHS Confederation, which represents statutory NHS bodies and service providers, has been more high profile than its predecessor bodies on policy matters. After an initial period of distrust, the Blair government began to involve the NHS Confederation more closely in policy development (Baggott, 2007). It grew in stature, and developed a strong relationship with the DH. This was partly due to a favourable political context, which facilitated the influence of managers, and to changes in the DH that led to the recruitment of NHS managers (see Chapter Three). Some, in contrast, argued that the NHS Confederation was too close to government and too pliant (see Baggott, 2007). Indeed, the NHS Confederation's broad support for government policies sometimes put it in a difficult position.

Other organisations representing parts of the NHS structure or areas of special interest should be mentioned. They include the National Association of Primary Care (which champions primary care provision and represents primary care professionals, and is now part of the NHS Confederation), the NHS Alliance (professionals, managers and others including lay people who have an interest in primary care and commissioning), NHS Clinical Commissioners (which represents CCGs), the Foundation Trust Network (a member organisation for foundation trusts), NHS Employers (which represents NHS bodies that employ staff, and is also part of the NHS Confederation), and the UK Public Health Alliance (which aims to provide a coherent voice on public health issues and includes practitioners, academics and campaigners). All these bodies are actively engaged in seeking to influence policy.

Other professions and health workers

Other professional organisations engaged in the policy process include dentists and pharmacists' associations, and organisations representing midwives and therapists. Other staff members are represented by large multi-industry trade unions such as UNISON, which speaks for almost half a million NHS employees including nurses, midwives, health visitors, healthcare assistants, administrators, ambulance workers and support workers. Another large trade union, Unite, includes within its membership around 100,000 NHS workers, including community nurses, health visitors, school nurses, mental health nurses, ambulance staff and speech therapists. The GMB, meanwhile, has approximately 60,000 members working in the NHS, including maintenance staff, technical and support staff and ambulance workers.

Commercial interests

The drugs industry

The drugs industry has several reasons for being active in the health policy process. The NHS is an important customer of the drugs industry, and therefore health policy decisions can affect sales and profits. Moreover, government regulates many aspects of the industry, including pricing, safety and marketing. The industry is also affected by government policy in areas such as trade and industry, employment, science and technology, research and development. Furthermore, as multinational corporations, drugs companies are active in the European and international policy processes (see Chapter Ten).

The UK drugs industry is economically and politically powerful. It is one of the most successful manufacturing sectors (Pharmaceutical Industry Competitiveness Task Force, 2001; ABPI, 2010). It is a major exporter, a significant employer, a major contributor to research and development, and makes a significant contribution to tax revenues. The overall value added to the economy by the industry has been estimated at approximately £6 billion a year in 2013 (see www.abpi.org.uk/Pages/default.aspx). These factors give the industry economic leverage, which, coupled with excellent political contacts, makes it an extremely powerful political force. Individual companies are well connected politically, both directly and through their trade body (the Association of the British Pharmaceutical Industry, ABPI) (Baggott, 2007). Contacts with government are strong. The industry has a good relationship with the DH, aside from occasional public disputes over drug pricing. The industry has good parliamentary links, and employs former civil servants who are knowledgeable about the corridors of power. It also has strong links with researchers and other professionals who advise government on policy and regulatory matters. Furthermore, it has built relationships with charities, health consumer bodies and patients' groups representing the interests of patients, users and carers (Baggott et al, 2005). Some commentators argue that this is unhealthy and may subvert these traditionally less powerful interests (Jones, 2008).

The drugs industry has a rather sinister public image (Collier, 1989; Moynihan, 1998; Abraham, 2002; Moynihan and Cassels, 2006; Goldacre, 2013). Its primary motive is to make profits. Although not necessarily acting against the public interest, there are instances where the industry has clearly acted against this (Health Committee, 2005b). Such activities include targeting of health professionals with marketing, sponsorship and inducements; selective publication of research findings on the efficacy of drugs, and in some cases, suppression of evidence on side-effects; and use of patients, professionals and the media to 'market' illness and drug treatments, a process labelled as 'disease mongering' (Moynihan, 1998; see also Chapter Five). It is believed that the industry exerts undue influence over regulators as well as prescribers and patients. Indeed, the regulatory regime has been criticised for being captured by the industry and not acting fully in the public interest (Abraham, 2002; Health Committee, 2005b). Individual cases, where drugs have later been found to have been associated with adverse events (including Thalidomide, Opren, Seroxat and Vioxx), have exposed the industry and its practices to wide media coverage, and have undermined its public image (Collier, 1989; Health Committee, 2005b).

The Blair government was seen as adopting a more adversarial approach on several issues – notably on drug pricing and the creation of NICE – creating tensions in the relationship with the industry. The coalition government was strongly supportive of the drugs industry, acknowledging its economic benefits and its role in health service innovation. Even so, at the same time it aimed to constrain the NHS drugs bill, and sought to ensure that medicines would be as widely accessible as possible (because of the political fallout of sick patients unable to get new and/or expensive drugs). As with previous governments, this approach has produced a generally close relationship, punctuated with occasional disputes.

The independent health sector

The creation of the NHS left a 'rump' of independent operators within the British healthcare system. The independent sector expanded from the 1970s onwards, partly due to Labour's attack on NHS pay beds (see Chapter Two). Additional opportunities arose from favourable conditions created by the Thatcher government that sought to encourage the sector. Subsequently, the Blair and Brown governments stimulated the independent sector by introducing schemes to give the private and voluntary providers greater access to the NHS market (see Chapters Two and Eight). The coalition built on this, creating more opportunities for independent providers to compete with the NHS.

Paradoxically, despite having unprecedented market opportunities, the traditional UK independent sector struggled to compete. The main beneficiaries of the pro-market health policies were the large insurance companies (which offer health insurance as part of a wider portfolio of products), private healthcare providers from overseas (for example, Sweden, South Africa and the US), and relatively new domestic players in the health market (such as Serco, Virgin and Circle) (Leys and Player, 2011).

Little is known about how exactly the independent sector has influenced policy. It appears to have been pushing at an open door, given the support of recent governments for greater competition and plurality of service provision. But there is more to it than this. The sector has aggressively lobbied for a greater slice of the action, cultivating support from within government (Leys and Player, 2011). Furthermore, its political leverage has increased in line with its expansion (Pollock, 2004, p 80).

There is now something of a 'revolving door' between government and the independent sector. Executives from the sector have been seconded to the DH to work on general policy as well as specific issues such as PFI and IT strategies (Leys and Player, 2011). Meanwhile, the sector employs former government personnel. Some key figures have moved between the sectors more than once. For example, Simon Stevens, the current chief executive of the NHS, previously worked for United Health Europe, a subsidiary of a US health corporation, and before that was a senior government adviser on health (Lister, 2006). The independent sector has good links with Parliament and works closely with several MPs and Peers (including former ministers), some of who are retained as advisers.

Other private contractors and suppliers

The NHS has always depended on commercial suppliers – medical equipment, instruments and devices are manufactured by private companies. This includes products ranging from expensive scanners through to small disposable items, such as syringes. The medical equipment industry is large, consisting of around 1,800 companies, and is worth £4.5 billion per annum (DH, 2004d). The government acknowledged its importance by establishing a joint industry–government task force to explore issues of mutual interest, including market access, international trade, research and development and regulatory matters.

Other private contractors have also benefited from policies that have given them additional business. These include management consultancies, marketing agencies and providers of 'outsourced' services (which began with the Thatcher government's policies in the 1980s; see Chapter Two). The Blair government encouraged private sector involvement in the building and maintenance of healthcare facilities, again building on the policies of its Conservative predecessor. Public–private partnerships (PPPs), and in particular, the private finance initiative (PFI), created huge opportunities for the private sector (see Chapter Eight). Consortia involved in such schemes, which were extremely lucrative, had a huge incentive to lobby for more contracts, and were influential in opening up more areas for commercial exploitation (Baggott, 2007).

Commercial interests and public health

Many industries have an interest in minimising the impact of health policies on their businesses. A classic example is the tobacco industry, which has tried to resist measures to curb smoking. The impact of other industries on health is more complex. The food industry plays an essential part in maintaining a healthy population, but certain practices, such as the marketing of high fat/salt/sugar products (particularly to children), mass production techniques and the use of harmful additives pose a threat to health (see Baggott, 2010a). The food industry has defended its practices and sought to minimise public fears (see Chapter Five). More recently, it has worked with government on initiatives to improve the nation's diet as part of a Responsibility Deal, although the outcome of this is as yet unclear. The alcoholic drinks industry (see **Box 6.1**) is in a similar position. Although its products are not always harmful, alcohol misuse seriously undermines public health.

Box 6.1: Political influence of the drinks industry

Historically, the alcoholic drinks industry has been regarded as a potent political force. When in Victorian and Edwardian times the drink question became a major national issue, the industry successfully defended its interests (see Greenaway, 2003). Although facing a mass campaign by the Temperance movement and a succession of hostile Liberal governments, the industry had friends in Parliament and was particularly influential within the Conservative Party. The imposition of wartime controls in the First World War eventually forced the industry to concede on many crucial matters of policy (such as the reduction of licensing hours).

In the 1970s and 1980s, concerns about the rising levels of alcohol consumption and misuse, voiced by professional groups, voluntary organisations and statutory authorities in policing, criminal justice, health and social welfare – coupled with wider public disquiet articulated in the media – led government to formulate an alcohol strategy. But the industry successfully lobbied against this, and the policy was significantly weakened (Baggott, 1990).

More recently, concerns resurfaced around 'binge drinking' and associated late-night public disorder in cities and towns. Chronic heavy drinking has also been acknowledged as a key public health problem. Pressure on government to act led to an alcohol strategy for England (PMSU, 2004). This was criticised for ignoring evidence on interventions that could reduce overall consumption (such as taxation and controls on availability; see Babor et al, 2003), and for giving a drinks industry organisation, the Portman Group, a key role in implementing the strategy (Drummond, 2004; Room, 2004).

The drinks industry has considerable economic leverage, is extremely profitable, generating large tax revenues, and is a major employer. The Portman Group, the major drinks companies and trade associations are close to government. They are effective in mobilising Parliament (for example, the All-Party Parliamentary Beer Group has strong support among MPs, and indeed, is the largest group of its kind in Parliament).

The industry ensured that government's policy did not harm its commercial interests. However, continuing public concern about alcohol misuse, and counter-lobbying by health, welfare and public order pressure groups, kept the issue on the agenda. This steeled the Blair government and later the Brown government into taking a tougher approach, with new legislation to regulate the industry's worst practices and measures to increase funding of alcohol harm prevention projects (Baggott, 2010b).

The coalition deferred to the industry, favouring a self-regulatory approach (as part of a broader policy of corporate social responsibility in public health; see Baggott, 2013). But it did back stronger policies, namely, a commitment to minimum pricing of alcohol (supported by public health campaigners as a means of reducing consumption and alcohol problems). However, a decision not to proceed with minimum pricing revealed the extent of the industry's leverage (see Gornall, 2014). The industry had frequent meetings with government on the issue, built strong support for its position in Parliament, canvassed media opposition to the plan, and was able to generate further opposition from right-wing think tanks.

Corporate interests in alcohol are powerful. They have excellent political contacts (see Hawkins and Holden, 2012), possess great economic leverage, and can persuade government not to adopt health policies inimical to their interests. Within the industry, there is a general dislike of government regulation and taxation. Even so, the industry is not a monolith, and some elements are more responsible than others. While preferring self-regulation, these businesses concede that tougher action from government may be necessary in some circumstances if only to protect the image of the industry and its products and to tackle the most unscrupulous competitors.

Voluntary organisations, charities and single-issue groups

Health consumer and patients' organisations

Some organisations seek to promote and represent the interests of patients, users and carers (Barnes et al, 1999; Wood, 2000; Baggott et al, 2005; Baggott and Jones, 2014). Most health consumer and patients' organisations are relatively small in terms of income and membership. Others have large incomes and thousands of members (such as the Multiple Sclerosis Society and Diabetes UK).

Health consumer and patients' organisations have extensive contact with decision-makers. They have regular contact with ministers, civil servants, Parliament and the media. There are increasingly taken seriously by other policy actors, such as the health professions and the drugs industry, which increasingly seek alliances with them. Even so, groups vary considerably in their policy activities and their influence over policy. The larger and wealthier organisations, those with research and lobbying skills, those willing and able to forge alliances with other stakeholders, and those able to bring the experience of patients, users and carers to the policy process in a coherent way, tend to be the most effective and influential.

Even so, the power of professional and commercial interests remains strong (Baggott et al, 2005; Baggott, 2007). This supports the conclusions of Alford (1975), Hogg (1999) and Salter (2003) about the underlying weakness of consumer, patient and public interests in healthcare systems, reflected in everyday decisions, in the structures and institutions of decision-making, and in the language and discourse of policy. One of their key weaknesses is a lack of economic leverage (unlike commercial interests). Also, their claims to knowledge have been less highly valued than the scientific and technical expertise of other policy actors, such as the health professions. There have been cases where professional groups and commercial interests have 'colonised' health consumer and patients' organisations or even created new groups to campaign on their behalf (to support the licensing of a new drug, for example; see Baggott et al, 2005; Health Committee, 2005b). Consumer and patient groups can also be manipulated by the government, which funds many of them, for its political ends. For example, they may be used to demonstrate support for government policies and to counter professional opposition (Baggott, et al, 2005; Baggott, 2007).

Other voluntary organisations

There is a significant body of other voluntary organisations that engage with the health policy process. These include research and service provider charities (such as the British Heart Foundation, Cancer Research UK, Macmillan Cancer Support, Mencap and Scope). Many have considerable resources and excellent political contacts. They are also experienced in the policy process, and have expertise that is highly valued by government. But this sector also includes small, charitable organisations that are not politically active and that concentrate on raising money for good causes and providing help for those in need.

In recent years the voluntary sector (including health consumer and patients' organisations) has become a more important player in the policy process. This is partly because it has become better organised, often forming alliances to campaign on issues or to provide a coherent response across a range of policies. An important body in the health policy arena is National Voices, which brings together over 200 voluntary organisations, and has campaigned on a range of issues. It lobbied successfully to strengthen the patient and public involvement (PPI) clauses of the Health and Social Care Act 2012 during its passage through Parliament. The government consults more extensively with the voluntary sector, and has created advisory groups for this purpose (in addition to holding ad hoc meetings with voluntary organisations to discuss their concerns). It should be noted that the standing of the voluntary sector has risen in recent years as the government has sought to increase its role as a service provider (see Chapter Eight). Although this has yielded opportunities for these organisations to increase their income and to strengthen political leverage and contacts, there is concern that voluntary organisations have become more financially dependent on government, and less willing to openly criticise policy. Moreover, not all groups have the capacity to engage with government by providing state-funded services or to get involved in the policy process, and there are fears that these developments could increase inequalities within the voluntary sector (Baggott, 2013).

Single-issue groups

Single-issue 'cause' groups have a clear public policy focus. They seek to move public policy in their chosen direction by demonstrating broad public support for action on a particular issue. An example is Action on Smoking and Health (ASH) and its adversary FOREST (Freedom Organisation for the Right to Enjoy Smoking Tobacco). Other interests also endorse and support causes. Professional organisations, such as the BMA and the Royal Colleges, have supported anti-smoking campaigns. Similarly, commercial interests, on the receiving end of protests, have funded or created 'front' organisations to promote their view on a particular issue, in areas such as food, tobacco and alcohol policy.

It is difficult to generalise about the influence of single-issue groups. Some have been very successful, particularly over the longer term. For example, ASH, formed in the 1970s (by the Royal College of Physicians), campaigned successfully for advertising restrictions (including a ban on tobacco advertisements and sponsorship) as well as a ban on smoking in enclosed public spaces. In the late 1990s the Bristol Heart Children's Action Group campaigned successfully for an inquiry into the standards of paediatric heart surgery at Bristol Royal Infirmary, that later had wide implications for policies on clinical governance, medical regulation and patient and public involvement. Subsequently another group, Cure the NHS (a small group of relatives/patients/community members) successfully campaigned for a public inquiry into the failings at Stafford Hospital, which had similarly wide ramifications for the NHS.

A number of generic campaigning organisations have flourished in the internet age. These have been credited with influencing policy across a range of issues, including health. For example, 38 Degrees, founded in 2009, has 2.5 million members who sign petitions, contact MPs, organise public meetings, and contact others to build public support (Moore, 2014). It also makes representations to government bodies and decision-makers. 38 Degrees campaigned against the Health and Social Care Act 2012 and against powers to close hospitals without full public consultation. It has played a key part in publicising issues, and has had some success in promoting changes to legislation.

Other organisations

A range of other organisations seeks to influence health policy. These include 'think tanks' (see Dorey, 2005; Ruane, 2005). Some specialise in health and care (such as the King's Fund and the Nuffield Trust), while others have a wide-ranging policy remit (for example, the Institute for Public Policy Research [IPPR], the Adam Smith Institute, Civitas, Reform, Policy Exchange, Demos, Catalyst and Social Market Foundation). The latter tend to be more ideological or associated with particular perspectives on welfare. It is difficult to generalise about the influence of think tanks. They can be highly influential, but much depends on how their ideas, findings and recommendations are taken up by others, including politicians, pressure groups and the media. The timing of reports is obviously important. If a policy is in the process of development, new ideas or findings can have a significant influence. Much also depends on the links between these organisations and policy-makers. Notably, several prime ministerial advisers have previously worked for think tanks, including Matthew Taylor (IPPR) and Geoff Mulgan (Demos) under New Labour, and Nick Seddon (Reform) for the coalition.

Highly respected health research bodies (such as the King's Fund) and think tanks with close links to those in government tend to be the most influential (see Ham, 2000). It should be noted that important policies have been generated from ideas provided by think tanks, including foundation trusts and the use of market incentives in the NHS (Ruane, 2005).

There is concern about the influence of think tanks (Shaw, 2014; Denham and Garnett, 2006). Many receive donations from other interests who may seek to influence reports and recommendations, such as businesses (or in some cases, trade unions) which have a vested interest in shifting policy in a particular direction. Some are very close to political parties, calling their independence further into question. The quality of their research methods and analysis has also been called into question, especially in relation to the more extreme ideological think tanks whose main purpose appears to be to legitimise radical policy options. However, some have built up a very solid reputation based on transparent and well-conducted research (such as the King's Fund and the Nuffield Trust, for example).

Other parts of the public sector

Health matters are of interest to a range of public bodies. Indeed, as we shall see in Chapter Eight, many such bodies are actively involved in implementing health policy. They also seek to influence policy. Examples include local authorities, police and fire services, schools and universities and environmental bodies. In most cases, public bodies operate through representative organisations. For example, the Local Government Association, which represents local authorities, has been heavily involved in lobbying on health and care issues. Professional associations and trade unions whose members work in public services also represent public sector perspectives. For example, groups such as the Association of Directors of Social Services, the Society of Local Authority Chief Executives, the Chartered Institute of Environmental Health, the Association of Chief Police Officers and the National Union of Teachers have commented on health policy issues related to their professional interests and expertise.

Individual campaigners, experts and academics

The various interests and organisations discussed so far are key players within health policy networks. However, individuals also play a role. This includes individual campaigners such as Jayne Zito, who campaigned for mental health reforms following the murder of her husband by a man suffering from mental illness. Another example is Julie Bailey, a formidable campaigner in the Mid Staffs scandal. But campaigners rarely act in isolation and, as these two cases illustrate, often establish groups (the Zito Trust and Cure the NHS respectively) to carry on their work.

Individuals also participate in policy processes, for example, as members of the public responding to consultations, or making representations on a particular issue organised by a group. Government undertakes consultations on a range of issues and individuals respond with comments and observations. It is often unclear whether this has any influence. However, individual experiences, especially where they reflect those of a wider section of the community, can have an impact. For example, patients' organisations do bring individual patients to meetings with decision-makers to exemplify problems facing service users, and it is believed that this has some effect (Baggott et al, 2005).

Individuals participate in policy processes as technical experts. This includes scientists and other academics. Government offers a range of opportunities for them to engage in consultations and calls for evidence. Individual experts are also appointed to advisory committees and undertake commissioned research on behalf of government. Academic researchers are perceived by policy actors as less influential in recent years. However, some individual researchers are highly regarded by both government and other policy actors, and can have an impact on policy initiatives.

Lobbying, 'pressure points' and resources

Those seeking to influence policy have a variety of options. Although their strategies and tactics will vary according to particular circumstances, there is some consensus on which opinion-formers and policy-makers to target (Baggott, 1995, 2007).

Central government

Those seeking to influence policy acknowledge the importance of participating in the institutions, networks and policy processes of central government (discussed in Chapter Three). Not surprisingly, the DH is seen as the main point of contact, except where other departments have specific health-related responsibilities (such as housing, road safety, health and safety at work). Even so, there is awareness of the increased role of Number 10 and the Treasury (see Chapter Three) with regard to health policy and the need to influence these core institutions.

Despite the acknowledged decline in civil service influence over policy in recent decades (see Chapter Three), the maintenance of close and long-term working relationships with civil servants remains a key aim for most who seek policy influence. Civil servants have considerable knowledge, understanding and expertise within specific policy areas. This enables them to act as an interface between government and outside organisations or individuals. This may involve listening to those affected by planned or existing legislation, identifying practical solutions to potential problems of implementation that they raise, and advising ministers and other colleagues of potential problems and solutions. Groups and individuals are also proactive in raising new issues and policies, which civil service contacts may feed into the policy process.

However, it is important to get ministers on side on the most controversial and high profile issues. Wherever possible, groups seek to build a constructive relationship with the Secretary of State. Relationships with junior ministers are also important because they operate on the Secretary of State's behalf, and liaise with groups on matters within their area of responsibility.

Ministerial advisers are important targets for lobbying (see also Baggott et al, 2005; Hawkins and Holden, 2012). Advisers often play 'intermediary roles' on behalf of ministers, which involves listening to the views of groups and negotiating possible solutions on behalf of ministers when necessary (see Chapter Three). Other advisers, such as the czars, are perceived as having influence over policy in their specific field of expertise (Baggott et al, 2005; Baggott, 2007; see also Chapter Three).

Information about meetings between ministers, senior officials and outside organisations and individuals is now publicly available. This reveals the extent and frequency of contact between government and interested parties. As an illustration, **Figure 6.1** shows contacts for a three-month period in 2011. This suggests that provider interests are frequently engaged at this level, especially state providers of health and social care, the NHS, local government,

Figure 6.1: External involvement in declared meetings with DH ministers and senior officials*, May to July 2011

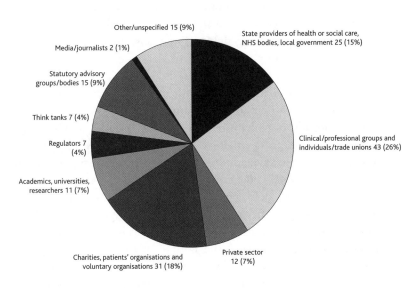

Total number of outside interests/organisations involved in meetings = 168**

Notes: * Ministers, Permanent Secretary, Chief Medical Officer and Chief Executive of the NHS.
** The total number of meetings recorded was 156; some meetings had more than one external participant.

Source of data: whoslobbying.com

clinicians, professional bodies and trade unions. The private sector was less frequently engaged in this period. It also reveals substantial contact between government and the voluntary sector. These figures must be treated with some caution, however. They only cover a relatively short period, and only relate to meetings at senior level (as opposed to routine contact with the civil service), and they don't cover informal contact.

Parliament and parties

Parliament remains a key target for lobbying, despite its marginal impact on policy (see Chapter Four). External groups and individuals are aware that parliamentary support is sometimes needed to draw the government's attention to a problem. Parliamentary activities (such as debates, amendments to Bills and questions) can be an important adjunct to a media campaign to propel issues on the agenda. Parliamentary pressure is particularly important when government is neutral or not committed to a course of action (for example, on cross-party issues). Parliamentary support is also required to gain concessions from government, for example, on legislation, although this is difficult when faced with a highly committed and disciplined government with a large majority.

Parliament is highly accessible to groups. As noted in Chapter Four, the level of interest in health matters is high among parliamentarians. External groups and individuals usually try to identify individual members likely to be helpful to them by tabling debates, motions, questions and other parliamentary activities. Some groups have databases, compiled using information from registers of members' interests and previous contributions to health debates, which enables the identification of 'friendly' MPs and Peers, and those hostile to their aims and campaigns.

In some cases, outside organisations will establish a panel of MPs and/ or Peers to liaise with on policy matters. These arrangements often evolve into APPGs (which can receive administrative and financial support from outside organisations; see Chapter Four). External bodies also target other parliamentary committees, such as public bill committees, which consider legislation and increasingly offer opportunities for groups and individuals to give evidence. Select committees (particularly the Health Committee) are also important targets. During the course of their inquiries, select committees receive oral and written evidence from a range of organisations and individuals (see Chapter Four). Policy actors believe these committees have the potential to create a more favourable climate for their policies, and argue that select committee 'endorsement' of policy recommendations can affect the direction of policy, particularly in the longer term (Baggott et al, 2005; Baggott, 2007).

When lobbying Parliament or government, most external bodies maintain a neutral stance with regard to party politics. Even trade unions and business interests are less partisan than was once the case; there are disadvantages with being partisan. If that party is out of office, there will be fewer opportunities to influence policy. Yet when that party is in power, policy influence is not guaranteed (as the trade unions have learned). This is why many external organisations seek endorsement for their policies from parties across the political spectrum, in an effort to improve the chances of implementation by future governments.

Media, public opinion and support

As shown in Chapter Five, the media contributes to the construction of health issues chiefly through definition and reinforcement of particular meanings and values. It can shape the political agenda by highlighting key issues. The media is especially potent as a negative force, discouraging specific policy options, although it can exert a direct and positive impact on policy.

It is testimony to the importance of the media in the health policy arena that external organisations and campaigners put so much time and resources into influencing it (see Chapter Five). Some find it easier to secure favourable coverage than others, however. Professional groups, particularly the medical profession, still command sympathetic media attention. In addition, some issues attract relatively more attention and more favourable coverage in the media (such as breast cancer and children's health) than others (such as mental health and the care of the elderly), although, as noted in Chapter Five, campaigners have challenged negative stereotypes with some success.

Some organisations and campaigners have used alternative ways of generating grassroots support. Direct action tactics, such as protests and boycotts, are increasingly used (Grant, 2005). Internet campaigns are now common, with direct action activities organised through email, Twitter, websites and mobile phone technologies (Moore, 2014). The health sector has had less experience of direct action than others (such as the environment, for example), but public protests against hospital closures and high-profile campaigns by patients to make new drugs more widely available indicate that this is changing (Mandelstam, 2006).

Access and influence

Good political contacts with decision-makers and opinion-formers are regarded as essential. As noted in Chapter One, it has been suggested that groups with good access to government that are regularly consulted on policy matters tend to be more influential than those lacking access and not regularly consulted. The former are regarded as 'insiders' and the latter, 'outsiders'. Doubt has been cast on this dichotomy. Strategies that rely heavily on good contacts with government may not be as effective as those deploying a wider range of tactics (an 'open' strategy), including contacts with the media and the mobilisation of public opinion (Whiteley and Winyard, 1987). In the health field, research by Baggott et al (2005) found that health consumer and patients' organisations that adopted an open strategy tended to be more successful than those that relied on good contacts with government. Further interviews with health policy actors (Baggott, 2007) confirmed that although contact with government is important, other pressure points, such as the media and Parliament, should not be neglected. Moreover, policy actors overwhelmingly emphasised that access to government does not equate with influence. Furthermore, it should not be assumed that 'outsider' groups, which focus on the media and mobilising public opinion, are without influence. Such groups may lack good contacts with decision-makers, but they can shape the political agenda, and thereby have an enormous impact on decision-making. For example, 'outsider' groups allied with social movements have been very effective in getting issues on the health agenda, changing the nature of public debate about these issues, and ultimately influencing decisions (see **Box 6.2**).

Box 6.2: Social movements and health

One must not ignore wider social movements in health, which have an impact on the underlying assumptions and values in health policy and practice. However, there is disagreement over what actually constitutes a social movement (see Byrne, 1997; Jordan and Maloney, 1997; Della Porta and Diani, 2005). Perhaps the best approach is to see social movements not as a distinct category of collective action, but as a complex array of activities that involves the following:

- Social movements challenge existing assumptions or ways of doing things from the outside rather than from the inside. One of the key attributes of a social movement is that it poses a challenge by those excluded from current arrangements (Scott, 1990; Tarrow, 1998). These may be socially excluded groups or those facing some form of discrimination (for example, minority ethnic groups, people with disabilities, women, lesbian, gay, bisexual and transgender [LGBT] people). However, many modern-day activists tend to come from higher socioeconomic backgrounds and are well educated, while members of the lower classes tend to be poorly represented.
- Social movements promote societal change rather than localised campaigns or policy-specific changes, although social movements are active on local and national issues and may have an impact on policies. However, their focus

is usually much wider, promoting values and principles (such as gender or racial equality, for example). Social movements tend to be ongoing (although particular movements may wax and wane over time).

- Social movements are not simply organisations. They encompass a range of activities, including the activities of informal groups and individuals, and are held together by common values rather than organisational structures. However, most social movements contain organisations that raise resources for campaigns and mobilise wider public support (such as Greenpeace and Friends of the Earth within the environmental movement).

- Social movements tend to adopt 'unconventional' tactics, such as protest and direct action rather than meetings with policy-makers. However, they and their constituent organisations also use conventional means (encouraging members and supporters to write to MPs, for example; see Ridley and Jordan, 1998). Furthermore, social movements do not have a monopoly on protest and direct action. Other, more conventional, pressure groups (such as trade unions and professional bodies) have also engaged in boycotts, strikes and protests from time to time.

- Social movements are concerned with politics and policies, but they are also concerned with the practices of everyday life. Indeed, theorists such as Habermas (1987) have pointed out that they can counter the 'colonisation of the lifeworld' by the state and other powerful groups such as the professions. Social movements therefore operate at the symbolic level and in cultural networks as much as in the political sphere (Melucci, 1989).

- Social movements are usually international in scope, not confined by the borders of nation states. They are related to broader global cultural and social debates.

- Social movements in the post-war period have been primarily concerned with lifestyle, environment and consumption issues rather than economic or material issues. People are part of a movement because they wish to express their values and identity rather than for any pecuniary motive. However, it is recognised that material concerns represent an important focus for many movements including those that seek to redress inequalities in society (such as the anti-poverty, women's, disability and racial equality movements).

Various social movements can be identified in the health field. Indeed, Brown and Zavestoski (2004, p 679) have defined health social movements (HSMs) as 'collective challenges to medical policy, public health policy and politics, belief systems, research and practice which include an array of formal and informal organisations, supporters, networks of cooperation and media.' They see HSMs as posing a challenge on several fronts, including political power, professional authority and personal and collective identity. They also identify three types of HSM: health access movements that address issues of access and provision of healthcare services; embodied health movements that focus on the personal understanding and experience of illness; and constituency-based health movements that address health inequality based on race, ethnicity, gender, sexuality and class.

Perhaps the most prominent examples are the childbirth movement and the mental health movement. In the field of maternity and childbirth, a social movement consisting of informal and formal organisations and individuals campaigned to de-medicalise childbirth and to restructure services to provide for a more women-centred approach (Declerq, 1998; Tew, 1998). This appears to have been fairly successful, leading to changes in government policy. However, in practice, implementation has been limited with women-centred services inhibited by resource constraints and professional and managerial conservatism (Garcia et al, 1998). Also, somewhat paradoxically, patient choice (and other factors such as fears of litigation) has driven an increase in medicalisation of childbirth as reflected in the increase in Caesarean sections to a level that has caused concern, even among obstetricians. With regard to mental health, the mobilisation of a users' movement drove efforts to create more humane mental health services, and challenged attitudes to mental illness within government, the health professions and in wider society (see Rogers and Pilgrim, 1991; Crossley, 2006). This had paradoxical consequences. The flawed implementation of community care created a public backlash paving the way for policies that reflected public safety rather than the needs of users (Rogers and Pilgrim, 2001). However, there are signs of improved cooperation between professionals and user groups in this field, which are increasingly working together on common issues.

These cases illustrate the difficulties of evaluating the impact of HSMs (see also Keefe et al, 2006). These problems are compounded by the kind of definitional issues raised earlier, by the multilevel impact of movements (on ideas, values, agendas, policies and practice) and the long-term nature of their struggle, which can mean that their impact should not be prematurely judged.

Resources

Aside from political contacts, other factors affect the likelihood that a group will exert influence over policy. The resources allocated to lobbying and campaigning is an important factor. The wealthier groups can afford to rent expensive offices close to Westminster and Whitehall (or in Brussels; see Chapter Ten); they can also employ specialist lobbying staff; and are able to commission research and publicity for their cause – the playing field is not level. Large professional membership organisations, trade unions, trade associations and companies have plenty of resources. Larger charities may also have big budgets, although their ability to lobby is sometimes constrained by their charitable status. Others, such as smaller single-issue groups, minority professional groups and most health consumer and patients' groups, are relatively resource-poor. They rely heavily on voluntary effort, and in some cases, a small number of administrators. Sometimes, however, the smaller organisations will be able to punch above their weight, particularly if they produce a well-argued case backed up with sound research (Baggott et al, 2005).

Skills

Some groups are able to employ specialist staff who have a thorough understanding of the political process and are experienced in dealing with government, Parliament and the media. In some cases these people have previously worked in government and have an inside knowledge of how the political process operates. The larger and wealthier organisations can afford specialist staff, and in some cases these form a self-contained policy unit (for example, in the BMA and RCN). The smaller groups tend to rely more heavily on volunteers to undertake policy roles. Where they can afford to employ officers, these are often less specialised, undertaking general administrative tasks alongside policy-related functions.

Expertise and knowledge

A key 'resource' possessed by groups is expertise and knowledge relevant to policy issues. Groups hold various types of knowledge. Some hold scientific and technical knowledge (about the cost-effectiveness of a particular intervention, for example), or they may hold practical or experiential knowledge (relating to the actual experiences of treatment or the workings of the health system). The distribution of knowledge and expertise varies across groups. Some have high levels of both types. The BMA, for example, possesses medical expertise and knowledge as well as the 'grassroots' experience of individual practitioners.

The government's demand for knowledge and expertise can change over time, and this can affect its relationship with particular groups. In recent years, for example, the government's preoccupation with healthcare costs, privatisation and marketisation has led it to become more dependent on those groups with financial and economic expertise related to healthcare, or which can help implement new modes of service delivery. Similarly, the government's aim to create a more 'patient-centred' healthcare system has enhanced the role of health consumer and patients' groups that can give an authentic account of the experiences of patients, users and carers (Baggott et al, 2005). The knowledge and expertise of those representing clinical and pharmaceutical interests is still regarded as extremely important by government, and continues to have a major impact on policy.

Economic leverage and sanctions

Groups that possess economic leverage or other sanctions are among the most influential. In the healthcare system the government is dependent on a range of organisations, notably those representing doctors and other professional groups, commercial organisations and, increasingly, private contractors. Ultimately, if these groups are unhappy with government policy, they can deploy sanctions. Examples include industrial action by staff, and drug companies moving their manufacturing operations overseas. Even the threat of such action can yield influence, although much depends on the government's resolve. Other groups have few sanctions. Managers have little leverage and lack public support. Moreover, as part of the management structure of the NHS, they are in a vulnerable position if they withdraw labour. Groups representing patients, users and carers also have few options to really damage government. Their main weapon is publicity – about issues such as inadequate standards, difficulties in access to services and the effect of budgetary decisions.

Alliances

An ability to work with other groups on issues of common concern is a major factor in determining policy influence. Alliances of groups tend to be much more powerful than the sum of their parts. Groups of professionals or workers can come together to fight on common issues. There now appears to be much more cooperation between professional organisations and trade unions on issues such as NHS reform and reorganisation, for example. In addition, professional and consumer/patient interests (and in some cases, commercial groups and single-issue groups too) can join forces on a particular issue. The campaign to ban smoking in public places in the UK, for example, was backed by a wide range of groups including the BMA, RCN, the British Heart Foundation, Cancer Research UK and ASH. There are many examples of coalitions that are lobbying for resources or treatments in a particular condition area (such as multiple sclerosis, breast cancer and Alzheimer's disease) that include health consumer and patients' groups, professionals and drugs companies.

Political consultants

Finally, wealthier organisations and individuals use specialist firms of political consultants to advise on how to influence policy, arrange meetings with decision-makers or opinion-formers, and even to influence policy on their behalf. There has been much controversy about these organisations. One concern is lack of transparency – it is difficult to track who is seeking to influence policy, and how decisions have been influenced. This lack of transparency is seen as encouraging 'sleaze' and corruption, undermining standards in public life and confidence in government. And as the services of political consultants are not cheap, there are fears about inequalities in influence, with powerful wealthy lobbies triumphing over less well-resourced groups and the public interest. These concerns have led to pressures to regulate lobbying, declaration of interests and relationships between policy-makers and those seeking to influence them (see **Box 6.3**).

> **Box 6.3: Regulation of lobbying**
>
> There has been much controversy in recent times about the influence of external interests or powerful individuals over policy-makers. This has arisen from concerns about conflicts between the public and private interests of ministers, MPs and Peers; the relationship between politicians, special advisers and civil servants and powerful external interests; the so-called 'revolving door' between government and certain organisations, especially business; and the activities of political consultants who advise and lobby on behalf of other interests.
>
> Parliament and governments have responded to public disquiet by introducing various codes and rules. For example, MPs and Peers must register pecuniary and other material interests on a regular basis, and declare any relevant interest when participating in parliamentary activities, such as debates. If there is a conflict of interest, the MP or Peer concerned must resolve it in favour of the public interest. Although payment for lobbying ('paid advocacy') is now banned, MPs and Peers may still be paid for advising external organisations. They are also allowed to earn money from external employment, investments and businesses.
>
> Under the Ministerial Code, ministers must relinquish control of financial interests while serving in office. Meanwhile, codes for civil servants and special advisers (who are, in effect, temporary civil servants) make it clear that they must not misuse their public position to further their private interests or those of others. Ministers, special advisers and the most senior civil servants must publicly declare gifts and hospitality. They have to log meetings with external organisations and individuals, and this information is publicly available. Furthermore, ministers, special advisers

and civil servants wishing to undertake paid work for an external body after leaving office must have their appointments scrutinised by the Advisory Committee on Business Appointments, which can make recommendations about any restrictions on their activities. The Committee may impose a waiting period before they can take up the appointment, and can recommend restrictions on any future lobbying activity (for example, that the ex-minister or official may not seek to influence former colleagues within a stated period). Notably, these recommendations cannot be enforced.

Further legislation – the Transparency of Lobbying, Non-Party Campaigning and Trade Union Administration Act 2014 (known as the Lobbying Act) – introduced controversial new rules in this field. One of the areas covered by the Act, the work of political consultants, has been criticised as too narrow. Although the Act established a statutory register of lobbyists, commercial organisations that engage in lobbying as an incidental activity are exempt. This means that trade associations, businesses, law firms and PR companies can evade regulation. The Act only covers a limited range of lobbying activities, that is, lobbyists' communications with ministers and the most senior civil servants (although there are powers to extend this to special advisers).

Another part of the Act has been criticised for limiting the legitimate freedom of outside organisations to campaign on public policy issues, such as charities, voluntary organisations, trade unions and professional associations. The Act regulates expenditure likely to influence elections. Organisations spending above a certain threshold must register with the Electoral Commission, and maintain records of expenditure. The Act has widened the definition of what counts as relevant spending, and it is feared that this will have a chilling effect on campaigning groups, discouraging them from raising policy issues, especially in the pre-election period. The law is underpinned by a tougher enforcement regime with severe punishments for breaching the new rules (including imprisonment for some offences). As the new rules also apply to joint campaigns, it is feared that they will discourage campaigns by alliances of groups and organisations.

Conclusion

It is very difficult to generalise about the influence of external groups and individuals over policy and their relationships with government. At any point in time, there is a huge amount of effort spent on influencing health policy, and the various constellations of groups and individuals will vary from issue to issue. Moreover, relationships between government and external policy actors can change over time (as can relationships between external organisations and groups). Despite this complexity and dynamism, it is possible to draw some conclusions about the role of groups in the policy process.

First, the medical profession remains influential. Although challenged by commercial, managerial and consumer/patient interests and other professional groups, the medical profession and its representative organisations continue to exert more influence over health policy than any other single group. Second, and related to this, the health policy network (see Chapter One) has become more crowded. The simple 'bilateral' relationships between medicine and the state have given way to a more complex set of relationships. Superficially, this is a more open 'issue network', but in reality, the traditionally powerful groups (medicine, and some commercial interests such as the drugs industry) remain in a pre-eminent position. Some 'stars' have risen – the private sector, sections of the voluntary sector – while others, such as nursing and management interests, have had a more mixed experience. Third, considerable inequalities persist between groups. Political resources – public support, economic leverage, status, possession of knowledge and expertise – are not evenly distributed. Furthermore, there is variation in the quality of political contact between groups with regard to the media, Parliament and government. Fourth, there is no simple prescription regarding strategy and tactics. To be an insider is not sufficient to guarantee influence over policy, while outsiders are not without influence. Groups should not neglect relationships with other arenas such as Parliament and the media that can help shape political agendas and provide rallying points for opposition to government policy.

Finally, while the focus on organised groups and interests is important, and provides much of the empirical data on the influence of interests and their relationships with policy-makers, one should not forget the role of diffuse and amorphous social forces, such as structural interests and social movements. These can exert influence over the context of health policy-making and the policy agenda in this field.

Summary

- The medical profession does not have a monopoly of influence over health policy. While the health policy network is more open and inclusive than previously, doctors' interests and their organisations remain highly influential within the policy process.
- Among the various other interests in health policy – other health professions, trade unions, commercial interests, health consumer and patients' groups, the wider voluntary sector and single-issue groups – some have grown in influence while others have had a more mixed experience.

- External organisations and campaigners possess various resources that they can bring to the policy process, which include status, expertise and economic leverage. These resources are not equally distributed, however.
- To be an insider group does not guarantee influence. Groups need to maintain contacts with several 'pressure points', including Parliament and the media.
- Changes in policy-making within central government (notably the involvement of Number 10 in health policy and the rise of special advisers) have been reflected in the strategies and tactics of pressure groups.
- Broader social movements can exert influence over the context of health policy and the health policy agenda.

Key questions

1. What are the main external interests in health policy? What influence have these groups had over health policy in recent years?
2. Has medical influence over health policy declined?
3. Does access to government equal influence over policy?
4. How, and to what extent, have health social movements influenced health policy?
5. What resources are important for external groups seeking to influence health policy?

seven

Health policy and the NHS

Overview

This chapter explores the implementation of health policy within the NHS. It focuses on the relationship between central government and the NHS, and the extent to which this has changed in recent years.

Implementation is a crucial part of the policy process (see Chapter One). In health policy, much of the task of implementation falls to the NHS. As this is a large and complex organisation, inhabited by conflicting and powerful interests, there is no guarantee that national policies will be implemented locally (Ham, 2004). This chapter explores policy implementation in the NHS and the activities of central government to ensure that policies are put into practice. When looking at policy implementation in the context of centralisation and decentralisation, one has to be aware of the multiple levers at the disposal of national policy-makers. This chapter explores the most significant of these, structure and organisation; priorities and planning; leadership and management; regulation; financial mechanisms and incentives; and culture and networks.

Structure and organisation

The NHS was originally constituted as a tripartite service: hospitals, owned and funded by the state, overseen by regional and local boards; state-funded family health services provided by independent contractors (such as GPs and dentists), administered by executive councils; and community and public health services run by local councils. The NHS in England has been reorganised many times (health service reorganisations in other parts of the UK are discussed in Chapter Nine). The original structure was reorganised in 1974. Public health and community health services were incorporated within the main NHS structure (Webster, 1996). The hospital boards were replaced by three tiers of health service management, at regional, area and district level, overseen by new regional and area health authorities. Executive councils were replaced by family practitioner committees (FPCs). This new structure attracted criticism, chiefly for being 'top-down' and over-bureaucratic (Edwards, 1993). The Royal Commission on the NHS (1979) subsequently recommended the abolition of one of the tiers below regional level (HM Government, 1979). In 1982, area health authorities and their management teams were abolished, and health authorities established at district level.

Further structural reorganisation took place following the White Paper, *Working for patients* (DH, 1989). Its aim, discussed in more detail later in this chapter, was to create a quasi-market in healthcare. This represented a different approach to reform. Unlike the previous reorganisations, there was no organisational blueprint (Harrison and Wood, 1998). Instead, the government combined organisational changes with new processes and incentives, with the intention that a new system would emerge. NHS bodies became 'purchasers' or 'providers' of healthcare. Purchasers included district health authorities (DHAs) and fundholding GPs (who, along with the other independent contractor professions, were managed by family health services authorities [FHSAs], which had replaced FPCs). The providers were established as new self-governing NHS trusts, removed from direct health authority control, and promised greater freedom to manage their affairs. They would earn their income through service contracts negotiated with the purchasers.

The creation of GP fundholders and trusts was done in stages, so the NHS structure was not transformed overnight. However, their emergence created pressures for further structural changes. In the mid-1990s, DHAs – whose purchasing role was increasingly transferred to GPs – were reduced in number and eventually merged with FHSAs to form unitary health authorities. In addition, many trusts merged, as some were too small to survive in the new health service market. Meanwhile, the regional health authorities (RHAs), which had divested most of their service provider functions, were abolished and replaced with regional offices of the NHS Executive, staffed by civil servants.

New Labour brought further organisational changes. The division between purchasers (by this time more commonly known as commissioners) and providers of healthcare was retained, but the GP fundholding scheme was abolished. New local bodies, known as primary care groups (PCGs), were created from clusters of general practices. They operated under the auspices of health authorities, and had a range of functions including the planning and commissioning of health services. It was envisaged that PCGs would eventually become primary care trusts (PCTs), free-standing bodies that could also take on service provision roles.

The move from PCG to PCT was expected to be voluntary and dependent on the local context. However, in 2002, all PCGs were converted into PCTs as part of a programme of 'shifting the balance of power' in the NHS to the local level (see below). Unitary health authorities were abolished, and 28 strategic health authorities (SHAs) created. This was accompanied by a reduction in, and then abolition of, regional offices. In 2006 there was yet another restructuring. As a result, the number of SHAs fell to 10 (becoming, in effect, RHAs), and PCTs to 152.

A further organisational change was the creation of foundation trusts. Foundation status was initially only available to those trusts that had received the highest performance ratings (discussed later in this chapter). Foundation trusts were promised certain freedoms to manage their affairs (including the ability to retain surpluses, borrow, sell assets, enter into private partnerships and to reward staff). In reality, there were constraints on their autonomy. They were subject to an independent national regulator (called Monitor) that could intervene if they failed to perform, and had to comply with certain national standards and frameworks, for example, on service quality. Restrictions were imposed on their ability to generate revenue from private sources. Furthermore, they were accountable to the local community through governing boards partly elected by local people and patients.

The coalition government also embarked on a radical restructuring, despite a commitment that implied it would not do this (see Chapter Two). SHAs and PCTs were abolished. Commissioning was undertaken by local CCGs and by a new national body, NHS England. All trusts were expected to become foundation trusts. The new government also proposed greater competition from the private and voluntary sectors, more choice and voice for patients, and the transfer of major public health functions to local authorities (considered in depth in the next chapter).

Why reorganisation?

Governments find it difficult to resist reorganising the NHS (McLachlan, 1990; Edwards, 1993; Klein, 1995; Edwards and Fall, 2005; Edwards, 2010). Reorganisation is a useful tool for politicians, as it highly symbolic. It shifts attention to the administration and management of the service, and can be used to deflect criticism of central government policies. Politicians, however, fail to think through the implications of their grand plans. Brown's observation, that 'reorganisation is normally undertaken in a spirit of over-optimism about the net advantages', remains true today (Brown, 1979, p 200).

The pace of reorganisation increased from the early 1980s, and even more dramatically from 1997 onwards (Webster, 2002; Tallis, 2004). Indeed, observers have used the term 'redisorganisation' to describe the perpetual restructuring that undermines the ability of the NHS to improve (Smith et al, 2001; Tallis, 2004). Reorganisation can lead to loss of skills and knowledge that it is difficult, if not impossible, to replace. It can be distracting and disrupt relationships within the NHS and with other agencies, and can reduce staff morale. Moreover, it incurs financial costs (arising from redundancy and relocation of staff, for example).

Notably, the coalition government fought hard to avoid publishing the risks and costs of its NHS reorganisation. The official figure was eventually revealed as £1.7 billion (NAO, 2013a). Others have estimated the costs at a much higher level, £3 billion start-up costs and £4.5 billion recurrent annual costs (Paton, 2014). In addition, the reorganisation may have undermined the government's principal policy aims. According to an evaluation of the coalition's record, 'it seems likely that the massive organisational changes that resulted from the reforms contributed to widespread financial distress and failure to hit key targets for patient care' (Ham et al, 2015, p 22). This report also noted that one of the key changes, the abolition of SHAs, made it more difficult for government to shape local health systems in ways that could have improved efficiency and service quality. It also highlighted the damaging effects of the complexity of the new structures created, which it likened to 'a Heath Robinson construct'.

Reorganisation has now become so discredited that critics have called for a moratorium (Smith et al, 2001; Audit Commission and Healthcare Commission, 2008). There have also been calls for evidence of the benefits and costs of reorganisation, to enable systematic evaluation of proposed changes (Edwards, 2010; Walshe, 2010). Others have argued that if reorganisation is pursued, it should be smaller-scale, evidence-based and piloted (Tallis, 2004). Indeed, there is support for organic change that builds on the strengths of existing organisations (Health Committee, 2006a).

Priorities and planning

In the early years of the NHS, little consideration was given to how services might be planned in order to meet existing and future needs (Webster, 1996). There was, moreover, no desire to intervene, as the Ministry of Health was a relatively weak department with low strategic capacity (see Chapter Three). From the 1960s onwards, however, central government tried to exert more influence over the NHS. The focus was initially on inputs: manpower and resources. This led to the publication of the Hospital Plan in 1962, and a community health services plan the following year (Ministry of Health, 1962, 1963; Webster, 1996; Mohan, 2002).

In the 1970s, a new planning system was introduced for the reorganised NHS. The government issued a national priorities document (DHSS, 1976). Each health authority (at every level of the NHS structure) produced a plan, for consideration by higher tier authorities. The overarching idea was to plan services more rationally, and to shift resources accordingly into services that had hitherto been neglected (the so-called 'Cinderella services', such as services for elderly people, people with mental illness and people with disabilities). Even so, the planning process remained persuasive rather than directive, and the government's priorities encountered considerable resistance at local level.

The Thatcher government attempted to simplify the planning process. Local health authorities were issued with a general statement of priorities rather than detailed guidance (DHSS, 1981). However, as the decade unfolded, central guidance became more prescriptive. An annual priorities document was produced, which set goals and targets for specific services. Health authority plans were subject to closer scrutiny by regions, and their plans in turn by the DH. The increase in central planning stemmed from a desire to strengthen line management in the NHS, discussed further below. In the 1990s, a centralist approach was further encouraged by initiatives such as *The patient's charter* and the *Health of the Nation* strategy (see Chapter Two), which provided a basis for targets (on health service standards and public health respectively).

New Labour's approach to planning was similar to its Conservative predecessor, but went much further (DH, 1997, 2000). Plans were developed by local health authorities and PCGs (and later, PCTs). Strategic plans were formulated by higher tier authorities (NHS regional offices and SHAs), and local plans were expected to be consistent with them. Meanwhile, the DH continued to set out national priorities. In 2000 it produced an overarching and comprehensive NHS Plan (see Chapter Two), which set out a range of policy objectives and targets (including waiting time targets). These targets became progressively more extensive and challenging, culminating in an 18-week maximum waiting time for hospital treatment following GP referral. In the meantime, further documents outlined policies on choice (see DH, 2003), system reform (DH, 2005), public health (DH, 2004b) and healthcare outside hospitals (DH, 2006a), setting out details of further policy aims and objectives. In addition, a range of national service plans and frameworks were devised, including the NSFs mentioned in Chapter Two, and a revised cancer plan.

The setting of targets was a key feature of New Labour's style of governance. Targets were applied across government and public services, and were embedded in PSAs (see Chapter Three). The NHS, as a major public service, was given hundreds of targets. Despite periodic efforts to streamline them, new initiatives invariably led to more. Under Brown, and following the Darzi Review that he initiated, New Labour's target culture relaxed a little. PSA targets still existed, but local decision-makers (in the NHS and local government) could now select performance indicators from a menu. However, national NHS 'must-do's' (for example, targets on waiting times and healthcare infections) remained.

There is a great ambivalence towards targets. On the one hand, they are credited with successfully highlighting key priorities and strengthening accountability (Baggott, 2007; Crisp, 2011; Thorlby and Maybin, 2010). Targets, bolstered by performance management (discussed further below) appeared to galvanise the NHS in key areas, such as waiting times (Propper et al, 2010; Mays et al, 2011) and reducing hospital infections (or at least those initially targeted: C. difficile and MRSA) (NAO, 2009). New Labour's targets culture also coincided with rising levels of public satisfaction with the NHS and improvements in key health indicators (such as life expectancy), with significant reductions in smoking rates, suicide deaths, cancer mortality and heart disease deaths (Thorlby and Maybin, 2010). Less positively, health inequalities widened, and some public health problems deteriorated (notably obesity, and to some extent, alcohol problems) (Baggott, 2010a). The NHS was criticised for not doing enough to improve productivity, increase patient choice and 'voice' (see below and Chapter Eight), and move care from hospitals into community settings (Wanless, 2007; Audit Commission and Healthcare Commission, 2008; Thorlby and Maybin, 2008; Mays et al, 2011).

Targets also have disadvantages (Baggott, 2007). As Crisp (2011), Chief Executive of the NHS under New Labour, conceded, there were too many targets, and some were badly conceived. Targets were associated with increased bureaucracy, arising from monitoring processes (King's Fund, 2011). Further criticisms of targets related to their unintended consequences. There was concern about the unforeseen effects of targets, and the scope for dysfunctional or even fraudulent behaviour, in the wider public sector as well as the NHS (Audit Commission, 2003; Select Committee on Public Administration, 2003). Negative consequences in the NHS include 'gaming', the deliberate manipulation of data and even the distortion of clinical priorities (PAC, 2002; Mannion et al, 2005a; Smith, 2005; Bevan and Hood, 2006; Crisp, 2011; NAO, 2014b). There are cases where patients have been harmed by targets, following manipulation of waiting times by trusts (File on 4, 2012). For example, Accident and Emergency (A&E) admission targets have been blamed for a practice known as 'stacking' where patients are kept waiting in ambulances outside hospitals (Ungoed-Thomas and Summers,

2012). This is not only potentially harmful to patients, but also restricts the capacity of ambulance trusts to respond to emergencies.

The coalition government was committed to moving towards outcomes-based measures of performance, and pledged it would get rid of New Labour's targets. Although it introduced outcomes frameworks (for public health, healthcare and social care), and scrapped some targets, it retained others. For example, inpatient, outpatient and A&E waiting time targets remained, with some modifications. Moreover, despite the initial emphasis on local autonomy, the coalition continued to set national priorities (through the NHS mandate; see Chapter Three). Systems of performance monitoring have continued via NHS England. Furthermore, the Secretary of State has continued to take NHS organisations to task when targets have been missed (Ham et al, 2015). Indeed, the coalition continued to intervene in the NHS, and the DH maintained a strong focus on operational matters (Ipsos MORI, 2013; Greer et al, 2014a).

Box 7.1: NHS performance under the coalition

According to a comprehensive analysis by researchers from the King's Fund (Appleby et al, 2015a, see also Appleby et al, 2015b), NHS performance held up well on several indicators in the first three years of the coalition, and then began to slip. This appears to have been due to two key factors: the implementation of the coalition's reforms, which destabilised the NHS; and the financial context of small, in real terms, annual increases in funding, much lower than in the previous decade.

The key indicators were:

- Patients' satisfaction remained high and rose across most services (but there was some variation between trusts). Overall public satisfaction with the NHS fell between 2010 and 2011 (from 70 to 58 per cent), but then rose (to 65 per cent in 2014).
- A dramatic fall in C. difficile and MRSA infections (more than halved between May 2010 and May 2015).
- Total number of (full-time equivalent) NHS staff increased marginally (by 2 per cent) under the Coalition.
- Problems with access to mental health services persisted.
- Some improvements in efficiency measures. Productivity rose 1.6 per cent per annum during 2010–12 (compared with 0.6 per cent per annum between 1996 and 2009). However, productivity rose at a much lower rate in the following year (Bjoke, et al, 2015).
- Spending increased in real terms between 2010 and 2015 (0.8 per cent per annum), but by a much smaller rate than in the previous decade.

- In the 2014/15 financial year, the combined deficit of NHS Trusts and Foundation Trusts was over £820 million. CCGs in contrast held a collective surplus of £151 million
- The percentage of patients waiting longer than 18 weeks for hospital treatment increased from the winter of 2012/13. The inpatient target (90 per cent of patients seen in 18 weeks) was missed for most of 2014 and by May 2015, 11.8 per cent of patients waited longer than 18 weeks. The outpatient target (95 per cent seen in 18 weeks) was missed for a time in 2014 and in early 2015. However, this target was met in May 2015 (when only 4.4 per cent waited longer than 18 weeks). The other main target, that 92 per cent of patients still waiting for treatment should wait less than 18 weeks from referral to outpatient or inpatient treatment, was met from 2012 onwards (although the percentage waiting longer than 18 weeks rose from 2013 and stood at 6.5 per cent in May 2015). Notably, the Department of Health authorised a 'managed breach' of these targets in 2014, which along with additional resources, enabled a backlog of untreated patients to be cleared.
- The percentage of patients waiting more than four hours in A&E rose from 2 per cent to 8 per cent between April 2010 and April 2015 (the coalition lowered the A&E target from 98 to 95 per cent of patients to be seen within four hours). In addition, the target that 99 per cent of patients would receive the results of diagnostic tests within 6 weeks was missed for 18 months in a row up to May 2015.
- One of the key cancer targets (85 per cent of urgent referrals from GPs to start treatment within 62 days) was missed from the last quarter of 2013/14 to April 2015 (when 82.3 per cent of patients were treated within this period).
- After a period of stability, there was an increase in delayed transfers from hospital care from 2013 onwards.
- There was a dramatic fall in the number of patients in mixed-sex hospital accommodation (from 2,200 to 350 a month by January 2015).

Leadership and management

Plans and targets are irrelevant without mechanisms to manage performance. Until the 1980s, NHS managers played an important but low-key role, acting as 'diplomats', sorting out 'turf wars' between professional groups and clinical specialties (Harrison, 1988; Harrison et al, 1992). They tended to be reactive rather than strategic, accepted the status quo, and were deferential to the medical profession. Senior doctors controlled their own territory. Although they engaged in forms of clinical leadership (through mentoring, teaching and research activity, for example), they were reluctant to engage in strategic or line management. Moreover, the medical profession was powerful at the local level, and able to block implementation of central policies and plans.

The Griffiths Inquiry, appointed by the Thatcher government, found an absence of clear management responsibility in the NHS (DHSS, 1983). It recommended a separate management board for the NHS at national level. The NHS Executive was subsequently established, distinct from the wider DH (see Chapter Three). This institutional separation of policy and management was later abolished by the Blair government (only to be revived by the coalition – see below).

Griffiths recommended that general management should replace consensus management (a system established in the 1970s to promote collaborative working across the different professions on NHS management teams). In future, a general manager would account for the management performance of each health authority or service provider. Griffiths placed great faith in performance reviews at all levels of the NHS, and the NHS was subjected to closer scrutiny, with increased use of metrics and targets.

Griffiths' recommendations heralded a more business–oriented approach to the NHS. It emphasised corporate responsibility (of staff to their host organisation) and upward accountability (of NHS organisations to higher-level authorities). The role of health authority chairs was strengthened and health authorities were subsequently refashioned as 'corporate bodies' (with senior managers sitting on boards alongside 'non-executive directors' and strengthening the role of chairs). In the 1990s, NHS regional offices staffed by civil servants replaced RHAs, strengthening the position of the centre. The introduction of the internal market in the 1990s (see Chapter Two, and discussed further below), despite its decentralist ethos, actually strengthened line management. The freedom of NHS trusts was limited in practice by a regime of central monitoring, regulation and direction (Mohan, 1995; Hughes and Griffiths, 1999).

The Blair government reinforced this centralising trend (Ross and Tomaney, 2001; Edwards and Fall, 2005; Baggott, 2007). It introduced a host of national inspectorates and standard-setting bodies, discussed later in this chapter. Central government took on new powers (under the Health and Social Care Act 2001) to intervene in health authorities, PCTs and trusts. Like previous governments, ministers intervened in health authority and trust appointments to reduce resistance at local level (although the Blair government established an NHS Appointments Commission to insulate ministers from allegations of political interference; this was later abolished by the coalition).

Central interventions were bolstered by the plans and targets discussed earlier. Managers faced sanctions if they failed to meet key targets, such as those on finance and waiting times (which became known as 'P45 targets';

see Greener et al, 2014, p 58). Moreover, health authority chairs and non-executives were threatened with removal if they did not comply with central directives. This 'targets and terror' approach (Bevan and Hood, 2006) had some impact, notably on waiting times (see above). Nonetheless, disquiet about the centralisation of management began to grow. From 2000 onwards, a new approach was enunciated, emphasising 'localism' (Milburn, 2001; see also Stoker, 2004). This proposed 'earned autonomy' – lighter regulation for those complying with central objectives. This regime promised greater autonomy, additional resources and less intrusive inspection of NHS bodies that performed well under a rating system. The 'localist' approach was reflected in other policies, such as the creation of foundation hospitals. The government's policy was outlined further in subsequent policy documents, which proclaimed a desire to shift the balance of power towards frontline staff (DH, 2001, 2002). This theme was echoed in subsequent policy documents (see DH, 2003, 2004a, 2005).

Policy actors in this period welcomed efforts to decentralise and devolve NHS management, but were cynical about central government's actual intentions (Baggott, 2007). A number of studies found that earned autonomy did not yield the benefits promised (Hoque et al, 2004; Mannion et al, 2005b). Autonomy was restricted by central targets. Incentives associated with autonomy were not sufficiently powerful to promote improved performance. Moreover, it appears that SHAs played a key role in acting as a conduit for central government (Storey et al, 2010). Their leaders were closely connected to the DH, and their main task was to cascade central directives to local NHS organisations, although they did perform an advocacy function for their regions, and fed information up the food chain to central government.

Anecdotal evidence indicated that central government continued to intervene in the NHS, especially where the political stakes were high. For example, ministers intervened in decisions by PCTs about independent sector treatment centres (ISTCs), in some cases removing those who objected from their positions (Carvel, 2004). Other examples of central direction included forcing PCTs to hive off their provider services so that they became purely commissioning bodies.

Under Gordon Brown such interventions continued in spite of revived localism rhetoric. The Darzi Review emphasised the need for clinically led changes to local services informed by public consultation. There was also a more flexible approach to targets, outlined above. However, national priorities remained, and local decision-makers were under no illusion that they were expected to implement them. Two examples stand out. In 2007, Brown ordered a 'deep clean' of hospitals, despite there being no evidence that this would actually reduce hospital infections (BBC News, 2007). In addition, a programme of establishing new primary care centres was implemented in each PCT area between 2008 and 2010. PCTs had no choice but to implement this programme, even if they believed there was already sufficient local service capacity, and that funds could be better spent. Many of these centres have since closed (Monitor, 2013).

Even so, PCTs and other local actors were not necessarily powerless in the face of central directives. Jones et al (2013) reported a number of coping strategies that enabled local agents to respond to central policies (see also Alvarez-Rosete and Mays, 2008; Exworthy and Frosini, 2008; Storey et al, 2010; Mays et al, 2011). These offered room for manoeuvre and could dilute the impact of reforms. These strategies included prioritising the most pressing concern, relabelling existing initiatives and using new policies as a lever to realise local objectives (see also Dixon and Jones, 2011). Jones et al (2013) found that existing local relationships could also limit the impact of reform (in this particular case, the implementation of market-based reforms).

The variable impact of reform across priorities, conditions areas (for example, disease and service groups), and geographical areas during the New Labour era was noted by Powell et al (2011). They found that implementation was important, and that the context in which reforms were introduced could make a difference to the outcome. A related point is that the quality of governance varies in NHS organisations (Storey et al, 2011). This affects their ability to implement central government policies (and their response to other policy instruments, such as clinical guidelines and regulatory directives).

It has been noted that the implementation of health policy in the New Labour period was affected by the lack of a blueprint for reform, which articulated the case for reforms and explained how the different components interacted with each other (Cabinet Office, 2007; Audit Commission and Healthcare Commission, 2008; Storey et al, 2011). An overarching narrative eventually emerged, but this was a 'post-hoc' justification provided for ministers rather than a means of strengthening policy implementation (Dixon and Jones, 2011).

The picture of a completely top-down NHS under New Labour is therefore inaccurate (Alvarez-Rosete and Mays, 2008). It is also at odds with the creation of foundation trusts. These organisations were able to defy local PCTs, commissioners and service planners, and tended to act in their own self-interest rather than in the interests of the local health services as a whole (Storey et al, 2010; Allen et al, 2012; Allen and Jones, 2011). At one stage the chief executive of the NHS (David Nicholson) had to remind foundation trusts that they were still part of the NHS (Carvel, 2008). Nonetheless, the radical intentions behind this reform were not fully realised. The government's ambitious target for all NHS trusts to become foundation trusts by 2008 was not achieved (just over half of acute and mental health trusts had become foundation trusts by 2010). Furthermore, as noted earlier, they were constrained in their financial freedoms and by national standards. Their local legitimacy was also weak, given the low turnouts at governing board elections and the low percentage of the public who joined as members (Allen et al, 2012). Accountability to local people was tenuous, not only because of limited participation, but also as a result of the weakness of their governing bodies (Storey et al, 2010; Allen et al, 2012). Researchers also found that foundation status made little difference to performance (Verzulli et al, 2011).

The coalition government was strongly committed to localism and greater autonomy for NHS organisations (see **Box 7.2**). It also wanted all NHS trusts to become foundation trusts by 2014 (a deadline it had not achieved by March 2015, when only 60 per cent of trusts were foundation trusts). The coalition gave foundation trusts greater freedom to generate their own resources by raising the cap on private income to 49 per cent of their turnover. It sought to limit ministerial responsibilities and powers in relation to the NHS while creating a statutory NHS body – NHS England – to achieve central objectives for the NHS set by ministers, allocate resources to the NHS, oversee local commissioning and directly commission some services (primary care, specialised services and some public health services). The initial thinking behind the creation of NHS England was that it would be a small body that would be largely non-interventionist. However, changes made to the Health and Social Care Act during its passage through Parliament (see Chapters Three and Four) restored, to some extent, ministerial responsibilities that the coalition had hoped to reduce, and increased NHS England's responsibilities and powers (Ham et al, 2015).

In the period prior to the reforms being implemented (May 2010 to April 2013), the coalition initially adopted a centralised approach to ensure that the NHS met government priorities and efficiency targets, and to manage the transition to the new organisational structures and processes. The stated intention was that this would then give way to a less interventionist approach. However, the early signs were that central government was still keen to intervene. For example, the Secretary of State, Jeremy Hunt, personally contacted chief executives of hospital trusts about missing A&E waiting time targets (Campbell, 2013). Furthermore, the DH amended the NHS mandate only a year after it was first formulated (Dowler, 2013a). The chair of NHS England made clear his concern about the extent of central intervention (Boffey, 2013).

Box 7.2: Taking the NHS out of politics?

It is claimed that the priorities of the NHS are too heavily influenced by the government's desire to get re-elected, reflected in politically driven targets on waiting times. It is also believed that the ability of the NHS to provide services on a day-to-day basis is inhibited by central micro-management to minimise media and public criticism.

Concern about political interference inspired a range of proposals to give the NHS greater independence from central government (see, for example, King's Fund, 2002; NHS Alliance, 2002; Edwards, 2007; Dixon and Alvarez-Rosete, 2008). Although varying in detail, these involve giving the NHS some form of independence from politicians with ministers retaining a role in setting overall objectives but not allowed to interfere in day-to-day management.

The coalition government aimed to establish the NHS on a more independent basis. It created a national commissioning board (NHS England) at arm's length from ministers, to oversee NHS planning and commissioning. In theory, ministers and the DH would confine themselves to setting overall NHS priorities and allocating overall resources, although in practice they have intervened in operational matters.

The problem with a more independent NHS is that it could be removed from democratic pressures and reduce public accountability. A possible compromise is to simultaneously strengthen accountability by strengthening patient and public involvement (PPI). Another idea is to extend local authority powers of oversight and scrutiny, or perhaps hand them a commissioning role in relation to NHS services (Glasby et al, 2006).

Another problem is that, as the NHS is funded mainly out of national taxation, the government is accountable to Parliament for this expenditure and is compelled to intervene. The NHS is unavoidably politicised in other ways. It is a large employer, its services affect many people in a significant way, and it is a major institution in the country. As Douglas Black (1987, p 38) wrote, 'it is not possible, as some wish, to take the health service out of politics – both the amount of money involved and the sensitivity of anything to do with health will keep the health service a major political preoccupation.'

Regulation

According to Storey et al (2011), regulation came late to the NHS. Regulation of long-stay hospital services followed a series of scandals in the late 1960s (Robb, 1967; Butler and Drakeford, 2005). In addition, there were long-standing systems of self-regulation operated by professional bodies, such as the GMC, although these were increasingly regarded as ineffectual.

But not until the new millennium did a significant growth in healthcare regulation take place (Walshe, 2003).

In 2000, the Blair government created a new statutory body, the Commission for Health Improvement (CHI) (Day and Klein, 2004). It was given a general duty to promote healthcare improvement, and was responsible for ensuring that NHS provider organisations introduced 'clinical governance', a system of quality assurance (discussed later in this chapter). CHI monitored NHS performance against service standards, set out by national bodies such as NICE (whose role is discussed later), in NSFs (see above), and elsewhere (for example, guidance from professional bodies). It also investigated serious service failures, and was given additional powers to inspect NHS bodies and recommend closure or suspension of services.

CHI produced information on performance, and was responsible for a system of star ratings (3, 2, 1, or no stars). Higher-rated organisations were promised greater autonomy; the lowest faced detailed scrutiny and intervention. This system was later replaced by an 'annual health check', based on measures of organisational effectiveness in using financial resources and providing quality care. Healthcare organisations were monitored against explicit core standards covering patient safety, clinical effectiveness and public health and their performance against government targets.

In 2004, CHI was replaced by the Commission for Healthcare Audit and Inspection (CHAI), known as the Healthcare Commission. The Healthcare Commission was established as a statutory non-departmental public body accountable to Parliament as well as health ministers. It acquired functions from other bodies (including the Audit Commission's responsibility for value for money in the NHS), and was given overall responsibility for assessing the performance of NHS organisations, reporting on the state of healthcare, regulating the private healthcare sector and promoting improvements in healthcare provision.

Yet another round of organisational changes in 2009 saw the Healthcare Commission merged with the Commission for Social Care Inspection and the Mental Health Act Commission to create a single quality assurance body, the Care Quality Commission (CQC). The CQC became responsible for registering all health service and social care provider organisations. The registration system was based on essential standards of quality and safety. Another regulatory body, the National Patient Safety Agency (NPSA), was created following concerns about adverse incidents in healthcare, to introduce a new system of incident reporting and to give guidance on how to avoid such events. It has since been abolished and its work taken over by NHS England.

The creation of these various regulatory bodies was inspired by a series of scandals, including the poor standards of paediatric surgery at Bristol

Royal Infirmary (The Bristol Royal Infirmary Inquiry, 2001), illegal and unethical organ retention at Bristol and at Alder Hey Hospital, Liverpool (Royal Liverpool Children's Inquiry, 2001), the case of Harold Shipman, the GP found guilty of murdering his elderly patients (The Shipman Inquiry, 2001, 2004), and many other individual cases of negligence and malpractice.

Professional self-regulation was also reformed (Allsop and Saks, 2002; Irvine, 2003; DH, 2006b). The Blair government introduced changes to make it easier to amend legislation concerning professional self-regulation. It introduced the UK Council for Healthcare Regulatory Excellence (CHRE) to oversee (and in some circumstances, challenge) self-regulatory bodies, promote cooperation between them, and, where necessary, require them to make new rules. In 2012, this body became the Professional Standards Authority for Health and Social Care. Meanwhile, the self-regulatory bodies reviewed and strengthened their procedures for dealing with complaints and maintaining high standards of practice. The GMC, for example, acquired new powers to suspend doctors or impose restrictions on them with immediate effect. It also introduced a system of revalidation for doctors – to demonstrate their fitness to practise.

An important part of the New Labour government's regulatory approach was the setting of clinical standards through NSFs and the activities of NICE. NICE was established in 1999 to provide evidence on the cost-effectiveness of healthcare technologies and medicines, develop clinical guidelines and support clinical audit. It was also given the task of checking the safety and efficacy of new clinical procedures, and acquired responsibility for the evidence base in public health (changing its name to the National Institute for Health and Clinical Excellence). In 2002, it became mandatory for NHS organisations to follow NICE technology appraisal guidance, although implementation varied (Sheldon et al, 2004; Raftery, 2006). NICE was accused of changing guidance in response to political pressure from government, the drugs industry and patients' organisations (Ferner and McDowell, 2006). It faced criticism for lacking transparency, basing judgements on a limited range of evidence, taking too much time to evaluate new treatments, and limiting clinical freedom by inhibiting treatments that might work in particular individual circumstances (see Consumers' Association, 2001; Health Committee, 2001).

With the creation of foundation trusts, yet another regulatory body was born. To meet criticisms that these bodies might undermine the principles of the NHS, the government created a national regulator, accountable to Parliament and to health ministers. This regulator, known as Monitor, was constituted as a non-departmental public body. Monitor was given responsibility for authorising the framework for each foundation trust, including conditions on the range of services it provided, the level of income from private practice, restrictions on borrowing and asset sales. It also authorised initial financial plans and governance structures. Monitor was given powers to intervene where foundation trusts breached their authorisation, for example, if they incurred high financial deficits or provided inadequate services. Its role has changed somewhat in recent years, as discussed below.

Problems with New Labour's regulatory system

The regulatory regime developed by New Labour was overwhelmingly centralist, with a strong emphasis on national standards, frameworks and processes (Davies, 2000; Walshe, 2003). Although national frameworks are important to ensure consistency and minimum standards across the NHS, a 'top-down' approach can be counterproductive, particularly where it is associated with over-regulation – which was a common complaint during this period (Storey et al, 2011).

The independence of the new regulatory regime was not guaranteed. Ministers could and did intervene in regulation. Some bodies (notably Monitor and CQC) were given greater constitutional independence. However, even these could be 'leaned on'. In the case of CQC and its handling of a series of scandals in the late 2000s, it appears that at the very least there was over-sensitivity towards political considerations.

A further criticism was that the system was fragmented, as revealed subsequently by the Mid Staffs Inquiry (see **Box 7.3**). Clarification of the role of regulators, and improvement in communication between them, was needed (Thorlby and Maybin, 2010; National Advisory Group on the Safety of Patients in England, 2013). A related problem was that constant organisational change in the regulatory arena was confusing and made it difficult for regulators to do their job. For example, CQC, heavily criticised for not acting sooner on allegations of poor care standards, struggled to implement its new responsibilities against a background of organisational upheaval (NAO, 2011). In particular, CQC inspectors were diverted from compliance duties to the registration of health and care providers, as required by the new regulatory regime. The organisation experienced a 6 per cent cut in its budget despite having a wider remit.

New regulatory regimes introduced by New Labour imposed substantial costs on the NHS (NAO, 2003; Walshe, 2003). Over and above the combined budgets of the regulators were hidden costs of institutional compliance. Moreover, the benefits of regulation were questioned (Walshe, 2003; Benson et al, 2004; Day and Klein, 2004; Gray and Harrison, 2004; Bevan, 2008, 2011; Storey et al, 2011). In particular, doubts were raised about the capacity of regulators to engage with practitioners, and their ability to improve service standards. Some aspects of regulation, notably star ratings, did appear to have an impact on reported performance (Bevan, 2011), although it was found that the ratings did not correlate with hospital productivity (Stevens et al, 2006). There is weaker evidence about the impact of annual health checks and clinical governance reviews. However, proper reviews conducted with inspections and based on good data were adjudged superior to the lighter-touch regulatory regime that superseded it. The latter approach was based too much on 'tick box' self-reporting, which made it relatively easy to fool regulators, as the Mid Staffs and other scandals revealed (Storey et al, 2011).

Box 7.3: The Mid Staffordshire scandal

From 2005 onwards, serious concerns about standards at Stafford hospital were raised by patients and relatives, and the hospital was also found to have relatively high mortality rates. Further investigations revealed evidence of extremely poor care (for example, A&E patients being triaged by unqualified staff, patients on the wards unable to access food and drink, left in soiled bed clothes, dirty wards, and a general lack of attention to patients' privacy and dignity). The Labour government refused to hold a public inquiry (which has greater powers to collect evidence), a decision reversed by the coalition. The public inquiry (into the trust responsible for the hospital, the Mid Staffordshire NHS Foundation Trust) reported in 2013. It was chaired by Robert Francis QC (who had led an earlier inquiry into the trust).

The Francis Report (Mid Staffordshire Inquiry, 2013) found that the culture of the trust was flawed, focused on financial issues, central targets and management processes rather than patients. The trust was blind to the problems identified, and ignored evidence of poor standards of care. It gave false assurances to regulators. Staff who raised concerns were ostracised. The regulatory system failed, with too much emphasis on self-reporting and compliance with bureaucratic procedures, and not enough attention on patients' experience. The Francis Report also found that national and local regulatory, scrutiny and commissioning bodies did not communicate with each other and had failed to take timely action. Professionals failed to challenge the dominant culture. Reorganisations were also blamed for disrupting processes that might have otherwise prompted a more effective response.

Francis's recommendations included actions to:

- foster a common culture that puts patients first;
- develop clear fundamental standards that should not be breached (with criminal liability for breaches that lead to serious harm or death);
- provide professionally endorsed compliance systems based on evidence;

- ensure openness, transparency and candour (that is, truthfulness) throughout the system;
- make healthcare regulators relentless in ensuring compliance with standards;
- ensure all who provide, lead and manage care are accountable;
- guarantee that the public are protected from those who provide substandard care;
- ensure that the recruitment, education, training and support of those who lead, manage and provide care inculcate shared values;
- continually improve ways of measuring and understanding the performance of healthcare providers;
- ensure that regulation is coherent and that regulators work together.

Francis made 290 recommendations, including a ban on gagging clauses in staff contracts, a statutory duty of candour (to ensure that staff and care organisations are open and honest with patients when things go wrong), changes to nurse training, regulation to ensure compassionate care, legal penalties for those providing misleading information to regulators, better leadership training, a process for disbarring leaders and managers who fail to achieve standards of conduct, clear metrics on service quality and patient safety and more sharing of information among those who monitor services, and more powers for the CQC, strengthening its capacity to undertake inspections.

The government accepted most of the recommendations. One of the main areas of disagreement was that although the government agreed to a statutory duty of candour for NHS and social care organisations, it did not implement this for individual staff. It also refused to create a single health regulator (effectively, combining Monitor and CQC), as recommended by Francis. Another area of contention was the government's refusal to introduce statutory regulation of healthcare assistants.

The Francis Report also made recommendations about scrutiny and patient and public involvement, and these are considered further in Chapter Eight.

Coalition and regulation

The coalition's NHS reforms (see Chapters Two and Four) necessitated a new system of market regulation. Following the Health and Social Care Act, Monitor's role was extended from foundation trust regulator to NHS market regulator. For the time being, however, Monitor continues to oversee foundation trusts (another body, the NHS Trust Development Authority [NHSTDA], does a similar job with regard to the remaining NHS trusts). With regard to its role as market regulator, Monitor is required to prevent anti-competitive behaviour (including mergers), and has investigatory powers. It works alongside the Competition and Markets Authority, which has a broader role in enforcing competition law. Monitor also sets the prices of NHS services, and determines which providers are permitted to provide NHS-funded services through a licensing regime. It has duties to ensure that patient choice of provider is realised, that services are integrated for the benefit of patients, and has powers to deal with failing providers. Monitor is also expected to work more closely than before with other regulators (for example, CQC and NHS England).

CQC has also undergone significant changes, mainly in the light of the Mid Staffs public inquiry. CQC and Monitor have a duty to work together to minimise bureaucracy, communicate and share information, and operate an integrated system of licensing and registration. Quality of care is now acknowledged as a trigger for intervention (by Monitor and the NHSTDA), where trusts and foundation trusts are failing, and CQC now plays a greater role in this process. In addition, CQC was given greater statutory independence from government and greater powers to intervene. It was also restructured into divisions headed by chief inspectors for hospitals, primary care and social care. Inspectors are expected to be specialists in the area they are reviewing, and there is greater clinical input into the inspection process. Procedures have been overhauled, with more reliance on inspection visits and evidence about quality and safety, and less on self-reporting and 'tick box' assurance processes. The coalition also took a renewed interest in Ofsted-style rating systems, aggregate measures of quality that echo the 'star ratings' approach of New Labour, despite concerns that they are simplistic and place an unnecessary burden on providers (Nuffield Trust, 2013).

NICE was also reformed, although the initial signs were inauspicious. The coalition introduced a new cancer drugs fund for people unable to access treatments through their local commissioners, which was seen as bypassing NICE judgements, thereby undermining its authority. In addition, the government placed faith in a new system of value-based drug pricing (where drugs manufacturers are paid according to evidence of a drug's effectiveness and benefits), believing this would obviate the need for NICE recommendations to be mandatory. But value-based pricing was slow to develop. Later, the government changed its mind, and made it compulsory for NICE appraisals to be included in local formularies (lists of drugs approved or selected for use and summaries of evidence about their effectiveness). Furthermore, NICE was strengthened – in 2012 it became a statutory non-departmental public body with greater independence from government. In addition, the legal basis of its quality standards was reinforced, and its remit extended to include recommendations on social care standards (and its name changed to the National Institute of Health and Care Excellence).

It should be noted that the DH was not a spectator in these regulatory reforms. It played a major part in the design of regulatory systems, through commissioning inquiries and reviews into NHS problems and failures, and then proposing new structures and processes of regulation. It also directly intervened to identify NHS providers that were not delivering care of sufficient quality. For example, in February 2013 the Secretary of State for Health and the Prime Minister initiated a review of trusts with higher than average death rates. This was undertaken by the NHS medical director (Keogh, 2013), and led to 11 being placed in special measures. It was intended that the special measures regime would be extended to GPs and adult social care providers.

Financial mechanisms and incentives

Centralised funding

One feature of the NHS has always been centralised: its funding. Because the NHS is funded overwhelmingly out of general taxation, National Insurance contributions and centrally fixed charges, there is little scope for NHS organisations to develop independent sources of finance. Aside from supplementary income-generating activities (such as car parking charges, asset sales and income from private patients), as well as endowments and charitable donations (which can be substantial for some prestigious hospitals), the NHS is dependent on income from central government. As health ministers are accountable to Parliament for the vast majority of NHS expenditure, they will be expected to achieve value for money. This creates political pressures to centralise health policy (see **Box 7.2**).

The amount of money allocated to the NHS has risen considerably over the years. The percentage of GDP spent on the NHS in the UK rose from 3 per cent in 1949-50 to 8 per cent in 2010 (Baggott, 2004; ONS, 2013). It has since fallen to 7.3% (in 2013, calculated from ONS, 2015). The NHS also took a greater share of public spending (10 per cent in the 1950s and 1960s, rising to 18 per cent in 2013-14, Keynes and Tetlow, 2014). Governments have varied in their generosity towards the NHS. The annual growth rate of UK public spending on health (adjusted for general inflation) rose 3.6 per cent between 1950/51 and 1996/97. It was lower than this (3.3 per cent) in the Conservative era between 1979 and 1997. Under New Labour the average annual growth was much higher, at 5.7 per cent. Under the coalition it was much lower (0.8 per cent per annum) (Vizard and Obolenskaya, 2015). When interpreting these figures it should be acknowledged that in most years the rate of inflation for health services is higher than the general rate. Furthermore, annual growth rates must be considered against the demand for healthcare, which is driven by technological changes and demographic factors (for example, an ageing population). It is estimated that annual real growth of 1.2–1.5 per cent is required to keep pace with demographic pressures alone (Vizard and Obolenskaya, 2015).

Although the amount of central funding gives the government considerable leverage, it was not until the 1960s that it was used to drive centrally planned service developments. The Hospital Plan, referred to earlier, was the first major attempt to stimulate local service developments (through a capital funding programme, which fell short of expectations). This was followed by efforts to alter the allocation of resources during the late 1960s. In the 1970s, the RAWP (Resource Allocation Working Party) formula was introduced with the aim of gradually shifting resources from areas of the country that were over-funded relative to their population needs to under-funded areas. During this period resources were earmarked for under-funded services, particularly the 'Cinderella services' mentioned earlier. Efforts to allocate resources based on measures of need have since continued, with each government modifying the funding formula to suit its particular needs. Meanwhile, central 'earmarked funding' has been used by all governments to promote key initiatives (for example, to stimulate new service developments and to reduce waiting times).

Another aspect of funding policy that deserves a mention is efficiency measures. Successive governments have pressured the NHS to make efficiency savings. This has strengthened central control as local health bodies are given financial targets against which their performance is measured. As already noted, the coalition adopted a tough approach on overall NHS spending, which has forced organisations to look at ways of cutting costs. The coalition adopted a programme introduced by the New Labour government, which aimed to save between £15 billion and £20 billion in costs between 2011 and 2015. The programme (known as QIPP, Quality Innovation Productivity and Prevention) involved a range of measures and initiatives, including pay freezes, rationalising 'back office' functions, more effective purchasing and procurement processes, asset sales, and service reorganisation and redesign. Although productivity increased after 2010, and reported savings from the QIPP programme were substantial, doubts were cast on the accuracy of the efficiency saving estimates figures and the sustainability of cost savings in the longer term (NAO, 2012a; Appleby, 2015a; Bojke, et al, 2015).

Internal market and commissioning

As noted above, although the Conservatives' internal market (see Chapter Two) was heralded as creating powerful incentives for change, the reforms were carefully managed and regulated. Competition was limited, and the incentives to change were not as dramatic as envisaged (Le Grand et al, 1998; Mays et al, 2000; Brereton and Vasoodaven, 2010). However, the internal market did have some impact. First, there was evidence of entrepreneurialism among fundholding GPs (Ennew et al, 1998), although due in part to the early entrants to the scheme being more business-like in their outlook than the average GP. However, there is little evidence linking fundholding to outcomes (mixed evidence on impact of referral rates, costs and patient satisfaction; see Brereton and Vasoodaven, 2010). Second, there were indications of increased efficiency in the hospital sector (Maniadakis et al, 1999). Greater competition was associated with lower costs, although the evidence was not strong (Söderlund, et al, 1997). Third, there was evidence of inequities arising from the reforms, notably differential access to hospital services between the patients of fundholders and non-fundholding GPs (Kammerling and Kinnear, 1996; Dowling, 1997; Propper et al, 2002). Fourth, although the impact of the market on quality of care was difficult to ascertain, some found that hospital competition might have had a detrimental effect (Propper et al, 2008).

As mentioned earlier, the Blair government abolished the Conservatives' internal market but retained the division between commissioners and providers of healthcare. GP fundholding ended and fundholders and non-fundholders were corralled into new local commissioning bodies, PCGs, and then subsequently into PCTs. Under the Shifting the Balance of Power initiative, PCTs acquired responsibility for over three-quarters of the NHS budget. In addition, a number of initiatives sought to strengthen commissioning. A weaker version of GP fundholding, known as practice-based commissioning (PBC), was introduced. This voluntary scheme allocated virtual budgets to GP practices to commission services. Patient choice was extended by allowing NHS patients to choose from a menu of potential secondary service providers, including the private sector. A programme to improve the standard of commissioning (World class commissioning) was also introduced.

Despite these efforts, commissioning remained weak and underdeveloped (Audit Commission and Healthcare Commission, 2008; Brereton and Vasoodaven, 2010; Health Committee, 2010; Thorlby and Maybin, 2010; Mays et al, 2011; Vize, 2013; Greener et al, 2014). PCTs were undermined by constant reorganisation (see above). Their discretion was limited by a range of factors, including the requirement to attain government targets. Politically, it proved extremely difficult for PCTs to dramatically alter funding flows to the acute and specialist providers (Deeming, 2004). They lacked capacity to commission services effectively, particularly key management and commissioning skills. Despite some improvements (arising chiefly from World class commissioning; Mays et al, 2011; NHS Confederation, 2013), capacity problems remained. PCTs were seen as lacking legitimacy, clinical engagement, public involvement and public accountability. They were weak relative to service providers, especially foundation trusts. Practice-based commissioning, meanwhile, was poorly developed and had little impact on efficiency or service improvement (Curry et al, 2008). Meanwhile patient choice of secondary providers increased, but fell short of expectations and varied geographically (Audit Commission and Healthcare Commission, 2008; Brereton and Vasoodaven, 2010). Nonetheless, in conjunction with competition and a new system of payment for care (discussed below), it may have had some limited impact on productivity and waiting times (Brereton and Vasoodaven, 2010; Dixon and Robertson, 2011).

Central government was blamed for introducing conflicting and contradictory policies, and for limiting the discretion of PCTs in practice, as well as destabilising them with constant reorganisation. However, others have suggested that the failures of commissioning in this period may be due more to the lack of fit between commissioning and NHS institutional features (Checkland et al, 2012a). They argue that commissioning was not embedded in social and institutional structures, which regarded it as alien, and that this inhibited its development.

Supply-side changes and payment by results

The New Labour governments embarked on a journey that would take policy back to the system inherited from the Conservatives (see Chapter Two). They introduced supply-side reforms, such as independent sector treatment centres (ISTCs), the franchising of NHS management (both discussed further in Chapter Eight) and foundation trusts (see above). Together, these reforms represented a significant change, although for some, nothing less than a redefinition of the NHS (Pollock, 2004).

A new system, called 'payment by results' (PBR), was launched in 2003/04 to reimburse providers for individual treatments supplied, based on the standard cost of a group of procedures (known as a 'tariff'). Trusts could no longer rely on large-scale 'block' agreements to generate income, but would have to 'sell' their services to PCTs, GPs and their patients. Reform was introduced gradually, until over 50 per cent of spending on acute hospital services and a third of NHS spending overall was covered by the scheme (Appleby et al, 2012).

PBR has been associated with reductions in costs and lengths of stay in hospital, which suggests greater efficiency (Farrar et al, 2006; Brereton and Vassodaven et al, 2010). However, it has been criticised on several grounds (Mays et al, 2011; Health Committee, 2011b; Appleby et al, 2012). It is branded as inflexible and unable to facilitate better health outcomes and greater efficiency. In particular, it is believed to encourage over-treatment in hospital settings (as hospitals are usually rewarded for undertaking more complex or increased activity). It has been criticised for increasing administrative and transaction costs (Audit Commission, 2005; Mannion et al 2006), which can offset any efficiency gains made. A more general point is that the inflexibilities of the PBR system may have inhibited PCTs from using commissioning to shift services out of hospitals into the community (although some PCTs did switch away from the national tariff to adopt local solutions to try and align resources to the development of new services). It is also blamed for inhibiting preventive interventions and integrated care.

Changes to PBR and additional schemes to reward quality, innovation and best practice were introduced in the last years of New Labour, inspired to some extent by the Darzi Review, which called for payments to be more closely linked to quality (DH, 2008; Appleby et al, 2012). These included CQUIN (Commissioning for Quality and Innovation), which enabled trusts to earn more income by achieving quality standards and improvements, best practice tariffs (to reward services that met best practice standards) and innovation payments (to fund new treatments and technologies). Evaluations of these various schemes suggest that they have not always achieved their intentions, and that their impact has been mixed (see, for example, McDonald et al, 2013).

The New Labour government placed great faith in competition as a means of improving health services. Evidence of the impact of its reforms is, however, contentious (for a discussion, see Brereton and Vassodaven, 2010; Mays et al, 2011; Greener et al, 2014). Some studies (Cooper et al, 2011; Gaynor et al, 2011; Bloom et al, 2014) suggest that greater competition in the hospital sector is associated with greater reductions in death rates, better management and increased productivity. These findings have been challenged on grounds that researchers have confused association with causation, and that they adopted a measure of quality (death rates) that is too crude (Pollock et al, 2011b). Another criticism is that the researchers failed to adequately explain exactly how competition produces improvements in quality (Bevan and Skellern, 2011). A further point is that positive outcomes may have arisen from other policies introduced at the same time (for example, increased funding, patient choice, regulatory changes and so on), and from improvements in clinical practice unrelated to competition.

The New Labour era also saw the use of incentives in other areas of health policy, notably primary care. GPs were given new incentives in the form of the quality and outcomes framework (QOF) introduced in 2004. QOF built on previous efforts to incentivise GPs, including payments to meet targets for vaccination and screening. Practices were awarded payments based on indicators of clinical and organisational performance. Researchers found that the impact of the scheme was mixed (Doran et al, 2008, 2014; Dixon et al, 2011; Greener et al, 2014). Although improvements occurred, as reflected in the achievement of targets, they may have happened anyway. There was evidence that areas not subject to additional payments were neglected (Doran et al, 2008). QOF did not improve public health outcomes (Guthrie et al, 2007; Dixon et al, 2011), although it did not increase health inequalities, as some feared (Ashworth et al, 2008; Doran et al, 2008). The coalition government reformed QOF. Under the new GP contract announced in 2013, 40 per cent of QOF funding was redirected. Most has been allocated to core GP funding, and the remainder to the management of vulnerable patients, especially those who are at high risk of being admitted to hospital.

Coalition changes to the NHS market

As already noted, the coalition initiated radical plans to extend commissioning, competition and choice in the NHS (see Chapter Two). Although these plans were amended during the legislative process (see Chapter Four), they nonetheless represented a major reform. The then chief executive of the NHS, Sir David Nicholson, said that the reform programme was so big 'you could probably see it from space' (cited by Greer et al, 2014a, p 3).

At national level, NHS England has important commissioning functions with regard to primary care, specialised services and some public health services. In these areas, commissioning is centralised, and in some respects, more so than under New Labour (although at the time of writing there are plans to give CCGs a role in primary care commissioning). NHS England also oversees local commissioning, and this gives it considerable leverage over CCGs. NHS England has regional and local offices which liaise with CCGs. Commentators have noted that NHS England has the potential to play a strong performance management role, and that its subnational structure recreates some former SHA/PCT functions (Gregory et al, 2012).

Meanwhile, the CCGs engage in needs assessment (with the health and wellbeing boards on which they are represented), develop plans and commission services for the local population for which they have responsibility. They are aided by commissioning support units, which provide a range of services including support for strategic development, financial analysis and contract management.

It is too early to assess the impact of the coalition's reforms as the system is still evolving. Research by Checkland et al (2012b) found there were considerable uncertainties in commissioning. In particular, it remained unclear how CCGs would resolve the need to be accountable upwards to NHS England and downwards to the public and member practices. Other issues included conflicts of interest in decision-making (see also Iacobucci,

2013) and the composition of CCG governing bodies. This research also found concerns about the capacity and capability of commissioning support units. Meanwhile, national policies are encouraging CCGs to adopt more local solutions and to experiment with new ways of paying for care, which involves moving away from a national tariff. But at the same time, CCGs are being pressed to meet national objectives that require closer collaboration with other bodies such as local government and the voluntary sector on issues including public health and integrated care (see Chapter Eight). In addition, there has been concern about central contracts for specialised services. These have been blamed for undermining patients' and clinicians' preferences regarding treatment, and for disrupting access to and continuity of care (File on 4, 2013). A more general problem is that commissioning is now highly fragmented between different organisations, and this could jeopardise effective care, particularly for patients needing several different treatments and services (Ham et al, 2015).

The coalition, like New Labour, placed great emphasis on competition, including encouraging the independent sector to compete with the NHS (discussed in Chapter Eight). As noted, Monitor's new role is to oversee the NHS 'market' and to tackle anti-competitive behaviour deemed not in the public interest. It also has a duty to promote integrated care. There are significant tensions between these roles. The anti-competitiveness rules have led to some merger plans being blocked (see, for example, Calkin, 2013). This also led to conflict between the various regulators (NHS England, Monitor and the Competition and Markets Authority) that have different perspectives on the role of mergers in promoting efficient and high-quality services. NHS England, for example, has warned that Monitor's fair competition rules could jeopardise services (Dowler, 2013b).

The coalition government initially placed even greater emphasis on choice, as a means of making the NHS and other health service providers more responsive to patients, and to stimulate competition. It pledged to extend choice for patients, including choice of a named consultant, of providers and GPs (Gregory et al, 2012). However, following Andrew Lansley's replacement as Secretary of State by Jeremy Hunt, the emphasis on choice waned.

There is little evidence that the coalition's focus on competition produced improvements in NHS performance (Gregory et al, 2012; Ham et al, 2015). This is perhaps not surprising given that the coalition's reforms did not come into operation until 2013 (although it did implement its predecessor's plans to allow more competition for NHS services from alternative providers under existing rules; see Chapter Eight). However, the balance of the evidence from previous efforts to introduce market reforms is that the coalition's policies were unlikely to bring about improvements in the quality of services or health outcomes. Indeed, they may have jeopardised both. In addition, market reforms are highly unlikely to achieve the level of efficiency gains needed, and may, in fact, lead to greater inefficiencies and waste (Allen, 2013; Paton, 2014).

Culture and networks

The health policy literature has focused on the top-down approach to policy-making. However, it is acknowledged that simply issuing directives from the centre, channelled via regional and local management, does not necessarily produce good policy outcomes and may even be counterproductive. In contrast, the literature on health service quality and safety emphasises the importance of organisational culture in producing better outcomes. The lessons of this work are somewhat uncomfortable for those who adhere to a top-down approach. Although central authority has an important role to play by setting a clear policy, standards and regulatory framework, the organisations commissioning and delivering care, and the people who work within them, are crucial to achieving improvements in safety and quality. The key messages from this research are that good governance is linked to performance, as indicated by better patient experience, higher quality ratings, lower mortality, fewer adverse clinical incidents, higher staff morale and less absenteeism (Mannion et al, 2005b; Storey et al, 2010, 2011; King's Fund, 2011, 2012; Chambers et al, 2011; NHSIII, 2011). Good governance incorporates a range of features, including decision-making based on good quality and timely information about processes and outcomes; transparency and accountability; an effective system of quality control and assurance; good quality input from non-executive directors; and clinical engagement. Organisations that perform well tend to have an inclusive style of leadership based on shared values that builds commitment among staff and stakeholders. This contrasts with the 'heroic' model of leadership, focused on individuals imposing change while pursuing performance targets as ends in themselves (King's Fund, 2011).

Concerns about the culture of NHS organisations were raised by revelations of poor quality and unsafe care at a number of hospital trusts from the mid-2000s onwards. The main focus was on the Mid Staffordshire NHS Foundation Trust, which eventually became the subject of a public inquiry (the Francis Inquiry; see **Box 7.3**). The Francis Inquiry linked the problems of the trust to its culture, and in particular to poor leadership, governance and management. The key lessons for the wider NHS were that more must be done to improve the culture of patient care, openness and transparency, clinical engagement, and leadership and management. These points were echoed by a further report commissioned by the DH (National Advisory Group on the Safety of Patients in England, 2013), the Berwick

Review, which made similar observations, and emphasised the importance of developing a learning culture in the NHS.

Openness and transparency

Most observers agree that in the past it was too easy to cover up management incompetence, clinical errors and poor care standards in the NHS. When such matters do come to light this tends to be as a result of courageous individuals ('whistleblowing' staff, patients and relatives) combined with investigative journalism and high-profile campaigns for official inquiries. This leads to political pressure, and if strong enough, government action.

The Mid Staffs scandal led to calls for new statutory duties on openness and transparency in the NHS. The government responded with new measures (see **Box 7.3**) including, following a recommendation from the Berwick Review, a new offence of wilful neglect and mistreatment (applying to formal healthcare and adult social care providers). CQC was reformed and strengthened. In addition, greater protection for whistleblowers was introduced (clarifying guidance on gagging clauses, extending the legal rights of whistleblowers to more categories of staff, and giving additional protection to those harassed by colleagues).

Clinical engagement

Doctors (and to some extent other professional groups as well) have long been able to resist initiatives, through direct opposition and by lack of cooperation with local managers (see Harrison et al, 1992; Harrison and Pollitt, 1994; Ferlie et al, 1996; McNulty and Ferlie, 2002). Doctors are notoriously difficult to manage, and have a high degree of autonomy, especially in technical matters (Fitzgerald and Dufour, 1997; Dopson and Fitzgerald, 2006). Despite attempts to regulate medical work more closely, implementation has been poor. The NAO (2013b) found that only 56 per cent of trusts aligned individual and trust objectives in all or most of their consultants' job plans. In addition, doctors dislike taking on management responsibilities, which they traditionally regard as low status. As a result, medical leadership and management is variable and underdeveloped, despite various efforts over the years to engage doctors in management (King's Fund, 2011; Dickinson et al, 2013a).

In recent years there has been a reiteration of the importance of engaging doctors and other clinicians in the management of healthcare organisations (Storey et al, 2010, 2011; King's Fund, 2013). The Darzi Review identified clinical input as vital to shaping the future organisation of health services and improving quality and safety (DH, 2008). It urged that clinical leadership be strengthened, and that clinicians should be more involved in service improvement and change. It concluded that quality should be the driver of the NHS, and recommended quality boards and medical directors at regional and national level to facilitate this. It also recommended clearer standards (set by NICE and overseen by a national quality board) and more public information about the quality of care (in the form of quality accounts published by healthcare providers).

Darzi also supported giving more responsibility and control to clinicians over the commissioning process. GP involvement in commissioning was part of the reforms such as of GP fundholding and PBC, and a key element of the coalition's reforms. Nonetheless, there have been concerns about the lack of specialist clinical input into commissioning. In response to this, clinical senates (comprising clinical experts to advise CCGs on commissioning) were established to accompany the coalition's reforms. In addition, CCG boards were required to include a hospital consultant and a nurse, and strategic clinical networks were established in each region to advise on specific issues relating to the organisation of care of particular groups of patients (for example, people with cancer). Even so, it should be noted that neither strategic clinical networks nor clinical senates have any statutory powers.

Over the years government have promoted systems of assurance and encouraged professions to audit clinical work. For example, the Blair government introduced clinical governance (Gray and Harrison, 2004). This involved establishing clearer lines of responsibility for care; a comprehensive programme of quality improvement; procedures for identifying and remedying poor performance; clear policies for identifying and minimising risk; and appropriate institutional arrangements within each trust. Some benefits arose from this. It was credited with getting providers to think about how to improve care. Clinical quality issues became more mainstream, and accountability for performance became more explicit as a result (Leatherman and Sutherland, 2003; NAO, 2003; Bevan, 2008). However, the system was expensive to operate, and covered both strong and weak performers alike. There was evidence of poor implementation of policies and variations between trusts and departments within the same trust. Failure in communication and learning both between and across organisations was found. It was also pointed out that the impact of clinical governance was limited to the 'top-down' and bureaucratic approach of inspections introduced by government that emphasised surveillance and compliance (see contributions in Gray and Harrison, 2004).

From this perspective, more can be achieved by a less punitive approach involving high-trust relationships with professions, involving them more closely in improving quality and standards (Leatherman and Sutherland, 2003; National Advisory Group on the Safety of Patients in England, 2013;

Ham et al, 2015). This approach emphasises the importance of informal and cultural aspects of professional work, and the need to create conditions to encourage self-improvement within the professions.

Learning organisations

Other initiatives placed greater emphasis on cultural change and collaboration. In the Blair era, 'NHS beacons' – examples of innovative practice – were publicised to spread good practice. Collaborative networks (Bate, 2000; Addicott et al, 2006) were established to challenge existing ways of delivering services. They formed part of national programmes connected to service plans and frameworks (such as the cancer plan, for example). These initiatives also emphasised the importance of involving local clinicians and other stakeholders (including social services and patients).

One of the key aims following on from the Francis and the Berwick reports is that much more needs to be done to improve lesson learning and the transfer of good and best practice within the NHS. This does not happen by chance, but can be facilitated by open, high trust and well-managed organisations. It is also essential that information systems enable learning, and that staff are not prevented from raising ideas, problems and potential solutions. Training is important here, as it can instil common values that support learning.

Codes and guidance

Various frameworks of conduct and practice underpin the culture of the NHS. These include codes of conduct for members of NHS governing bodies and practice guidance for various professional groups, formulated by regulators and professional bodies. An example is the GMC's guidance for doctors, *Good medical practice* (GMC, 2013) that sets out what is expected of doctors with regard to knowledge, skills, performance, safety, quality, maintaining trust, communication and working with others. The NHS Constitution, which sets out what staff, patients and the public can expect from the NHS, is another example of a framework aimed at influencing behaviour (DH, 2015).

Such frameworks are important because they set out a consensus on what should be happening, but their value in improving the quality and standards of management and practice is difficult to assess. They tend to lack teeth. Even so, they can be given greater force, for example, when reinforced by employment contracts, or where a breach of standards may be used as evidence of professional misconduct.

Conclusion

Most commentators agree that the longer-term trend has been the centralisation of key elements of policy and the increasing use of 'command and control' in policy implementation (Greer et al, 2014a; Greener et al, 2014). Other ways of improving policy implementation have been recognised, notably organisational learning, trust building and cultural approaches. However, these have been secondary to the top-down bureaucratic model. Meanwhile, there has been a clear attempt to pass responsibility down the structure of the NHS, by seeking to divide policy from management. While there may be good reasons for devolving responsibility – especially where power is also devolved – the persistence of command and control means that this has largely been an exercise in shifting blame away from central government to the local NHS.

As we have seen, governments have resorted to reorganisation as a tool for strengthening their grip on implementation. This has proved counterproductive, inhibiting the ability of the NHS to respond effectively to future challenges. Some have called for an end to root-and-branch reorganisation. A more measured approach would be to allow reorganisation where there is a proven case, and where evidence supports this (Greener et al, 2014).

Summary

- Central government has centralised many aspects of health policy, and this process has increased markedly in the past 20 years. Centralisation has been accompanied by a process of decentralising responsibility to the local level of the NHS.
- The NHS has undergone many reorganisations. Such constant reorganisation can be counterproductive and costly.
- Central government has taken a more active role in setting plans and targets for the NHS in recent decades. Although planning is regarded as important, crude targets are seen as counterproductive.
- Management reform has been an important feature of the NHS since the 1970s. Managers are regarded as key players in implementing government policies.
- There has been a large increase in regulation and inspection in the NHS, reflected in the creation of new regulatory bodies. There have also been efforts to strengthen self-regulation by the professional bodies.
- The medical profession remains powerful within the NHS.
- Improvements in the NHS depend, to a large extent, on cultural changes within the professions and in healthcare institutions.

- There have been calls to take the NHS out of politics, but these ignore the fact that the NHS is highly politicised due to its funding and organisation, and the prominence of health on the political agenda.

Key questions

1. Why has the NHS been reorganised so often?
2. Can the NHS be taken out of politics?
3. How important is cultural change to the implementation of policies? How can cultural change be promoted within the NHS?
4. Has the NHS become more centralised? If so, in what sense?
5. Name the key regulatory bodies in health services, and specify their particular functions.

eight

Partnerships and health policy

Overview

This chapter explores the role of other organisations and stakeholders involved in the implementation of health policy. It discusses key players and their involvement in health and care provision: local government, the private sector, the voluntary sector, and communities and citizens. It also focuses on partnership working and efforts to improve collaboration in this field.

Health policy is not a matter for the NHS alone. The implementation of health policies depends heavily on other organisations that provide health and social care services, support people with health problems, and promote health and wellbeing. These include local authorities, the private sector and voluntary organisations. This chapter examines the need to form effective partnerships with these organisations (see Chapter One). It also examines the role of patients and the public in health policy and implementation.

Local government and health

Historically, local government played a major role in the improvement of health and the provision of healthcare and related services (Snape, 2003; Baggott, 2010a). When the NHS was created, local councils ceded their hospital services but retained other health service responsibilities including ambulance services, school health services, home nursing and other community and public health services. Local authorities also kept their role in funding and providing social care. However, the interface between local authority social care and the NHS was, and has remained, problematic (Glendinning et al, 2005; Health Committee, 2012; Wistow, 2013). This led to poor coordination of services for those with multiple needs (including children, elderly people, people with mental illness, those with learning disabilities and people with long-term conditions).

There were regular calls for better working arrangements between local authorities and the NHS. These included recommendations to transfer health services to local government (Committee of Inquiry into the Cost of the National Health Service, 1956; Royal Commission on Local Government in England, 1969a, 1969b). Governments rejected these ideas and opted instead for reorganisation in 1974. Local government health responsibilities were transferred to the NHS, leaving local authorities with responsibility for social services and environmental health. The reorganisation was meant to address problems of collaboration, particularly between hospitals, primary care and community health services. However, it reinforced existing divisions between social services and health services. New planning arrangements (in the form of joint consultative committees and planning teams) and financial incentives (a system of joint finance) were introduced to support NHS/local government collaborative ventures. These were widely regarded as unsuccessful.

Although the main focus of concern was on the relationship between social services and health services, the interface between the NHS and local government on public health matters was also poor. Despite official policy documents calling for closer cooperation between these bodies to prevent illness and to promote health (DHSS, 1981; DH, 1987, 1992), little was done to ensure this.

New Labour and partnership working

Efforts to strengthen partnership working in health in the last two decades must be seen in the context of structures and processes introduced by New Labour to enhance the leadership role of local government. They were also linked to new joint working arrangements overseen by central government as a means of achieving key national targets, set out in public service agreements (PSAs).

New Labour endorsed the idea of local authorities as community leaders and 'place shapers' rather than simply service providers (Department of Communities and Local Government, 2006). Local authorities (particularly the county councils, single-tier or 'unitary' authorities and the London boroughs) were expected to lead local partnerships of other public sector agencies and private and voluntary organisations. Overarching partnership bodies, local strategic partnerships (LSPs), were established under the leadership of local authorities in England, while similar bodies were created in other parts of the UK. LSPs were charged with formulating sustainable community plans and developing local area agreements (LAAs), which set out goals and targets. Local authorities were also expected to have a leading role in comprehensive area assessment (CAA), introduced in 2009. Under CAA, the performance of local public services in a particular area was measured in the round, with a greater focus on outcomes achieved and future improvement. This approach was taken further by other initiatives, including a pilot project, Total Place, which enabled local areas to explore new ways of addressing specific problems by bringing together different agencies and funding streams.

Local authorities also acquired new powers to promote or improve the economic, social and environmental wellbeing of their communities. Some acquired additional responsibilities, such as health scrutiny (see **Box 8.1**).

Box 8.1: Local health scrutiny

Health scrutiny was introduced in 2003 (Coleman and Glendinning, 2004). Local authorities with social services responsibilities were required to establish health overview and scrutiny committees (HOSCs) to scrutinise the planning, provision and operation of health services. HOSCs, consisting of councillors and co-optees, were given two main functions: to undertake reviews of local health issues and healthcare services and to make recommendations; and to be consulted on substantial changes in NHS services (referring such matters to the Secretary of State for Health if dissatisfied).

Although welcomed as an addition to existing local authority scrutiny functions, a number of shortcomings have been identified. These include a lack of relevant technical knowledge in health, limited powers, and insufficient support and resources for their role (Johnson et al, 2007; Boyd and Coleman, 2011). Health scrutiny did not provide a strong mechanism for holding the NHS to account (LGA Health Commission, 2008; Mid Staffordshire Inquiry, 2013). Moreover, HOSCs have not always interacted effectively with other agencies that can highlight problems (for example, PPI bodies – see below). Although HOSCs have had little influence in changing NHS plans and services, and have been fairly weak in securing accountability, they have at least opened the NHS to external perspectives. HOSCs have often taken a broader perspective on health, exploring public health and wellbeing issues such as obesity, alcohol, abuse, teenage pregnancy and health inequalities, and raising the profile of these issues on local agendas. They have also explored cross-cutting issues across the NHS, social care and public health, strengthening the case for collaboration.

The health scrutiny functions of councils were revised by the coalition government. The scrutiny function was conferred on the authority as a whole, giving it greater flexibility in determining arrangements. Councils may retain HOSCs or adopt a different approach, such as delegation to other committees. Indeed, many councils operate scrutiny committees that cover health as part of a wider thematic policy remit (such as 'health and wellbeing' or 'health and adult care'). Their scrutiny powers were extended to all NHS-funded services, including independent providers of primary care, social care and hospital care, as well as local authority public health services. Moreover, commissioning bodies, such as NHS England and CCGs, and the new health and wellbeing boards, come within the scope of local health scrutiny.

Powers and procedures relating to the scrutiny of substantial changes in NHS services were also amended. NHS bodies were required to establish clear timescales for consultation, notifying health scrutiny bodies and the public. Circumstances when normal consultation procedures would not apply were clarified. The power of referral to the Secretary of State was vested in the council as a whole (although it can delegate this power). The new process also placed a greater onus on all parties to make reasonable efforts to reach agreement on changes.

Under New Labour, policies placed greater emphasis on partnership and collaboration in health and care (see DH, 1997, 2000, 2006a). Organisational changes aimed to improve the relationship between health services and local government. The creation of PCGs (and later, PCTs) was expected to produce closer ties with local government. Local authorities were represented on these organisations. From 2006, most PCTs were coterminous with upper tier local authorities (those with social services responsibilities), which, it was believed, would improve collaboration. PCTs acquired key public health leadership roles and were expected to work closely with local authorities on health improvement as well as social care. In addition, local authorities were given a greater role in NHS planning. Initially, they were required to participate in the formulation of local health improvement plans. In 2007, local authorities and PCTs were given joint responsibilities to produce a joint strategic needs assessment (JSNA) for their area. The government also encouraged joint appointments for senior posts (for example, local directors of public health) and joint commissioning by PCTs and local authorities.

Public health

The Blair and Brown governments saw local authorities as crucial to the public health agenda, including the reduction of health inequalities (DH, 1999b, 2004b, 2006a). They introduced initiatives that sought to strengthen partnership working in this field (see Baggott, 2013). These included: Health Action Zones (HAZs), which brought local agencies together to tackle specific health problems in areas of high need (Judge and Bauld, 2007); regeneration programmes (for example, Neighbourhood Renewal Programmes); and other community-based programmes (for example, Sure Start, which sought to improve the health and wellbeing of pre-school children). In addition, the DH funded a range of collaborative health promotion initiatives on issues such as smoking cessation, sexual health, alcohol misuse and obesity (for example, the Communities for Health programme).

It is difficult to assess the impact of these various programmes because of the large number of initiatives, the presence of organisational and procedural changes, and the poor quality of evaluation (Health Committee, 2009; Hunter and Perkins, 2014). There does appear to have been some improvement in partnership working overall, although much variation between areas persisted (see Audit Commission, 2009a; Healthcare Commission and Audit Commission, 2008; Hunter and Perkins, 2014). In terms of outcomes, however, a systematic review found no evidence that partnerships improved health, reduced disease or narrowed health inequalities (Hunter et al, 2011).

Social care

The health and social care interface was a major preoccupation of the New Labour government. Specific guidance on health and social care collaboration was issued (DH, 1998b) alongside joint national priorities (DH, 1998c). In addition, the Health Act 1999 established a new statutory framework that reiterated duties of cooperation on health and welfare for NHS bodies and local government. This Act also enabled the NHS and local government to pool budgets, transfer funds and delegate commissioning and provider functions to each other. The system of joint consultative committees and planning teams was abolished. Joint work on health and social care was also underpinned by NSFs (see Chapter Seven), which set out how best to meet health and social care needs for several groups, including elderly people and people with mental illness. Joint investment programmes were also established for these groups, setting out needs, service provision, future plans and investment needed. In addition, some of the HAZ schemes, mentioned above, focused on improving the coordination of services for groups with multiple health and social needs.

Other initiatives introduced by New Labour included an expansion of intermediate care (a range of integrated services to provide faster recovery from illness, prevent unnecessary acute hospital admission, facilitate timely discharge and support independent living). This required greater cooperation of health and local government bodies (and involved working with others such as the private and voluntary sectors). In addition, care trusts were created to deliver both health and social care services for groups such as older people, people with mental illness, and people with learning disabilities (Glasby and Peck, 2003; Miller et al, 2011). Although heralded as a major initiative, only a small number of care trusts were established, largely because of political and practical barriers to integrating services in one organisation. Another new policy was 'cross-charging' of local authorities, when patients could not be discharged from hospital due to a lack of social care facilities. This was to incentivise councils to invest in social care services and reduce the number of delayed discharges.

These policies were supported by guidance that sought to clarify joint responsibilities for health and social care between the NHS and local authorities. It was envisaged that services would be increasingly provided by joint health and social care teams, who would undertake holistic assessment of needs and produce integrated care plans for those needing health and social care. In addition, a range of programmes encouraged joint working on health and social care for specific groups. For example, Partnerships for Older People Projects (POPPs), led by councils in partnership with PCTs and the voluntary and private sectors, promoted local innovations such as multidisciplinary teams, support workers and intermediate care services.

Subsequently, the Darzi Review (DH, 2008) called for a patient-centred approach based on closer working relationships between health and social care agencies. Darzi proposed piloting integrated care organisations, bringing together professionals from community services, hospitals, local authorities, and others. A programme was launched, aimed at improving the health and wellbeing of patients using a range of health and social care services.

Given the number and diversity of these initiatives, it is extremely difficult to evaluate their impact. However, it appears that relationships between the NHS and local government on social care issues began to improve after 1997 (Glendinning et al, 2003). More specifically, Health Act flexibilities were used extensively, including pooled budgets (Phelps and Regen, 2008; Audit Commission, 2009b). Joint commissioning of health and social care was encouraged (Dickinson et al, 2013b). Cross-charging was associated with a significant decline in delayed discharges, but other factors were at work (for further discussion, see Glasby and Dickinson, 2014). Intermediate care services reduced inappropriate admissions to acute or residential care and saved costs (Cameron et al, 2014), but other services, in particular those aimed at supporting discharge from hospital, could increase costs (see Glasby et al, 2008). A number of areas attracted wider interest for bringing agencies together (for example, Torbay and Somerset; Peck et al, 2002; Thistlethwaite, 2011). Some established care trusts, enabling a higher degree of formal integration (Miller et al, 2011). Although local efforts were useful, as an illustration of what could be achieved and of the barriers to change, evaluations indicated that lessons were often complex and outcomes ambiguous (see Peck et al, 2002).

There was insufficient evidence to clearly demonstrate that these initiatives had improved outcomes for patients and service users (Audit Commission, 2009b; Glasby, 2012; Wistow, 2013; Cameron et al, 2014; see also **Box 8.3**). However, some research found that users identified key aspects of services relevant to outcomes, including co-location, multidisciplinary working, specialist partnerships that understood specific needs, and extended partnerships that provided a gateway to other health and care-related services, such as housing (Petch et al, 2013).

Despite efforts to improve partnership working on health and social care in the New Labour era, this was undermined by several factors (Audit Commission, 2009b; NHS Future Forum, 2012; Glasby, 2012; Health Committee, 2012; Wistow, 2013; Glasby and Dickinson, 2014). First, the turbulence caused by constant reorganisation of both the NHS and local government disrupted relationships. The transfer of community services from PCTs (arising from an initiative of 2008) was particularly disruptive (see Edwards, 2014). Second, too much emphasis was placed on organisational structures and processes, and not enough on cultural factors. Indeed, both organisational and professional cultures can be resistant to new ways of working (Hudson, 2002; Hultberg et al, 2005).

A third problem was that different systems operating in the NHS and in local government continued to inhibit partnership working. For example, different financial systems produced disincentives to collaborate, while information systems inhibited the sharing of information. Fourth, centralisation in the NHS and in central/local government relations adversely affected local partnerships (Glendinning et al, 2003, 2005; Snape, 2003). Centralisation undermined local capacity and initiative by driving local agencies to respond to their own hierarchies rather than local priorities. Finally, planning and commissioning focused on services rather than people or places (Dickinson et al, 2013b; Wistow, 2013). Joint commissioning and partnership arrangements displayed a tendency to become ends in themselves rather than the means of improving outcomes.

Partnerships and the coalition

Although the coalition government continued to emphasise the importance of partnership working, it dismantled much of New Labour's partnership infrastructure. LAAs and CAAs were abolished. LSPs, having lost their core functions, were dismantled or reformed. Government Offices of the Regions (which predated New Labour, but had become crucial to its monitoring of local partnerships, agreements and targets) were also abolished. However, the coalition built on the spirit of its predecessor's initiatives, such as establishing pilot programmes to pool funds to deal with multiagency problems – Whole Place community budgets addressed a variety of problems including welfare dependency, skills gaps, worklessness, the integration of health and social care, support for people with long-term conditions, domestic abuse and anti-social behaviour. A further initiative, City Deals, devolved central budgets to local authorities to enable them to develop local economies and an infrastructure, which was expected to strengthen partnerships between parts of the public sector and between the public and private sectors. These agreements have increasingly covered larger geographical areas and have been extended to other functions and responsibilities, including, in one case so far, health and social care budgets. In 2015 the government agreed to devolve health and social service budgets to the Greater Manchester region (Hudson, 2015), and it is likely that similar agreements will follow in other areas. The coalition also introduced specific changes in the two key areas of collaboration: public health and social care.

Public health

The coalition government brought radical changes to public health, which had widespread implications for partnership working. The first key measure was the establishment of a new body, Public Health England, to undertake national functions, monitor health trends, provide expert advice and support, and oversee the local public health system. A new duty was placed on local authorities (the upper tier authorities, mentioned above) to improve public health. Statutory responsibilities for commissioning most local public health services were transferred to these authorities (including, for example, giving information about healthy lifestyles, providing facilities for the prevention of illness and reducing health risks from the environment). Some of these services were mandated (which means local authorities must provide them) – for example, public health advice to CCGs and the provision of information and advice to support health protection. In addition, a public health outcomes framework was devised, setting out key indicators for local authorities in this field. The transfer of functions was accompanied by the relocation of the local director of public health and public health teams from PCTs to those local authorities undertaking the new responsibilities. In addition, a ring-fenced grant was established for local authority-commissioned public health functions and services (£2.66 billion in 2013/14).

Health and wellbeing boards (see **Box 8.2**) were established as committees of local authorities, to lead partnership working on the formulation of local health and wellbeing priorities, through the JSNA and new joint health and wellbeing strategies (JHWS). JSNA and JHWS became the joint legal responsibilities of CCGs and local authorities. Health and wellbeing boards were expected to reduce health inequalities and promote integrated working between health and social care services, as well as promoting closer working with health-related services, such as housing. In addition, duties were imposed on health and social care commissioners, including duties to have regard to JSNA and JHWS when commissioning services (see **Box 8.2**).

There was much support for the return of public health responsibilities to local government (LGIU, 2010; Health Committee, 2011a; Communities and Local Government Committee, 2013; Tudor Jones, 2013). It was argued that local authorities would be able to take a holistic approach to health across different departments, and promote better collaboration between them. It was also believed that these additional duties and powers could extend the 'place shaping' role of local authorities, and ensure that health issues would feature on council agendas. By placing key health responsibilities in elected local authorities, accountability for health services could also be strengthened. Furthermore, it was thought that the introduction of statutory health and wellbeing boards would formalise, and thereby strengthen, partnership working in public health (as well as helping to integrate health and social services, discussed further below).

However, some saw this transfer of functions as a threat to existing partnerships, dislocating good relationships where they currently existed. It was believed that the transfer of public health functions would cause further fragmentation in some services, for example, sexual health (Health Committee, 2011a). There were particular concerns about the effects of the reforms on collaboration between councils in two-tier council areas. In these areas, important health-related functions such as environmental health and housing lay with lower tier district councils, outside the immediate remit of the authorities acquiring the new public health functions and staff (the county councils). It was argued that the contribution of district councils was undervalued, and that they should have been given a more explicit public health role (see Health Committee, 2011a; Kuznetsova, 2012).

Added to this were doubts about the capacity of local government to take on new public health roles, especially in the context of austerity and the relatively small amount of ring-fenced funding allocated. Some believed that councils would redesignate projects as 'public health', enabling them to divert resources to them (Public Health for the NHS, 2012). Furthermore, there was concern that the transfer of directors of public health to councils would weaken public health functions. Some suspected that the directors would not have sufficient influence within the council (Health Committee, 2011a). Moreover, it was feared that they would be prevented from speaking out on key public health issues, especially where their employing council had a conflict of interest. The government responded by giving the directors 'chief officer status', and introducing regulations and guidance about the appointment, employment conditions and dismissal of directors of public health and other public health staff.

Following these concessions, the transfer of functions to local authorities was implemented with little controversy. Even so, the impact of the changes was mixed. Although some councils made great strides, others were much slower off the mark (Tudor Jones, 2013). Concerns about public health funds being mis-spent were reignited by a *British Medical Journal* investigation, which found that local authorities had allocated public health funds to services such as leisure services and trading standards (Iocabucci, 2014). Even so, at least these investments had the potential to improve health and wellbeing. Capacity remained a problem, however. One in six director of public health posts were vacant or had a temporary incumbent (Paine, 2014). Turnover of senior public health staff was revealed by a survey of directors of public health undertaken by the Association of Directors of Public Health (ADPH, 2014). Worryingly, this report also found that a small minority of councils actively resisted or avoided public health commitments. It fuelled concerns about the lack of seniority of directors (less than half stated that they reported directly to the council chief executive or equivalent post). On a more positive note, the survey reported that their role had expanded into other areas including emergency planning, housing, trading standards, social care, environmental health, community and neighbourhoods. Moreover, 80 per cent of respondents stated that their council had a clear vision for public health, and 15 per cent reported that their council invested more than the ring-fenced budget.

Much attention focused on the newly created health and wellbeing boards and their relationships with other bodies. Reviews of their activities (Humphries et al, 2012; Kuznetsova, 2012; Humphries and Galea, 2013; Communities and Local Government Committee, 2013; Tudor Jones, 2013) identified a number of key themes.

First, health and wellbeing boards' weak statutory powers meant that 'soft power' was very important to their success (soft power means operating through partnerships and using persuasion to build consensus around objectives and actions). It appeared that most local authorities were committed to this role, indicated by their board being chaired by a senior elected member. It was noted that although health and wellbeing boards identified priorities, they had yet to come to terms with the challenges facing local health and care systems.

Second, there was scope for improvement in the relationships between health and wellbeing boards and commissioners. Health and wellbeing boards were particularly weak in relation to NHS England (which commissions national public health services, specialised services and primary care).

Engagement with GPs and with secondary care providers was also in need of improvement. Relationships with CCGs, however, were reported as very good and improving.

Third, health and wellbeing boards in two-tier authorities faced greater challenges than in single-tier areas. More positively, some county councils actively sought to involve district councils fully in public health strategies and initiatives.

Fourth, engagement with their communities proved a difficult task for health and wellbeing boards, and the new bodies did not have a high profile. It was argued that they needed to work more closely with communities and those speaking on their behalf, such as voluntary organisations and the local Healthwatch (see below on PPI).

Box 8.2: Health and wellbeing boards

The coalition government established statutory health and wellbeing boards in local authorities with social services responsibilities (that is, county councils, unitary authorities and London boroughs). Health and wellbeing boards must include the director of public health, director of children's services, director of adult social services, representatives from each CCG in the area, at least one elected representative, and a representative from the local Healthwatch (see below). A representative from NHS England must also sit on the board (when JSNA and JHWS are being formulated). Other members may be co-opted, including representatives from district councils, other council departments, the voluntary sector and other service providers.

Health and wellbeing boards seek to encourage bodies that provide health and social care services to work closely together and in an integrated manner to improve the health and wellbeing of the local population. They advise on, assist with and support the use of existing legal powers to pool and delegate budgets. They have a brief to promote closer working between health-related services such as housing, and the health and social care system. They are also expected to help reduce health inequalities. Their key functions are to lead the process of JSNA and JHWS formulation (which involve CCGs, NHS England and local authorities). Health and wellbeing boards must be involved by CCGs in the preparation and revision of commissioning plans. CCGs, NHS England and local authorities have a legal obligation to have regard to JSNA and the JHWS of each area for which they commission services.

Health and wellbeing boards are responsible for pharmaceutical needs assessments (which inform decisions about NHS-funded pharmacy services). They have also acquired additional responsibility for new budgets to promote integrated working between health and social care bodies – the Better Care Fund. Local authorities are legally permitted to delegate other council functions to health and wellbeing boards (but not health scrutiny).

Social care

The coalition government continued to emphasise closer working between health and social care services. It intended to promote integrated care (see **Box 8.3**), building on some of the initiatives introduced by New Labour.

First, the coalition clarified, consolidated and extended the law on social care. The Care Act 2014 set out the general responsibilities of local authorities (including promoting individual wellbeing, prevention of problems leading to people needing care and support, providing information and advice and promoting diversity and quality in provision of social care). It placed responsibility on councils to promote the integration of care and support with health and other services (including housing). Importantly, it also set out new duties of cooperation for local authorities and their partners with regard to care and support. The other main provisions of the Act included a single consistent route to establishing entitlement to publicly funded services, the introduction of a new cap and thresholds concerning individual payments for care and entitlement to state support, and measures relating to the support of carers.

Second, additional funds (around £2 billion a year) were allocated to social care, half from the NHS budget. This funding was subsequently increased to £3.8 billion per annum from 2015/16. This pooled budget – renamed the Better Care Fund – was ring-fenced and placed under the aegis of health and wellbeing boards. As already noted, these bodies had been given a duty to encourage integrated working and to support flexible arrangements to pool or delegated budgets. This approach was widely supported (Health Committee, 2012, 2014; NHS Future Forum, 2012; Commission on the Future of Health and Social Care in England, 2014).

Third, the Health and Social Care Act 2012 placed specific duties on NHS bodies with respect to integrated care. NHS England was given a duty to ensure that health services would be provided in an integrated way to improve the quality of care and reduce health inequalities. It was also required to ensure the integration of health services with social care and/ or other health-related services. NHS England has a further obligation to encourage CCGs to pursue integration leading to the above improvements (and CCGs have similar duties to ensure integration for these purposes). Furthermore, Monitor, the regulator of competition for NHS services (see Chapter Seven), has a duty to enable integrated working when undertaking its functions.

Finally, the coalition endorsed integrated care in a number of initiatives and announcements. These included the publication of *Integrated care and support* (DH, ADASS, CQC, 2013), a collaboration of national organisations including the DH, Association of Directors of Social Care, Association of Directors of Children's Services, CQC, NICE, Monitor, NHS England and the Local Government Association. Linked to this initiative, 14 integrated care pioneers were established, covering areas from Barnsley to Worcestershire, to provide examples of how health, social care and other services could work together seamlessly to meet the needs of local people. In addition, integration was emphasised in strategic policy documents, including the NHS mandate (DH, 2013a; 2014).

While the coalition's commitment to integrated care and joint working was broadly welcomed, there was much criticism of the impact of austerity budgets on social care funding. Local authorities implemented severe budget cuts. The NAO (2014a) discovered an 8 per cent cut in adult social care spending by local authorities between 2010/11 and 2012/13. Local authorities increasingly rationed care to those with the highest level of needs. Eighty-five per cent of adults lived in areas that arranged services for people with substantial or critical needs only (NAO, 2014a). Concerns were expressed that insufficient resources could jeopardise efforts to establish integrated care services (Health Committee, 2012, 2014; Commission on the Future of Health and Social Care in England, 2014; PAC, 2014b). Services that could reduce the burden on hospitals by preventing admissions or expediting discharge were under-resourced relative to demand and needed more investment (NHS Benchmarking Network, 2013). This underpinned calls for an overall financial settlement for health and social care that reflected the level of need (see Humphries, 2013; NHS Confederation, 2012; Commission on the Future of Health and Social Care in England, 2014).

The Better Care Fund also attracted criticism (Hawkes, 2014; Health Committee, 2014; PAC, 2015). It was feared that the additional funds taken from the NHS would reduce its capacity to deal with current demands. As a result, people with long-term conditions could face difficulties in getting timely access to healthcare, and their conditions might deteriorate, adding to the strain on the health and social care system. Although there was much support for the ring-fenced fund, and for handing the role to health and wellbeing boards, there was some disquiet about their capacity and their lack of focus on integrated care (Humphries, 2013).

One of the main obstacles to implementing integrated care was the government's NHS reforms (NHS Future Forum, 2011, 2012). The Health and Social Care Act 2012 established the foundations for a more competitive and pluralistic NHS, with greater private and voluntary sector provision. This was an extension of both New Labour and previous Conservative government policies. Although not entirely new, many saw the radical nature of the 2012 reforms as a threat to the ethos of partnership and collaboration that underpins integrated care. Competition was seen as causing two potential problems. First, it was associated with a low level of trust, which undermines collaboration. Second, the creation of more providers would be likely to exacerbate problems of fragmentation, making integration more difficult. Furthermore, the PBR system (see Chapter Seven) was seen as a barrier to developing community services that are essential to the development of integrated care. As PBR applied predominantly to acute and emergency care, it was believed these services had an incentive to increase activity, while community-based services, funded mainly by block contracts, would be disincentivised (Marshall et al, 2014; Health Committee, 2010). There were calls to make the payment system more flexible so as to create stronger incentives to integrate care and strengthen community-based services (Appleby et al, 2012; Health Committee, 2014; Ham and Walsh, 2013). The government and health service regulators did respond to these concerns by introducing some flexibilities (see Monitor, 2014) and encouraging their application at local level (especially by the new integrated care pioneers).

One of the key points was that future health and social care services must integrate around the needs of the patient (NHS Future Forum, 2012; Commission on the Future of Health and Social Care in England, 2014; Independent Commission on Whole Person Care, 2014). There was also a wide consensus that integrated care must focus on improving outcomes. Related to this, a number of commentators pointed out the need to ensure that regulatory and performance management frameworks also focused on outcomes and were consistent with each other (NHS Future Forum, 2012; Ham and Walsh, 2013). There were particular concerns that Monitor, despite the statutory requirements mentioned above, might not place sufficient emphasis on integration and the outcomes that it may achieve.

Box 8.3: Integrated care

There has long been concern that health services, social care and other health and care services need to work together more effectively to meet the needs of people, especially those with complex and multiple needs. These considerations have been given additional weight by several related trends. These are: the ageing population (the percentage of people in the UK aged over 85 is set to double between 2010–30), which is likely to increase the overall health and care needs and the complexity of these needs (House of Lords Select Committee on Public Service and Demographic Change, 2013); the rise in the number of people with long-term conditions, who account for 70 per cent of total spending on health and social care (Health Committee, 2014); and the rise in co-morbidity (people with more than one illness or condition), which means that there is a need for better coordinated and person-centred care. The urgency is heightened by the difficulties of the current system of health and care to cope with demand, and the prospect of static or declining health budgets in the future.

As RAND Europe/Ernst & Young LLP (2012) reported, the concept of integrated care is used in many ways and there are many terminologies (for example, managed care, collaborative care, seamless care and case management). As a result, it covers many different approaches, including co-location of care, the sharing of information about patients, single assessment processes, integrated management of disease in chronically ill people and others. Added to this, there are different types of integration: normative integration (where integration is based on shared values); systemic integration (based on implementation of rules and policies); organisational (coordinating structures, governance systems and relationships between organisations); administrative (aligning back office functions, budgets and financial systems); and clinical (coordinating information and services and integrating patient care within a single process) (Shaw et al, 2011; see also Fulop et al, 2005; Armitage et al, 2009; RAND Europe/Ernst & Young LLP, 2012; Goodwin, 2013). Furthermore, integrated care can focus narrowly on improving healthcare, or it can extend to social care and beyond (including housing and other services that support health and care).

Nonetheless, there is much consensus around three things. First, the principal focus of integrated care should be about meeting the patient's needs (NHS Future Forum, 2012). Second, we must be clear about the aims and objectives of integration. And third, the evaluation of integrated care projects has been problematic. Many benefits have been claimed for integrated care, including better quality care, improved outcomes and greater cost-effectiveness (NHS Future Forum, 2012; Health Committee, 2014; Independent Commission on Whole Person Care, 2014; Ham and Walsh, 2013; Commission on the Future of Health and Social Care in England, 2014). Although integrated care projects have yielded benefits, systematic reviews and programme evaluations have produced more cautious conclusions.

A review by Cameron et al (2014) found that evaluations of joint and integrated working identified improvements in health and wellbeing, reductions in inappropriate admissions to acute or residential care, and showed that intermediate care can reduce costs. But it also concluded that the evidence base remains weak, especially regarding cost-effectiveness (see also Nolte and Pitchforth, 2014). Meanwhile, the RAND Europe/Ernst & Young LLP (2013) study of the integrated care pilots in England found that although staff were positive about the changes, patients did not experience improvements, and there was a deterioration in important aspects of care (for example, people reported less involvement in decisions about their care). In addition, the study found no reduction in emergency hospital admissions (although planned admissions and outpatients visits fell). The Nuffield Trust's evaluation of various integrated care initiatives also found that emergency admissions did not fall (Bardsley et al, 2013). Meanwhile, a report from the Centre for Health Economics at the University of York (Mason et al, 2014) found that empirical studies of integrated care fell short of high expectations, and seldom led to improved outcomes. This report also noted that coordinated approaches to care appeared to reveal rather than resolve unmet needs, potentially adding to financial pressures on health and care systems.

In summary, achieving integration is not a simple matter, and it takes time and resources (see Ham et al, 2013; Ham and Walsh, 2013). Strong leadership and competent management are necessary but are not always sufficient conditions for successful integration. Much depends on achieving cultural change, particularly with regard to enabling the creation of innovative approaches to complex problems.

Independent sector

Recent governments have extended partnerships to include the independent sector, which includes private 'for profit' businesses (hereafter, the private sector) as well as voluntary organisations, charities and other third sector bodies (see the next section). This attempt to build partnerships with organisations outside the public sector has mirrored the expansion in the independent sector's contribution to health and social care, a trend encouraged by successive governments since the 1980s.

The state accounts for 80 per cent of healthcare spending in the UK, and only a minority of people (around one in ten) have private health insurance (Arora et al, 2013). However, on the supply side, the picture is more complex. Independent sector bodies provide more services on behalf of the NHS than previously. In addition, NHS organisations and professionals receive significant private income. With regard to social care, where public funding has historically played a smaller role, the process of increasing the independent sector's provider role has almost reached completion. In 2012, only 6 per cent of all residential and nursing home places were in the state sector (compared with 64 per cent in 1979) (Fotaki et al, 2013). Furthermore, the percentage of home care services provided by the independent sector rose from 5 per cent (1993) to 89 per cent (2012). These trends have resulted from a deliberate policy of forcing local authorities to concentrate on planning, needs assessment and commissioning, and to reduce their provider role, replacing it with a provider market dominated by independent sector suppliers.

As we saw in Chapter Two, the Conservative governments of the 1980s and 1990s actively promoted the privatisation of health services, although this was mainly confined to ancillary and support services. The NHS was urged to involve the private sector in planning and joint projects. It was also encouraged to use spare capacity in the private sector to reduce waiting lists. New Labour continued and extended the policies adopted by the Conservatives. It embarked on an ambitious hospital capital programme using PFI, which the Conservatives had begun to apply to the health sector.

PFI schemes (and similar projects in primary care) have remained controversial, mainly due to cuts in services due to the financial burden of PFI, and the huge profits made by private companies involved (Pollock et al, 2011a; PAC, 2012; Treasury Committee, 2011; Vecchi, 2013). The coalition government was initially very critical of PFI, but decided to revamp it with some minor safeguards (renaming it PF2).

PFI was one of several strands of a pro-independent sector policy that developed under New Labour. A concordat was agreed between the Independent Healthcare Association and the DH (2000) as a framework for collaboration. PCTs were told by the DH to make full use of the capacity in the independent sector, reinforced by imperatives to reduce waiting times. A programme of independent sector treatment centres (ISTCs) involved overseas health corporations (Pollock, 2004; Leys and Player, 2011). These were established to undertake high-volume surgical procedures on behalf of the NHS. The scheme cost £1.7 billion between 2003–10 and was criticised as poor value for money (Slater and Beckford, 2011; Leys and Player, 2011). It was also alleged that ISTCs fragmented services (Turner et al, 2012) and undermined NHS services by diverting revenues away from them (Health Committee, 2006b). Allegations that ISTCs produced lower quality care than the NHS was not, however, borne out by the research (Chard, 2011).

In addition, a new system of franchising for NHS trusts was introduced. This enabled independent organisations to take over the management of trusts deemed to have performed badly. Although rarely used, a decision made late in the lifetime of the Labour government paved the way for the takeover of Hinchingbrooke NHS Trust (in Huntingdon, Cambridgeshire) by the Circle Health Partnership. The takeover, completed in 2012, was a disaster. The hospital's debts continued to increase. It was also the subject of a criticism from CQC about its care standards, which led to it being placed in special measures. In 2015, Circle exercised a clause enabling it to end the contract early.

The creation of foundation trusts by New Labour gave NHS service providers more freedom to engage in partnerships with the private sector. The amount of privately funded work that foundation trusts could undertake was, however, capped at their pre-foundation trust status level. The coalition raised this to a maximum of 49 per cent of total income, with board governors deciding on any annual increase of 5 percentage points or more.

In addition, the Blair government set a target for expanding the private sector's share of NHS work even further, stating that the private sector could provide up to 15 per cent of operations by 2008. The use of the private sector was encouraged in others ways; for example, the right of NHS patients to choose and book hospital treatments was also extended to include at least one private supplier. New Labour also embarked on a further round of contracting out and privatisation in its latter years. Independent provision of primary care was promoted by the introduction of alternative primary medical services and by changes in the GP contract which left some services (notably out-of-hours primary care) open to independent sector provision. A number of larger businesses moved into this field, including Serco and Virgin (although Serco has since withdrawn from NHS clinical contracts following losses and criticism of some of its services; see NAO, 2013c). Similarly, the policy of divesting PCTs of their community health services created further opportunities for the independent sector. Although 80 per cent of community health providers were eventually transferred to NHS bodies, the remainder ended up in the hands of private businesses and social enterprises. New Labour continued to explore ways of contracting out services, identifying several services for competitive tendering, including pathology. Furthermore, New Labour's policy of 'any qualified provider' sought to extend patient choice for elective care to all providers registered with the CQC.

Together these policies led to an increase in NHS spending on non-NHS providers, by 62 per cent between 2006/07 and 2011/12 (Arora et al, 2013). The proportion of the secondary care budget accounted for by non-NHS providers rose from 9 to 12.3 per cent, almost wholly due to ISTCs and other commercial contracts. The voluntary sector, meanwhile, increased its share of secondary care, but from a low base. However, there was considerable variation in the proportion of NHS work done by the independent sector across different geographical areas. There was also much variation across different treatments. For example, following this period of growth, almost one in five elective hip and knee replacements funded by the NHS were performed in the independent sector (Arora et al, 2013). Late in the day, New Labour heralded a shift in policy when, in 2009, the Secretary of State for Health stated that the NHS should be the preferred provider of services, but this did little to change things.

After the coalition came to office these policies were extended further. Existing regulations were used to open up the NHS to competition from independent providers. A new statutory framework was established to promote commissioning, competition and market testing by the Health and

Social Care Act 2012 (see Chapters Two and Seven). Although the original Bill was heavily amended, this did not satisfy the most vociferous critics. For example, they pointed out that price competition was still permitted at a local level in certain circumstances (Fotaki et al, 2013). Controversy returned in 2013 when the government introduced its competition regulations (which fleshed out the provisions of the 2012 Act). Critics argued that the regulations would force commissioners to open services to competition. The government made further concessions by clarifying the rules regarding commissioning and the provision of integrated care, and the circumstances where a commissioner could award a contract to a single provider.

Nonetheless, the majority of contracts (56 per cent) issued since the new regulations came into force in April 2013 were awarded to the independent sector, although it has less than 50 per cent share by value (File on 4, 2014). It was also reported that many CCGs' fear of falling foul of market competition rules led them to err on the side of caution and open services to tender (West, 2014; Welikala and West, 2015). So competition rules remain a powerful driver, and much depends on their interpretation. Notably much depends on the approach taken by Monitor, the NHS market regulator, which is staffed primarily by people from a business management or commercial background (PAC, 2014a). Furthermore, there are additional concerns about the future impact of international and European competition rules on the commissioning of NHS services (see Chapter Ten).

There is much suspicion of the motives of the independent sector, and especially commercial organisations that seek to make a profit for the benefit of investors (Ruane, 2002; Pollock, 2004; Leys and Player, 2011). There is a strong belief that the private sector will make money at the public's expense where it can, by overcharging for its services, as occurred in both PFI and ISTCs, for example. There is also a fear that it will seek to 'cherry pick' the most profitable areas of healthcare provision, and leave the public sector with the higher cost and complex forms of care. Such profit-seeking behaviour may also increasingly apply to parts of the public sector if foundation trusts, which now operate on a much more commercial footing and are allowed to generate more private income, focus excessively on income generation.

When criticising NHS changes, critics often draw on the experience of social care, which, as noted earlier, has been subject to increasing competition from the independent sector. According to some observers, this process has been very damaging, focusing on reducing costs (see PAC, 2014b; Fotaki et al, 2013). This has undermined the quality of services, promoted the casualisation of staff, and in some cases, has led to instability and even the collapse of providers (as in the case of Southern Cross in 2011), all of which has had adverse consequences for users.

There is a belief that the type of ownership is crucial to the achievement of quality care. The balance of the evidence is that 'not-for-profit' hospitals, nursing homes and other healthcare organisations provide better quality care than 'for profit' organisations (Devereaux et al, 2002; Rosenau, 2003; Himmelstein et al, 1999; Comondore et al, 2009). However, the evidence is not conclusive (Eggleston et al, 2006; Comondore et al, 2009).

In England, poor quality services provided by the 'for profit' sector have been highlighted in the media. A major case of systematic patient abuse – the Winterbourne View scandal exposed by the BBC in 2011 – was under private ownership (CQC, 2011; DH, 2012). There have also been other cases where private sector providers have not followed required procedures to monitor quality, reduced staffing, or otherwise cut corners to save money (see File on 4, 2013). Other cases have involved allegations of fraud or misrepresentation (see, for example, Britten, 2012; NAO, 2013c).

A range of other concerns has been raised about private sector involvement. These include lack of transparency, weak accountability and inflexibility resulting from contractual issues. Private companies are not subject to Freedom of Information legislation, and they can refuse to give details they deem commercially sensitive. A commissioning body can require information from a contractor, but only about contractually specified details. NHS-funded private providers are now subject to health scrutiny, but commercial sensitivity can still be used as grounds for refusing information requests.

Another criticism is that government often ends up subsidising or bailing out private operators. Companies have received subsidies when participating in waiting list initiatives and establishing ISTCs. In addition, private facilities have been bought out by the NHS when facing problems with finances or quality standards (Molloy, 2013). The private sector is also subsidised when it uses NHS trained staff. Although some private hospitals are involved in junior doctor and nurse training, this represents a fairly small contribution compared to what the sector gains from taxpayer funding of clinical and other staff training.

Partnership with the voluntary sector

The voluntary sector is highly differentiated and complex. It includes large organisations and small informal groups, and incorporates various legal entities. It is therefore unsurprising that a commonly agreed definition has been elusive. To make matters even more difficult, the labels used to describe the voluntary sector have changed over time. In the New Labour era, the term 'Third Sector' was in vogue, to capture a broader range of non-governmental bodies (including mutuals, cooperatives and social enterprises). Under the coalition, the term 'civil society' was used, to emphasise the importance of individual community action and volunteering. Underpinning most labels and definitions, however, is that the voluntary sector is distinct from government and from the private sector. Its voluntary and autonomous status distinguishes it from the former; its not-for-profit status demarcates it from the latter. However, in practice these distinctions are blurred.

The voluntary sector has a long history of involvement in health and social care. Although the creation of the NHS removed large areas of healthcare from the voluntary sector, the latter continued to play a significant role in providing care, information and support. Voluntary organisations have flourished in areas such as maternity and childbirth, children and young people's health, the care of the elderly and disabled people, support for those with long-term conditions, care and support of people with learning disabilities, and in mental health and palliative care. They have been engaged in raising funds for research. Voluntary organisations have also been involved in public health issues through community development and health promotion activities, and by campaigning for policies and interventions to improve health and prevent illness. In addition, they can act as a voice for patients, service users, carers, vulnerable and disadvantaged groups and local communities (Baggott et al, 2005).

During the post-war period, central government increasingly acknowledged the value of the voluntary sector. The Conservative governments of Thatcher and Major were keen to promote the voluntary sector, especially in public services, as part of their policies to stimulate alternatives to state provision. New Labour built on this, introducing the voluntary sector compact in England (Home Office, 1998), which set out shared principles and undertakings by both the government and the voluntary sector (Scotland, Wales and Northern Ireland developed their own compacts). This was accompanied by new funding mechanisms to strengthen the capacity of voluntary organisations.

New Labour also provided more opportunities and support to help voluntary organisations compete for public service contracts. There was particular encouragement for social enterprises, businesses with primarily social objectives whose profits or surpluses are mainly reinvested rather than paid to owners or shareholders. Local authorities were encouraged to formulate their own compacts with the voluntary sector, involve voluntary organisations in decisions about policies and services, and give them opportunities to bid for public services.

The coalition government adopted the rhetoric of the 'Big Society' (Cabinet Office, 2010). This had five themes: to give communities more powers; to encourage people to take an active role in their communities; to transfer power from central to local government; to support voluntary organisations, mutual organisations and social enterprises and especially to help them run public services; and to publish government information about social problems and public services. However, sceptics saw this as a cover for public spending cuts and privatisation (Hudson, 2011). The coalition revised the national compact, with a stronger focus on public service delivery, commitments and outcomes. It continued to emphasise the role of voluntary organisations as potential contractors, but cut support to the voluntary sector. Bodies established by New Labour to advise government on voluntary sector issues and oversee policy implementation were abolished. Some funding schemes were cut or discontinued, although new ones were established (such as the Big Society Bank). However, the broader context of public sector funding cuts – to reduce the budget deficit – boded ill for voluntary organisations reliant on state funding (NEF, 2010; Kane and Allen, 2011).

Health and care voluntary sector

In the field of health and social care, policies advocating a role for the voluntary sector were strengthened from the 1960s onwards. A financial support scheme for voluntary groups in the health and welfare field was introduced in 1968. Voluntary organisations were increasingly represented on NHS bodies. National policy guidance urged local NHS bodies to collaborate with and consult the voluntary sector on health and care issues and service planning (Wyatt, 2002).

Under New Labour, a strategic agreement between the DH, NHS and the voluntary sector set a framework for relationships in this area (DH, 2004c). A National Strategic Partnership Forum was established to take forward the initiative, including the promotion of local partnership agreements. New Labour's retention of the division between commissioners and providers yielded further opportunities for the voluntary sector. Voluntary organisations contributed to commissioning, the assessment of needs, the representation of user, carer and public perspectives, and the monitoring and evaluation of the quality of services. With regard to wider public health issues, programmes such as Sure Start, New Deal for Communities, the Neighbourhood Renewal Fund and HAZs emphasised the importance of partnership with voluntary organisations. LSPs were also expected to engage with the voluntary sector (see Taylor, 2006).

The coalition government also emphasised the importance of the voluntary sector in health and care. For example, it envisaged that, where appropriate, voluntary groups would be represented on the new health and wellbeing boards and would support JSNA and the production of JHWS. As noted earlier, the coalition's NHS reforms continued and extended the policy of competition for health and care provision services, enabling the voluntary sector to bid for contracts. The coalition, like the previous government, was particularly keen to encourage social enterprises. Social enterprises fitted neatly with its desire to promote enterprise as well as voluntarism. Under both New Labour and the coalition, these organisations were promised investment and support from government (Addicott, 2011).

Key issues for the voluntary sector in health and care

The voluntary sector has become a more significant provider of services in public health, healthcare and social care (ACEVO, 2010; Baggott, 2013). Its income from secondary healthcare commissioners grew by almost half between 2006/07 and 2011/12 (Arora et al, 2013). However, during this period, the sector's share of this market actually declined. The 'for profit' private sector, in contrast, saw a threefold increase in its income from NHS-funded secondary care, from a larger base. By 2011/12 the voluntary sector's income from the NHS was around a tenth of the private sector's.

The voluntary sector continues to be constrained by capacity problems (Curry et al, 2011). Although various schemes have built capacity and given support, voluntary sector funding is limited, and in recent years, many organisations have faced cuts. There are significant inequalities in capacity and skills, both within the voluntary sector, and between the voluntary and private sectors. In particular, smaller voluntary organisations are at a disadvantage when bidding for contracts (ACEVO, 2010; Curry et al, 2011), and may be drawn into subcontracting arrangements that allow exploitation by larger voluntary organisations or private operators (Reynolds and McKee, 2012).

Despite efforts to encourage NHS and local government bodies to contract services to the voluntary sector, and improvements in relationships between statutory agencies and voluntary organisations, considerable obstacles remain. For example, there are often major differences in perspectives, values, cultures and processes that impede the contracting out of public services to the voluntary sector (ACEVO, 2010; Addicott, 2013). Meanwhile, there is much scope for improving engagement between the voluntary sector and statutory health bodies. According to one survey (NAVCA, 2015), 51 per cent of charities stated that CCGs engaged with them. Less than a third (32 per cent) felt able to influence health and wellbeing boards. Other research (Humphries and Galea, 2013) found that just over half of health and wellbeing boards contained representatives from the voluntary sector.

Some voluntary organisations are better able to engage with statutory organisations and exert influence. Larger charities are heavily involved in supporting commissioning, and can even influence the design of service provision (see Holder, 2013). Again, this suggests that inequality between voluntary organisations remains an issue. It also underlines the problems of capacity within the voluntary sector (see also Hunter et al, 2011). Despite the willingness of voluntary organisations to engage in activities such as planning, consultation and service development, there has been a failure to appreciate that these various roles impose significant costs, not fully covered by current levels of financial support. Moreover, given the increasing demand for their involvement, one can understand how voluntary organisations get overloaded. 'Consultation fatigue' is a common complaint (Craig et al, 2004).

The autonomy and independence of voluntary organisations could be compromised by taking on a greater role in state-funded provision. Providing services on behalf of public bodies can lead to voluntary organisations compromising their advocacy role. This is unpalatable for voluntary organisations, but unless they have alternative sources of income and a high public profile, they are in a weak position. As voluntary groups work more closely with government, particularly providing services under contract, they could become heavily dependent on their patronage, and more easily manipulated into legitimising decisions that are not in the interests of users.

Furthermore, the representative role of voluntary organisations is itself problematic (Alcock and Scott, 2002; Craig and Taylor, 2002; Baggott et al, 2005). There are major inequalities within the voluntary sector that mean that some voices are stronger and more influential than others. Genuine partnership with the voluntary sector means providing opportunities for weaker, marginalised and less well-resourced groups to participate. Otherwise, differences in the willingness and ability of groups to participate will, by default, advantage representatives of the better resourced, politically astute organisations. As a result, the diversity of views across the voluntary sector as a whole may not be captured.

Finally, there are concerns about the role of social enterprises. Recent governments have been uncritically in favour of these organisations. However, a variety of organisational forms can sail under the convenience flag of social enterprise. It is feared that they may be a vehicle for public services to be apportioned to organisations that benefit private interests (Marks and Hunter, 2007). There are also worries about the fragmentation of services that might result, the long-term viability of social enterprises, and their limited accountability and transparency (Addicott, 2011). More evidence is needed on their role, contribution and impact (Roy et al, 2014).

Public and patient involvement

In recent decades, there has been much greater acknowledgement of patient and public perspectives on health and care (Baggott et al, 2005; Hogg, 2009; Coulter, 2011; Foot et al, 2014). This has led policy-makers to declare that services must be 'patient-centred', and that service users (and where appropriate, their families and carers) must have a greater role in their care and treatment, including greater choice. It is also acknowledged that policy-makers, planners and service providers must take into account the views of patients, users, carers and the wider public when making policies and arranging or delivering services. Furthermore, there has been increasing emphasis on the responsibilities of citizens, both in terms of their use of health and care services, and as agents in the promotion and protection of their own health and of their communities.

There is, however, a variety of perspectives on the purpose and effectiveness of patient and public involvement (PPI) (Foot et al, 2014). Furthermore, a range of competing terminologies co-exist (Baggott et al, 2005; Wait and Nolte, 2006). It is acknowledged that PPI is a very loose term for a complex multidimensional collection of activities and processes. In this section, three aspects are considered: PPI bodies; surveys and feedback; and involvement in care and treatment. These are now briefly outlined, focusing primarily on health and care in England (the other countries of the UK are covered in Chapter Nine).

Patient and public involvement bodies

Ever since the creation of the NHS, health authorities and boards have included lay representatives (that is, people who are not clinicians or NHS managers). This was later augmented by the establishment of PPI bodies (see **Box 8.4**). The current system, Healthwatch, was established by the Health and Social Care Act 2012.

Box 8.4: The system of patient and public involvement in England

Community Health Councils (CHCs) were established in England and Wales in 1974 (along with similar bodies in Northern Ireland and Scotland; see Gerrard, 2009; Hogg, 2009). CHCs were statutory bodies, established in each district. They undertook a range of roles, monitoring local services and producing an annual report, obtaining and providing information about services, and assisting with complaints. They also had the right to be consulted on substantial changes in health services.

In 2003 CHCs were replaced by Patient and Public Involvement Forums (PPIFs), established in PCTs and trusts. PPIFs were also statutory bodies. Their main function was to monitor services from a patient-citizen perspective. The complaints support role of CHCs was allocated to a new Independent Complaints Advocacy Service (ICAS). Meanwhile, Patient Advice and Liaison Services (PALS) were created in

---

every PCT and trust to support, inform and advise patients, relatives and carers, particularly where they had queries or concerns. CHC functions with regard to consultation on major service changes were transferred to HOSCs (see **Box 8.1**). In addition, a national organisation was created (Commission for Patient and Public Involvement in Health, CPPIH) to advise, assist and support the PPIFs and represent their views.

In 2008, CPPIH was abolished, and the PPIFs replaced by new bodies, Local Involvement Networks (LINks). Each LINk covered a local authority social services area (and was funded by the local authority). Although not statutory bodies, LINks retained similar statutory powers and duties of the PPIFs. These powers were extended, to cover social care providers, the NHS and independent sector providers of state-funded healthcare. The functions of LINks were to promote and support the involvement of people in the commissioning, provision and scrutiny of health and social care, to enable people to monitor and review the commissioning and provision of local services, to obtain the views of people about their needs and experiences, to present these views to commissioners, providers, managers and those scrutinising services, and to make recommendations about service improvements.

Further reform occurred following the coalition's plans to reorganise the NHS. In 2013, local Healthwatch organisations replaced LINks. Like LINks, they are funded by upper tier local authorities (whose geographical area they cover), and focus on health and social care matters. Local Healthwatch organisations are constituted as non-statutory bodies (their functions can be undertaken by charities and social enterprises – see below), but have legal powers and duties. Their functions are similar to the previous bodies, and include promoting public involvement, articulating the views of local people, monitoring services, issuing reports and making recommendations for improvement. In addition, they must make their views known to a new national body, Healthwatch England (see below), and support it in the exercise of its functions. They are formally represented on health and wellbeing boards, and are involved in the formulation of JSNA and JHWS. They must also advise and inform local people about access to health and care services and about the choices available. They may also provide or commission local independent complaints advocacy services (the national ICAS scheme ended in 2013). Alternatively, local authorities, which acquired the responsibility for funding and commissioning ICAS, are permitted to commission this service directly from other organisations. Local Healthwatch organisations were established as social enterprises (the definition of social enterprise in this case including charities as well as profit-making bodies that reinvest at least half their profits in securing benefits for the community). Local Healthwatch may also subcontract its functions to other bodies.

A new national body, Healthwatch England, was created in 2012, as a subcommittee of the CQC. The key functions of Healthwatch are to advise the Secretary of State for Health and other bodies (including CQC, Monitor and NHS England) on the views of health and care service users, to be consulted by these bodies on specific issues (for example, the Secretary of State must consult Healthwatch England when setting out the mandate for the NHS), and to recommend that CQC carry out specific investigations where problems have been identified. Healthwatch England provides advice and assistance to local Healthwatch organisations. It also monitors and issues guidance on the local authority commissioning of local Healthwatch.

In addition, NHS bodies have statutory duties to consult and involve the patients and the public. New Labour revised and extended existing duties, creating a general duty to involve patients and the public in health service planning and provision. This legislation was superseded by the Health and Social Care Act 2012, which set out specific duties on NHS England and CCGs to involve patients and the public in the commissioning, planning and provision of services. Additional duties were imposed on NHS England to monitor and report on CCGs' arrangements to involve the public and patients (with additional duties on CCGs to heed guidance issued by NHS England, to publish their arrangements for PPI, and to report on their activities). In addition, health and wellbeing boards must involve the public in their work, both via the local Healthwatch, and directly.

Foundation trusts also involve staff, patients and local people. These constituencies are able to join foundation trusts as members and vote in (and stand for) elections to their governing bodies. The governing body does not run the trust, however. It appoints the chair and non-executive directors of the trust's management board, seeks to hold the management board to account, works with it to produce future plans, and represents the views of the trust's members.

Surveys and feedback

Service users and the wider public can be involved through surveys of public opinion and patient experience, specific consultation events and meetings. Feedback on services is increasingly provided online, on social media as well as through specialist sites (Foot et al, 2014). Patients' views on the efficacy of treatment are collected through PROMs (Patient Reported Outcome Measures). The Friends and Family Test (FFT) provides a simple (and perhaps simplistic) measure of patient satisfaction based on whether patients would recommend that friends or family should be treated at the same facility (Picker Institute Europe, 2014).

Mechanisms of complaint and redress in health and care are also important in relation to accountability, and can generate pressure for policy development and service improvement. The Health Ombudsman has already been mentioned (see Chapter Three). New Labour introduced PALS (see **Box 8.4**) to help resolve issues raised by patients and relatives. Meanwhile, ICAS supported those wishing to take matters further. The system for formal complaints in the NHS was reformed in the 1990s and again in 2003. In both cases, the aim was to provide a system that would be fair to all parties, independent, timely, streamlined, and that would lead to better quality services. Amid rising levels of complaints and high-profile cases where complaints of poor quality care had being ignored, the coalition launched a further review of the complaints system (Clwyd and Hart, 2013). One of the main problems is the presence of different channels for complaints, and there have been calls to integrate the various systems to avoid confusion (see Healthwatch, 2014).

Involvement in care and treatment

Recent governments have sought to use choice and markets as a means of making services more responsive to users (see Chapters Two and Seven). While choice is valued by patients and service users (Dixon et al, 2010; Dixon and Robertson, 2011), in practice, these initiatives have been restricted by lack of relevant information, availability of clinicians and overall resources. Meanwhile, initiatives in social care have given people their own budget for care and support. Direct payments, enabling users to pay directly for community care services, were introduced in the late 1990s (Carr and Robins, 2009). Subsequently, the introduction of personal budgets took this a stage further, setting an overall budget for an individual's needs, and supporting them in making decisions about commissioning care and support. Personal budgets appear to have improved quality of life and social care outcomes, as well as other indicators (financial position, choice and control, and participation in community life) (Glendinning et al, 2008). In a further move, personal budgets were piloted in healthcare for people with long-term conditions, with mixed results (Forder et al, 2012).

At the time of writing there are moves to extend personal health budgets and to integrate health and social care budgets for some service users. The Health and Social Care Act 2012 imposed a duty on NHS England and CCGs to enable choice, and on Monitor to protect and promote it. The Care Act 2014 promoted choice by placing a duty on local authorities to ensure that a variety of providers of social care services existed, requiring local authorities to inform people about the choices of different types of services and providers available.

There has been much emphasis on strengthening the participation of patients, users and carers in individual care and treatment (Foot et al, 2014). The notion of shared care is based on an appreciation that patients and users (and carers) have experience, skills and knowledge that can contribute to improved outcomes (Nunes et al, 2009; Coulter and Collins, 2011). Indeed, those who have experienced long-term conditions are often considered 'expert patients'. These patients often self-manage their own illness as well as contribute to treatment decisions, which can potentially save resources by preventing unnecessary hospital admissions. Government, the NHS and voluntary organisations have supported schemes to support patients' involvement in their own care (for example, Expert Patients' programmes). In addition, patients often support themselves and others through self-help groups (Borkmann and Munn-Giddings, 2008).

The involvement of carers and families is widely regarded as a positive development. According to Carers UK (2014), there are 6.5 million people providing informal care in the UK. Carers can also play an effective role in decisions about care and treatment (Pharoah et al, 2006), but there are barriers to their involvement (Ridley et al, 2014). Carers need greater support to enable them to undertake their role. New Labour introduced a Carers' Strategy (HM Government, 1999a, 2008), which proposed improvements in information, support and access to services, and provided some additional funding. Legislation was introduced to give carers a right to their own needs assessment. This strategy was relaunched by the coalition (HM Government, 2010b). Subsequently the Care Act 2014 extended legal rights to carers' needs assessment and support, and this has been followed with new commitments to prioritise support for carers (HM Government, 2014; NHS England, 2014).

Has patient and public involvement improved?

As shown, various initiatives have targeted citizen participation in health and care. However, there has been a significant gap between the rhetoric of support for greater PPI, and the reality of everyday health and care policy and service provision. The key criticisms across all these areas of activity have been as follows (Hogg, 2009; Foot et al, 2014).

First, despite all the initiatives, patients, carers and the public have limited influence over policy and services. Although PPI has been a stated priority for many years, in reality, it is not. It is under-resourced, and has lacked leadership at all levels. Professional and managerial power remains prevalent. This is not say that people have no say or influence whatsoever – there are occasions when the dominant forces in health policy are challenged, for example, when a major scandal is uncovered. But these are rare.

Second, some groups of patients and citizens lack the resources to engage with decision-makers. Efforts have been made to involve 'hard-to-reach' groups (including minority ethnic groups, disadvantaged people and those with communication disabilities). Attempts have also been made to overcome bias arising from listening to the same kind of people, those with the time, skills and resources to get involved. Even so, considerable barriers and inequalities remain.

Third, there is too much emphasis on the formal structures of PPI. Although important in providing channels to hold health and care bodies to account, they are not a substitute for informal channels and everyday encounters between lay people and those who provide services. Indeed, day-to-day interactions are crucial in shaping the culture of involvement in which the formal structures should be embedded. If people feel they have no say in these individual encounters with health and care services, they are unlikely to have much confidence in the formal systems of representation and accountability.

Conclusion

This chapter has shown that the implementation of health policies depends on effective working relationships between the NHS and other agencies, both statutory and independent. Despite a more strategic approach to partnership and evidence of good examples of joint working, the picture remains one of limited success, with a mixture of good and poor practice. In particular, it appears that the cultural aspects of partnership – the need to share vision and commitment – must be given greater weight, rather than simply concentrating on 'top-down' organisational structures and processes. Another key point is that the opening of the NHS to greater competition has created the potential for more fragmentation, making it more difficult to secure collaboration and integration. The chapter has also indicated that partnership must also extend meaningfully to patients and the public, and their representatives. They have an important role to play in the success of health policy initiatives and more must be done to involve them.

Summary

- Recent government policies have emphasised the importance of joined-up government and improved partnership working involving NHS organisations, local government and the private and voluntary sectors.
- Efforts to improve coordination between the NHS and local government, on public health and social care, have had limited success.

- More radical approaches, involving the transfer of functions between NHS and local government bodies, have become more common.
- Government policies to strengthen competition in health and social care have created additional challenges for partnership working, not least of which are the contrasting aims and principles of the private 'for profit', voluntary and public sectors.
- The voluntary sector is an important player in health and social care, and in public health. It is both an advocate of policy and a provider of services. Efforts to strengthen partnership with the sector must recognise this 'dual role'.
- Much more needs to be done to involve the public, patients and carers in the commissioning, planning and delivery of health services. These efforts must address the cultural and political barriers to their involvement.

Key questions

1. What kinds of partnership exist in the health policy arena?
2. Should local government take over responsibility for commissioning all health services?
3. What are the strengths and weaknesses of health and wellbeing boards?
4. In what sense is the 'for profit' private sector now a partner in health and care provision?
5. Is the voluntary sector in danger of becoming merely an 'arm' of the state in health in health and social care?
6. What can be done to strengthen PPI?

nine

Health policy in Scotland, Wales and Northern Ireland

Overview

Health policy varies across the different countries of the UK. New devolved governance arrangements have increased the scope for such policy variation. This chapter discusses these constitutional changes in the context of health policy. It examines health policy and policy processes in Scotland, Wales and Northern Ireland. It also compares policy outcomes and explores the scope for policy learning.

Differences in health policy between the countries of the UK existed before the introduction of devolved governance in the late 1990s (see Levitt and Wall, 1984; Webster, 1996; Stewart, 2004; Woods, 2004). The NHS in Scotland was governed by separate legislation and fell within the responsibilities of the Secretary of State for Scotland and the Scottish Office. Although broadly adopting the policies of the UK government, Scotland had some leeway in how it organised the NHS. In 1974, for example, it established unified health boards responsible for family health services as well as hospital and community health services. Wales, meanwhile, began to enjoy a measure of administrative devolution for the NHS in the late 1960s, extended further in 1974 when responsibility for all health services was delegated to the Secretary of State for Wales (Webster, 1996). Until the early 1970s, Northern Ireland had responsibility for health services under Home Rule arrangements. It had its own Parliament and government. These arrangements were suspended due to civil conflict in the Province (known as 'the Troubles'). Northern Ireland was from then on subject to direct rule from the UK government.

However, a high degree of administrative devolution was allowed in the field of health policy, under the stewardship of the Northern Ireland Office.

Political and cultural differences were also relevant prior to devolution. For example, Scotland is regarded as having powerful medical elites (Greer, 2009). Scotland and Wales both have strong socialist traditions, embedded within their political cultures. Such factors may explain discernible differences in policy implementation on issues where the UK government was not strongly committed or was disinterested (Woods, 2004). For example, both Wales and Scotland were able to prioritise public health in the 1980s, a time when the UK government was less engaged with these issues (Greer, 2009). Indeed, in some areas of policy and organisation, the countries of the UK demonstrated innovative approaches. Examples include the pioneering approach to services for people with learning disabilities in Wales (Drakeford, 2006), Scotland's experience of managed clinical networks in promoting collaboration, and the establishment of joint health and social service boards in Northern Ireland.

Devolution

Although it is impossible to give here a detailed account of the history and politics of devolution in the UK (see Bogdanor, 2001; Mitchell and Mitchell, 2011), a brief outline of recent changes is necessary. An elected Scottish Parliament was established in 1999 and was granted wide competencies and powers, including the right to make primary and secondary legislation on a wide range of matters, including health, education, justice, rural affairs and the environment. Other areas of policy are reserved for the UK Parliament and include defence, immigration and foreign policy. The Scottish Parliament was also given powers, as yet unused, to vary basic Income Tax levels by up to 3 percentage points. Scotland's fiscal powers were extended in 2012 to include setting Income Tax rates (from 2016), powers to set new taxes, and devolution of other existing taxes.

The Scottish government (until 2007, the Scottish executive) exercises executive power on behalf of Parliament and is accountable to it. It is headed by a first minister who works alongside Cabinet secretaries and ministers (including a deputy first minister) with various departmental and cross-government responsibilities. These positions are held by members of the Scottish Parliament (MSPs) drawn from the governing party (or parties). The secretaries and ministers direct and oversee the work of the directorates, staffed by civil servants, which implement the policies of the Scottish government.

Although Scotland has acquired substantial self-governing powers, a strong body of opinion in the country desires independence from the UK. This policy has been pursued by the Scottish Nationalist Party (SNP), which has governed in Scotland since 2007. In 2014, a referendum was held on Scottish independence, which produced a narrow majority against independence. The strength of the nationalist vote, however, coupled with the SNP's spectacular performance at the 2015 General Election (winning all but three seats in Scotland and becoming the third largest party at Westminster), increased pressure for greater devolution of powers. At the time of writing, proposals to extend these powers are being considered under the auspices of an independent body, the Smith Commission (see www.smith-commission.scot).

In Wales, a National Assembly was elected in 1999. Initially, it could only pass secondary legislation in certain policy areas (including agriculture, environment, health, housing, education and local government) within the constraints of primary legislation passed by Westminster. Following the Government of Wales Act 2006, the Welsh Assembly acquired limited powers to initiate legislation. Its law-making powers were further extended following a referendum in 2011, giving the Welsh Assembly the power to make primary legislation in 20 areas of policy competence. A review subsequently recommended more devolutionary powers over policy and fiscal matters, along Scottish lines (Commission on Devolution in Wales, 2014). So far, only the fiscal measures have been enacted (in the Wales Act 2014), and some of these require approval (by the UK Parliament or a Welsh referendum) before they can come into force.

In contrast to Scotland's Parliament, the Welsh Assembly was given parliamentary and executive functions. It later distinguished these functions by designating a Welsh Assembly government to exercise executive power on its behalf, with the Assembly holding it to account (Jeffrey, 2006). This separation is now formalised, and the executive body is now known officially as the Welsh government. The Welsh government consists of a first minister, nominated by the Assembly, who appoints Cabinet ministers and deputy ministers. All are Assembly members drawn from the party (or parties) able to form a government, They direct and oversee the Welsh government administration, which implements policy.

As earlier noted, Northern Ireland had previously possessed legislative and executive powers, until the 1970s. In 1999, following the Good Friday Agreement of the previous year, devolved powers were restored. A new elected Assembly with primary legislative powers, and a 'power-sharing' executive (containing representatives from multiple political parties) were established. These arrangements were suspended on several occasions amid growing distrust between the sectarian political parties, notably between 2002 and 2007, during which direct rule was re-instated. Devolved government has continued since 2007.

UK governments have also explored regional devolution within England. The only instance of political powers being devolved so far is in London, with the Greater London Authority (consisting of a directly elected mayor and the London Assembly). The London mayor has a specific duty in law to promote the health of Londoners, and has acquired responsibility to prepare a health inequality strategy and to reduce health inequalities. Although he has no statutory powers, funding or functions regarding health or health services, he is able to influence the NHS and other bodies by forging partnerships and highlighting specific health problems and possible solutions. The mayor has powers in some areas (such as transport and economic development), which can be used to improve public health, but for the most part, the mayor operates by exhortation, in particular by identifying problems, setting out strategies and providing a lead for other agencies (Hunter et al, 2005). In recent years there has been interest in devolving powers to other regions and cities, including health and social services (see Chapter Eight).

It is not surprising that observers describe devolution in the UK as 'lopsided' (Jeffrey, 2006). Devolved governments vary in their powers and responsibilities, and also differ in their political culture and organisation. It is therefore difficult to generalise about the impact of devolution, even in a specific policy area such as health.

Devolution and health

Health policy is an important arena for devolved governments (Woods, 2002, 2004; Jervis and Plowden, 2003). Health expenditure accounts for a larger proportion of the devolved budgets of Scotland, Wales and Northern Ireland than the UK as a whole, largely because they have fewer areas of budgetary responsibility (Timmins, 2013). These countries also face bigger health problems than England (as measured by rates of illness, mortality rates and other health indicators).

Greer (2009) commented that the extent of policy divergence since devolution has been an uncomfortable surprise for many. Observers have found significant policy innovation in many policy areas, including health (Keating, 2005; Adams and Schmuecker, 2006). Lessons can be learned from different approaches. However, policy variation is often rhetorical. Leaders of devolved governments and assemblies are keen to emphasise their differences from England, as reflected in Welsh First Minister Rhodri Morgan's call for 'clear red water', distancing the Welsh government from Westminster (Morgan, 2003). Actual policy differences may be smaller (see Adams and Schmuecker, 2006). Indeed, as Smith and Hellowell (2012) have argued, the similarities of the four systems are greater than the differences. In all four parts of the UK, health services are funded mainly by public expenditure from general taxation, largely delivered by public providers, are comprehensive and mostly free at the point of use. Moreover, there are countervailing pressures that promote convergence across the UK, and that have constrained policy options for devolved governments.

Nonetheless, most attention has been on policy diversity. Differences can occur as a result of several factors (see Keating, 2005; Adams and Schmuecker, 2006; Jeffrey, 2006; Greer, 2009):

- *Different political cultures and parties* (Adams and Schmuecker, 2006; Timmins, 2013). Scotland and Wales have a stronger socialist tradition than England and Northern Ireland. Northern Ireland is dominated by sectarian political parties. In Wales and Scotland, competition for office has been between parties on the left of the political spectrum (between Labour and the nationalist parties), who have a strong commitment to state intervention and the public sector. This contrasts with England, where competition is between left and right (and arguably between parties of the centre and the right). In Wales and Scotland, political debate tends to be about the nature of state intervention rather than the classic 'state versus market' debate, producing greater potential for policy differences with England.
- *Different electoral systems and coalition governments* (see Keating, 2005). The use of proportional representation in elections for the devolved assemblies avoids the exaggerated majorities usually produced by Westminster 'first past the post' elections. This means that governing parties in Scotland and Wales tend to adopt a consensual approach to policy-making. Given the left-oriented nature of party competition and political debate noted above, this reinforces the potential for policy differences with England, especially when the Conservatives hold power in Westminster. Divergence is further encouraged where, as in both Scotland and Wales, parties on the left have entered into coalitions in order to form a government. True, the UK government was run by a coalition between 2010 and 2015. While this may have moderated some aspects of policy in England (as indicated by the Liberal Democrats' efforts to dilute some aspects of the Health and Social Care Bill), it did not alter the direction of travel.
- *Different policy networks* (Greer, 2009). Differences in policy networks – the clusters of interest groups that engage with government on policy – reinforce the impact of electoral and party factors. In both Scotland and Wales, policy networks have tended to promote consensus and stability, and have advocated distinctive policy approaches, detailed later in this chapter.
- *Constitutional autonomy.* Devolution arrangements have placed few levers or controls in the hands of the UK government. The Scottish Parliament has one of the widest 'competences' of any devolved government in Europe (Keating, 2005), and is expected to extend its powers. Wales now has greater

powers of self-government. The Northern Ireland situation is more difficult to assess because it has enjoyed substantial formal powers, but these have been suspended in times of crisis. Notably, the UK government has made little or no attempt to set minimum standards in areas that fall within the competence of the devolved governments (Adams and Schmuecker, 2006).

- *Financial discretion.* The devolved governments receive funds in the form of block grants from the UK government. This can largely be spent at the discretion of the devolved government. This gives the UK government little influence over how funds are spent, and has been described as 'uniquely permissive' (Keating, 2005).

But these factors are counterbalanced by others that produce convergence:

- Although the competences of devolved assemblies and governments are widely drawn, the UK government has reserved powers in a number of important policy areas. Even in policy areas where devolved assemblies can legislate, certain matters are still reserved. For example, in health, these areas include regulation of medicines and professional standards. In addition, some professional contracts are agreed at the national level, including those of hospital consultants and GPs. Furthermore, the UK government retains responsibility for key policy areas that have an impact on health. The most important of these is social security, which (with the exception of Northern Ireland) can restrict devolved governments' ability to devise policies for vulnerable groups such as elderly people, mentally ill people and those with learning disabilities (see Keating, 2005; Fawcett, 2005). In addition, the UK still operates a common foreign policy, a common market in goods and services, and a single labour market, all of which promote convergence. The tax system is also fairly uniform, although, as noted above, some flexibility has been agreed for devolved governments.
- The EU is also a force for convergence (Greer, 2004; Woods, 2004; Keating, 2005; see also Chapter Ten). It sets a common regulatory framework across all member states, which affects devolved governments. As will become clear in the next chapter, EU institutions have taken an increasing interest in health policy. On EU matters, the devolved governments tend to liaise very closely with Whitehall in order to produce a common front (see Jeffrey, 2005).
- Inter-government coordination (IGC). Although IGC is formalised on matters relating to the EU, it is otherwise weak (Adams and Schmuecker, 2006; Greer and Trench, 2010). Joint ministerial committees do coordinate policy across the governments of the UK, including health policy, but are regarded with marginal importance (Woods, 2004; Greer and Trench, 2010). For the most part, coordination and conflict resolution is undertaken

informally through officials from the various devolved governments, or through political channels, via ministers. The latter approach was relatively effective when the Labour Party simultaneously governed Wales (initially as a coalition partner with the Lib Dems, and then as majority party), Scotland (in coalition with the Lib Dems), and the UK as a whole (Jeffrey, 2006). But more recently, governments in the UK have been run by different parties (between 2010 and 2015 there was a Conservative–Liberal Democrat coalition in Westminster, an SNP government in Scotland, a Labour government in Wales and a Sinn Fein/Democratic Unionist Party-led governing coalition in Northern Ireland).

- A further constraint is public opinion (Greer, 2005). Although public opinion in Scotland, Wales and Northern Ireland broadly supports devolved governance, it remains attached to notions of equality and solidarity (Adams and Schmuecker, 2006) that have strong resonance in the health field. Indeed (and despite some re-branding of the NHS in Scotland and Wales), the public and the media still regard the NHS as a national institution, and will not tolerate inequities in services between the different parts of the UK. Hence, Scottish and Welsh governments faced enormous public pressures to change policy in light of the waiting time health targets adopted in England (Bevan and Hood, 2006; Drakeford, 2006).

- England continues to dominate policy development and debate. In part this is a legacy, reflecting stronger capacities for policy-making in Whitehall prior to devolution. It is also a reflection of the power of the London-based media, and the pressure group system, which, despite some refocusing on the devolved governments and assemblies, remains strongly oriented towards Whitehall and Westminster. Other factors underpinning this continued domination have been identified (Keating, 2005; Adams and Schmuecker, 2006), including the fact that England still has the vast majority of the UK population (around 85 per cent), and remains the dominant economic power within the UK. Another unifying factor is that the UK Department of Health is much larger and better resourced than its counterparts in Scotland, Wales and Northern Ireland. The devolved governments sometimes follow its lead when there are no major differences, and benefit from its resources and work (Greer and Trench, 2010). There is also some reliance on the expertise of English regulatory bodies (such as NICE and CQC).

- The final source of convergence is that health systems within the UK are facing similar pressures and problems (Smith and Hellowell, 2012; Timmins, 2013): austerity in public finances, rising demands for healthcare, increasing public health problems and inequalities, the imperative to improve care quality and safety, the quest for greater efficiency, the need to coordinate health and social care, and so on. Although specific approaches adopted differ in style and content, the menu of realistic policy options is restricted and inhibits divergence.

Devolution and health policy in Scotland

Policy-makers and processes

Health and social care in Scotland falls within the ministerial responsibilities of the Cabinet Secretary for Health, Wellbeing and Sport, a senior member of the Scottish government. The minister is supported by a Minister for Public Health and a Minister for Sport, Health Improvement and Mental Health, responsible for these areas of work. Scottish health ministers are accountable to the Scottish Parliament for the NHS (branded as NHS Scotland) in much the same way as the Secretary of State for Health is at Westminster. Moreover, they are responsible for a number of special health authorities and agencies (including the Scottish Ambulance Service and Healthcare Improvement Scotland, discussed further below).

Ministers must answer PQs and respond to parliamentary debates. There is also a parliamentary committee (Health and Sport Committee) that scrutinises policy and administration in health and social care. This Committee has a wider remit and greater formal powers than its counterpart at Westminster. As well as investigating policy issues and commissioning its own research, it scrutinises legislation, and can bring forward its own legislative proposals. It can also consider petitions within its remit, submitted by members of the public.

The Scottish government is smaller than the UK government and has fewer responsibilities. This facilitates a more 'joined-up' approach to policy-making (Stewart, 2004). It also encourages a more informal policy style, a point discussed further below. Smaller government can have disadvantages, however. The Scottish government is said to lack capacity in policy-making, partly due to the historical legacy of administrative devolution under the Scottish Office, which focused on implementation rather than policy formation (Keating, 2005). Nonetheless, it has tried to strengthen capacity by reorganising administrative structures and focusing on the delivery of key objectives. In 2007, the SNP government replaced the departmental structure of the Scottish executive with directorates. The health and social care directorates, overseen by a director of health and social care (who is also the chief executive of NHS Scotland) are: health and healthcare improvement; healthcare workforce and performance; health finance and information; health and social care integration; children and families; Commonwealth games and sport; CMO and public health;

and Chief Nursing Officer, patients, public and health professions. Each is headed by a director, and the last two directorates are led by the CMO and Chief Nursing Officer respectively. The rationale behind this change was to produce a stronger emphasis on strategic objectives while strengthening future policy development.

Another key development was the adoption of a new national performance framework. In 2007, the Scottish government set out five strategic objectives (see Scottish Government, 2015). A national performance framework for all five national objectives was established, alongside high-level 'purpose targets' and national outcomes. To measure progress, national indicators were also set. Health featured strongly in this framework. One of the strategic objectives was 'helping people to sustain and improve their health, especially in disadvantaged communities, ensuring better, local and faster access to healthcare.' 'Increased healthy life expectancy' by 2017 was one of the purpose targets. 'Longer healthier lives' was identified as a national outcome. Health indicators constituted over a quarter of the original national indicators. The performance framework has since been modified, and there are now 16 national outcome targets and 50 national indicators. The current indicators cover a range of issues, including smoking, emergency admissions and mental wellbeing.

In addition, the Scottish NHS has its own performance framework. HEAT targets, annually agreed by the Scottish government, cover four areas: **H**ealth improvement; **E**fficiency and governance; **A**ccess to services; and **T**reatment appropriate to individuals. HEAT sets objectives to be achieved by a particular deadline. Examples include increasing the number of child healthy weight interventions, meeting threshold targets for A&E waiting times and achieving discharge deadlines for hospital patients. The extent to which targets have been achieved is discussed further below.

Policy participants have commented on the consensual and inclusive nature of the Scottish policy-making process (Baggott, 2007). This is partly due to the nature of Scottish political debate, which, as earlier noted, means debates are less ideologically polarised between left and right. The electoral system adopted (a form of proportional representation) also plays its part by increasing the probability of coalition and minority governments. Even when a majority government is formed, its majority is generally smaller than under the first past the post system of elections.

The predominant consultative and consensual policy style is particularly noticeable in relationships between government and pressure groups. The limited policy-making capacity of Scottish government has placed value on constructive relationships with such groups with the knowledge and expertise to contribute to policy development and implementation (Adams and Schmuecker, 2006). Professional groups, and in particular, the medical profession, enjoy a close relationship with government and exert great influence (Greer, 2009). In general, devolution has affected the pressure group system in Scotland. Groups have responded with 'territorial differentiation'. They have reoriented their lobbying efforts and organisational structures towards the new devolved governing bodies (Keating, 2005; Jeffrey, 2006). In the health policy arena, organisations representing health professionals and workers now have separate structures for dealing with devolved governments, including UNISON, RCN and some Royal Medical Colleges. Health charities have also introduced changes to reflect devolution. For example, the Parkinson's Disease Society now has a team of officers working full time on Scottish issues (and a similar group working on Welsh matters).

Structures and organisations

The current structure of the NHS in Scotland differs significantly from England. Fourteen geographically based health boards are responsible for both the planning and provision of primary care, community health and hospital services. Social services are provided by 32 local authorities. Local authorities are represented on health boards. In addition, Scotland experimented with direct elections for health boards, but this proved unsuccessful in improving democracy and accountability, and the policy was abandoned (Greer et al, 2014b).

Scotland has made considerable efforts to join up and integrate health and care policies, especially for groups that require preventive interventions, healthcare and social care (such as elderly people, for example). In 2007, the Cabinet Health Secretary acquired responsibility for adult social services. In 2003, community planning partnerships (CPPs), led by local authorities, were created to plan and coordinate public services and partnership working between local agencies (including the NHS, private and voluntary sectors). Part of their remit is to draw up local plans that include health improvement, reducing health inequalities and improving social care. In addition, community health partnerships (CHPs) were established in 2005, under health boards, to coordinate different health providers. In some areas social care providers were included in these arrangements (and named community health and care partnerships, CHCPs). Following evidence that levels of service integration were being met (Watt, 2010; Audit Scotland, 2011, 2013), CHPs and CHCPs were replaced by a more integrated system of health and social care partnerships (HSCPs), for which the health boards and local authorities are held jointly responsible. Health boards and councils must establish local arrangements to plan, resource and deliver integrated services for health and social care, and have to meet joint outcomes (see Steel, 2013 for further discussion of integrated care in Scotland).

A number of other NHS Scotland bodies should also be mentioned. Healthcare Improvement Scotland inspects and regulates healthcare organisations. It is similar to the CQC, although differs in a number of ways. It provides more support in quality improvement, and provides clinical standards and guidelines (tasks undertaken by NICE in England). However, unlike CQC, it does not regulate social care (in Scotland this task is undertaken by the Care Inspectorate). Healthcare Improvement Scotland incorporates other bodies, such as the Scottish Medicines Consortium (SMC), which makes recommendations to NHS boards on whether newly licensed drugs should be made available by the NHS in Scotland. Other key advisory bodies within Healthcare Improvement Scotland are: the Scottish Health Technologies Group, which provides advice on the clinical and cost-effectiveness of healthcare technologies, and the Scottish Intercollegiate Guidelines Network, which develops evidence-based clinical guidelines for NHS Scotland. Another relevant body is the Scottish Health Council, which was established in 2005 to promote patient focus and public involvement in the NHS. This body is constituted as a subcommittee of Healthcare Improvement Scotland, but has its own identity. It has local offices in each health board area, and provides support for independent scrutiny panels that consider major changes in local NHS services in Scotland.

Policies

Devolution has affected the way Scottish policies have developed, distinguishing them from other parts of the UK, notably England. Differences include the following (see Stewart, 2004; Greer, 2009; Steel, 2013; Timmins, 2013; Bevan et al, 2014):

- A strong emphasis on collaboration, both within the NHS and between health and social care, which has been embodied in key reports and documents (Kerr, 2005; Scottish Government, 2007a, 2007b), and through structures and networks such as CPPs, CHPs, CHCPs, HSCPs and managed clinical networks.
- Free long-term personal care for the elderly. Scotland decided to use public funds to cover the cost of personal as well as nursing care, as recommended by the Royal Commission on Long-Term Care (DH, 1999a). This is a major departure from the policy pursued elsewhere in the UK, where only free nursing care is funded by the government (see **Box 9.1**).
- Abolition of NHS charges. In Scotland, eye and dental checks are free. This contrasts with the rest of the UK (although entitlements to free checks are wider in Wales than in England and Northern Ireland). Prescriptions are also free. This policy was adopted first by Wales in 2007, then by Northern

Ireland in 2010, and Scotland in 2011. Prescription charges remain in England, although there are exemptions for children, elderly people and for people with some chronic medical conditions (for example, cancer or epilepsy). In Scotland (and Wales) parking charges at NHS hospitals have been abolished, except where there is an existing contractual requirement to charge (for example, at PFI hospitals).

• Mental health reform. Scotland engaged in a root-and-branch reform of mental health legislation in 2003. These pioneering changes were based on human rights principles, were broadly welcomed and introduced in a spirit of consensus (Darjee and Crichton, 2004). In contrast, attempts to change the law in England and Wales were much more controversial and were blocked by professional bodies, patients' groups and mental health charities because of their lack of attention to patients' rights. The UK government subsequently amended existing legislation in 2007, thus avoiding radical reform (although Wales has since passed additional rights legislation using its devolved powers).

• Scottish health policy has placed a higher priority on public health and health promotion than England (Scottish Office, 1991, 1992; Scottish Office, 1999; Scottish Executive, 2000, 2003a, 2003b, 2004). Specifically, Scotland was ahead of England in adopting a strategy on health inequalities, as well as programmes promoting healthy eating and physical exercise. It introduced joint public health plans for the NHS and local government at an earlier stage. Scotland introduced a smoking ban in public places earlier than the rest of the UK. It was also the first part of the UK to adopt a policy of minimum unit pricing for alcohol, although this measure is currently the subject of proceedings in the European Court to test its legality. In 2014, both the Northern Ireland Executive and the Welsh government backed this policy, whereas the UK government, after initially endorsing the measure in 2012, subsequently dropped it.

Box 9.1: Free personal care in Scotland

The provision of free personal care has been a popular policy (Bell et al, 2007; Independent Review of Free Personal and Nursing Care in Scotland, 2008; Audit Scotland, 2008). Although broadly well-implemented, some problems have come to light, including inconsistencies in charging and eligibility between different local authorities, the operation of waiting lists, and weaknesses in future planning (Audit Scotland, 2008). There have also been negative consequences for younger disabled people needing care who are not covered by the scheme (Bell et al, 2007). In addition, the policy has faced criticism for its costs, which rose from around £220 million in 2003/04 to over £450 million in 2012/13 (National Statistics, 2014). In the context of public expenditure constraints imposed by the coalition government in Westminster, which had a knock-on effect on the devolved government budgets, this fuelled fears that the system may be unsustainable. The SNP government has continued the policy and provided additional resources, but there are increasing calls to dilute the policy by introducing charges and/or stricter eligibility criteria.

As suggested earlier, much policy variation on health matters has occurred as a result of not pursuing or discontinuing policies formulated in England, such as the commissioner–provider split, the creation of foundation trusts and PBR (Stewart, 2004; Woods, 2004; Bevan et al, 2014). The Scottish government has had a more distant relationship with the independent sector. It did not adopt a programme of ISTCs as in England, nor has it opened the NHS in Scotland to the same degree of competition. Indeed, private commercial companies are banned from holding primary care contracts and hospital cleaning and catering contracts (Smith and Hellowell, 2012). However, NHS patients can be treated in private hospitals as a short-term means of reducing waiting times. There have also been longer-term NHS contracts with the independent sector in some areas of specialist care. PFI-style arrangements have been used for capital projects in the Scottish NHS, but not as extensively as in England. With regard to social care, the picture is very similar to England, as the majority of residential care is now provided by the independent sector, which also increasingly provides home care services (Audit Scotland, 2012).

Scotland has also shifted on some issues. Although a performance management regime was introduced for the Scottish NHS, unlike England, it avoided giving institutions a simple 'star rating' based on performance (which England subsequently dropped). However, following criticism of the performance of the NHS in Scotland, new waiting time targets were introduced in 2004 for inpatient treatment and outpatient consultations. Targets for reducing delayed discharges and emergency inpatient admissions of elderly people were also set. Specific waiting times for diagnostic services and for treatment for specific conditions were introduced (for cataracts, for example).

The national performance framework, introduced in 2007 and described earlier, led to a more comprehensive and systematic approach. Health targets and indicators are now linked into a broader system of performance management, which incorporates the health dimension into other public policy areas (for example, by encouraging walking and cycling in transport policy). The Scottish waiting time targets and standards have become progressively more challenging since they were introduced, and are now broadly similar to England, although there are some notable differences. The Scottish NHS retained access targets for general practice, dropped in

England by the coalition government. Scotland also introduced a challenging treatment time guarantee whereby 100 per cent of patients must wait no longer than 12 weeks from when the patient has been diagnosed and agreed to inpatient or day case treatment. It should also be noted that targets are not enforced in the same way through 'targets and terror' (see Chapter Seven). Even so, Scotland has not escaped the adverse consequences of the target culture – a major scandal occurred in the Lothian region where waiting lists were manipulated to meet targets (File on 4, 2012).

Devolution and health policy in Wales

Policy-makers and processes

The policy process in Wales bears some similarities to Scotland, but exhibits important differences. Like Scotland, Welsh political debate is to the left of England, and is similarly underpinned by competition between parties of the left rather than on a left–right axis (Drakeford, 2006; Timmins, 2013). Like Scotland, the electoral system for the Welsh Assembly uses a form of proportional representation, which inhibits large governing majorities. This, coupled with the creation of the Welsh Assembly as a corporate body, promoted an informal and consensual approach to policy-making (although, as noted, there is now a formal distinction between the Welsh government and the Assembly). Informality is further encouraged by the small, close-knit nature of Welsh political culture and institutions (McLelland, 2002). A consultative approach is, as in Scotland, partly a consequence of the lack of policy-making capacity of Welsh institutions and their reliance on outside expertise.

The Labour Party currently governs Wales. It remains a more traditional 'old Labour' Party than its counterpart in England, and its leaders have made great efforts to distinguish Welsh policy from that of England, as reflected by the 'clear red water' rhetoric mentioned earlier. The Welsh Assembly lacks the legislative and fiscal powers of the Scottish Parliament, although these have been extended. Wales also lacks the strong professional policy networks of England and Scotland (Greer, 2009) – notably, medical elites are not as powerful as in Scotland, and this has allowed other players to exert influence, such as trade unions and local government interests.

Within the Welsh government, the Minister of Health and Social Services is responsible for the health policy and the NHS, supported by a deputy minister who focuses on social care services. Ministers oversee the Department of Health and Social Services, which implements policy, manages and supports the delivery of health and social care services. The Department is divided into divisions, including: corporate services and partnerships; workforce; finance; nursing (headed by the Chief Nursing Officer for Wales); the CMO/Medical Director's division; and social services and integration. Its administrative head is the director general of health and social services, who also holds the post of the chief executive of the NHS in Wales (known as NHS Wales). Health services are delivered through a number of all–Wales bodies and local health boards (see below). Social care is the responsibility of local authorities.

Parliamentary scrutiny of health and related matters in Wales is undertaken by the Health and Social Care Committee, a subject committee of the Welsh Assembly. Its membership is drawn from all parties, approximately in proportion to their representation in the Assembly. Its functions include scrutiny of legislation, holding ministers and health and social service bodies to account, and scrutinising health and social service budgets. It also undertakes reviews of issues and policies (see, for example, Health and Social Care Committee, 2013), and makes recommendations on future policy and service development.

Structures and organisations

The current structure of the NHS in Wales was established in 2009 (Longley et al, 2012). Prior to this, health services were commissioned by 22 local health boards, whose boundaries were coterminous with local authorities. Most health services other than primary care were provided by NHS trusts. The new structure created seven larger local health boards responsible for both the planning and delivery of hospital, community and primary health services. Three All Wales organisations continue to operate as NHS trusts: Welsh Ambulance Service (which includes NHS Direct Wales), Public Health Wales (the expert national public health body) and Velindre NHS Trust (which provides a range of specialist services at local, regional and national level, including cancer services and the Welsh Blood Service, and which hosts a number of other national organisations, discussed below). Specialist care is commissioned by the Welsh Health Specialised Services Committee (accountable to local health boards).

Other bodies also support and/or regulate the NHS in Wales. The NHS Wales Shared Services Partnership provides support services (such as employment services, legal advice, counter-fraud services, procurement, specialist estates and workforce development services). It is an independent organisation, but owned and directed by NHS Wales, and hosted by Velindre NHS Trust. Other services hosted by the Velindre NHS Trust include the NHS Wales Informatics Service and the National Institute for Social Care and Health Research Clinical Research Centre. Hosted organisations have their own board and are not directly accountable to the Trust but to the

Welsh government. Wales has its own healthcare regulator, Health Care Inspectorate Wales. The regulation of social care is undertaken by a separate body, the Care and Social Services Inspectorate.

Wales has its own system of patient and public involvement. Community Health Councils (CHCs) (which were abolished in England in 2003) were retained in Wales and given more powers to inspect and review health services, assist patients with complaints and to be consulted on service changes. With regard to the setting of standards and assessment of cost-effectiveness of interventions, Wales relies heavily on guidance and advice from NICE. However, there is an All Wales Medicines Strategy Group that advises the Welsh government on medicines management and prescribing, including the use of new drugs.

Integration

The integration of health services, social care and public health has been a major priority in Wales for some years. This is underpinned by joint statutory duties on local health boards and local authorities. From 2003, both were required to formulate joint health, social care and wellbeing strategies for their area. These (and other local plans) have been superseded by a single integrated wellbeing plan that covers a wider range of community and public service issues for each local authority area. It should also be noted that in Wales, local authorities have representation on health boards (unlike CCGs in England). Another factor has been the development of multiagency locality networks, involving GPs, community health services, social care and other relevant agencies (Longley, 2013). These networks provide a foundation for local service planning. Their aim is to plan, coordinate and develop out-of-hospital services (including home-based care), and to promote the integration of health and social care services.

The organisation of the NHS has largely supported a collaborative approach (Welsh Assembly Government, 2005), bolstered by the 2009 reorganisation. There was concern, however, that the reorganisation meant that health boards and local authorities no longer had the same boundaries (which tends to improve, although does not guarantee, collaboration). Even so, the boundaries of the new health boards do not cut across different local authority areas, and on balance, the reorganisation appears to have been conducive rather than harmful to collaboration.

Policies

Traditionally, the Welsh and English NHS have had strong similarities. However, the efforts of the Welsh Assembly and government to pursue a distinctive approach have widened policy differences. The main variations can be summarised as follows (see Drakeford, 2006; Longley et al, 2012; Longley, 2013):

- Welsh health policy has long prioritised public health, health inequalities and health promotion to a far greater degree than in England. Public health priorities were established in the late 1980s, earlier than England. Welsh policy-makers have also emphasised more strongly the importance of socioeconomic factors in ill health (Welsh Office, 1989, 1998; Welsh Assembly Government, 2002, 2003, 2009; Welsh Government, 2014). Wales has pioneered some specific policies (notably, it was the first country of the UK to commit to a ban on smoking in cars where children are present). It is also at the forefront of moves to introduce 'Health in All Policies', requiring all public bodies to contribute to health objectives. Wales also established a national public health service before England.
- As noted above, health policy-makers in Wales have placed great emphasis on partnership, collaboration and integration. Joint plans for health and wellbeing (including social care) were introduced earlier than in England. There have also been efforts to join up health and social care. However, in practice, partnership working has not operated as intended, and there remains scope for improvement (NLIAH, 2009; Longley, 2013).
- As noted, Wales retained CHCs, the local patients' watchdogs in the NHS, which were abolished in England (see above).
- Prescription charges in Wales were initially abolished for people under 25 and frozen for those who had to pay them. Free prescriptions were extended to all in 2007, a move since followed by Northern Ireland and Scotland. Wales has more generous exemptions from dental examination charges than England and Northern Ireland (but not Scotland). A free eye care service exists in Wales for groups at risk of developing serious eye diseases. Most Welsh NHS hospitals, as in Scotland, do not charge for parking.

Wales took a different approach to performance management in the NHS than England. It did not introduce star ratings. Targets were set for health services, but were not as demanding as in England or Scotland. For example, while *The NHS Plan* for England in 2000 set out to reduce waiting times to six months for inpatients, the corresponding Welsh target at the time was 18 months. However, criticism of the performance of the Welsh NHS with regard to waiting times led to tougher waiting time targets in the mid-2000s (Wales Audit Office, 2006). Although these were tightened further, the main access target was less challenging than England (that at least 95 per cent of patients waiting to start treatment must have waited less than 26 weeks from referral to treatment). However, this was supplemented by a second target which sought to ensure that all patients would be treated within 36 weeks. In 2014, a new approach was proposed, focusing on clinical outcomes rather than achievement of time-based targets.

The NHS planning framework in Wales is now focused much more on improving performance. There are regular quality and delivery meetings with NHS organisations, and measures to address poor performance, including development teams to improve local services and regional intervention to reconfigure hospital services. The approach has come closer to England, following criticism of access and quality of services (Longley, 2013). The Welsh government sets out annual requirements and standards, which includes targets covering service quality, access, efficiency and mortality reduction. Some targets are set centrally in line with national priorities; others are agreed locally. But although there has been a much stronger emphasis on targets and performance indicators in recent years, it is generally understood that these are still not enforced as strictly as in England (Bevan et al, 2014).

Even so, the Welsh government continues to reject reforms adopted in England. It has resisted adopting the English system of PBR, although there has been some support in Wales for greater incentives in the health system, including the development of standard tariffs for services. The Welsh government was also opposed to extending patient choice along English lines. Wales rejected foundation trusts and subsequently opted for integrated health boards. PFI has been used in Wales, although restrictions were imposed that made the schemes less attractive to consortia (for example, by excluding lucrative services from contracts). Some services (such as cleaning, for example) have been brought back into public provision. Furthermore, in 2007 the Welsh government ruled out PFI for future health services. Meanwhile, the private health sector has not been used for NHS-funded operations to the same extent as in England, due to the hostility of the Welsh government.

Devolution and health policy in Northern Ireland

Policy-makers and processes

Health policy in Northern Ireland is the responsibility of the Department of Health, Social Services and Public Safety (DHSSPS), which is responsible for health services, public health, social services, fire services and emergency planning. The Department is headed by a minister who sits on the Northern Ireland executive and is a member of the Assembly. The minister is supported by civil servants, including the permanent secretary of the Department, who is also the chief executive of the health and social care system. The

Department has a dual structure consisting of administrative divisions (for example, healthcare policy, resources and performance, social services policy, health estates investment and the Office of the CMO) and professional groups (medical, social services, dentistry, pharmaceutical, and nursing, midwifery and allied professions). It should be noted that the professional groups advise other departments and agencies on health matters, as well as the DHSSPS.

The Department is a policy and strategic body. According to a recent report (Donaldson et al, 2014), it is now more focused on policy support for the minister, and less involved in the central direction of the NHS and social care bodies. At the time of writing, central government reforms in Northern Ireland are being considered, and it is likely that the Department will change its name to reflect its wider role in promoting public health and wellbeing across government.

The Department is held to account by a statutory committee of the Northern Ireland Assembly, the Committee for Health, Social Services and Public Policy. This examines the departmental budget and scrutinises legislation. It initiates inquiries and makes reports on issues within the departmental remit, and considers matters referred by the minister.

Structures and organisations

Since 1973, Northern Ireland has had an integrated structure for health and social services (Heenan, 2013). The current structure, dating from 2009, consists of a health and social care board, which oversees the health and social care system, and allocates funding, implements performance management and service improvement, and supports the work of local commissioning bodies and holds them to account (Gray and Birrell, 2013; O'Neill et al, 2012). There are five local commissioning groups, constituted as committees of the health and social care board, each covering a specific geographical area. These are responsible for assessing health and social care needs, planning services and securing delivery. Services are provided by five health and social care trusts that cover the same geographical areas as the local commissioning groups. In addition, the Northern Ireland Ambulance Trust provides service across the country.

There are a number of other Northern Ireland-wide bodies as well, including the Business Services Organisation, which provides a wide range of support functions and specialist professional services to health and social care organisations. The Public Health Agency was established in 2009 to improve health and wellbeing, protect health, support commissioning and policy development and undertake research and development functions. Other Northern Ireland bodies include the Regulation and Quality Improvement Authority, which regulates and inspects all statutory and independent health and social care services, including children's social services. The Patient and Client Council represents the views of the public on health and social care services, and seeks to ensure that these views are taken into account by health and social care organisations, promotes PPI in planning, commissioning and delivery of health and social care, assists people with complaints, and promotes the provision of advice and information to the public about health and social care services.

Policies

Under both direct rule and devolved arrangements, health policy-making in the province has been cautious and gradual (Greer, 2005; Heenan, 2013). In periods of direct rule, UK ministers did not want further controversy by introducing radical reform. The result was often a delayed and diluted imitation of English reforms. Under devolved government, the preoccupation with sectarian politics and maintaining the peace left little space for domestic reform, such as health and social care (Keating, 2005). A consequence has been that Northern Ireland has tended to lag behind the rest of the UK in introducing reforms.

As already noted, Northern Ireland adopted an integrated approach to health and social care. In addition, its population and geographical size gives greater scope for collaboration compared with the other, larger countries of the UK (O'Neill et al, 2012). However, despite evidence that it has conferred some advantages over other parts of the UK, notably in mental health and older people's services, the structural integration of health and social care has not fulfilled its potential (Hudson and Henwood, 2002; Heenan and Birrell, 2006; Heenan, 2013). A recurring problem has been the dominance of healthcare – and hospital-based care (Heenan, 2013). Nonetheless, the principle of integration remains entrenched, and the 2009 structural reforms helped to reinforce it (Gray and Birrell, 2013). Each new trust was responsible for all health and social services in their area (some pre-reform trusts provided hospital services only). Subsequently other reforms (emerging from the Compton Review, discussed below) aimed to improve integration by recommending shifting resources and workload from hospital to community and primary care. For example, integrated care partnerships have been established to bring together local health and social care services more effectively. According to Heenan (2013), however, there is a danger that these new networks, which are clinically led, may focus on integration between hospital and primary care at the expense of integration between health and social care.

Northern Ireland has pursued a more vigorous public health policy than in England, understandable perhaps given its higher levels of ill health and the role of socioeconomic factors, such as poor housing, unemployment and social division. Public health interventions have been explicitly linked to wider social welfare and social inclusion programmes. A major public health strategy, *Investing for health* (DHSSPS, 2002), emphasised stronger partnership arrangements between the NHS and local government. It also introduced demanding targets for reducing health inequalities. Although this approach contained much potential, and achieved better overall levels of health, inequalities persisted (DHSSPS, 2010). Moreover, efforts to work across agency and departmental barriers were frustrated by a silo mentality (see also O'Neill et al, 2012).

A policy review led to *Making life better*, a new 'whole system' framework for public health (DHSSPS, 2014). This set out collaborative action to influence factors that shape lives and choices, and a framework for action at central government, regional and local level. The key themes are: giving every child the best start; equipping people through life; empowering healthy living; creating the right conditions; empowering communities; and developing collaboration. The framework includes various cross-government commitments, intended outcomes and indicators. It also outlines a governance framework including a strategic ministerial committee, a departmental officials group, a regional project board and local partnerships. Planning and reporting mechanisms have been introduced alongside additional public health funding.

With regard to health services, English policies, such as working more closely with the private sector (with the exception of some PFI schemes), patient choice, foundation trusts and market-style reforms, have not been on the Northern Ireland agenda. However, Northern Ireland has not been completely isolated from health policy reforms elsewhere. It introduced access targets in the mid-2000s, which were subsequently made more challenging. The current targets cover similar issues as other parts of the UK, although there are differences in detail. For example, the current inpatient and day case targets in Northern Ireland are that 80 per cent of patients must wait no longer than 13 weeks, and that no one should wait over 26 weeks. There is also a range of targets for social care, assessment and hospital discharge. The DHSSPS also set out a comprehensive range of objectives for policy and service development alongside a new planning system, with a stronger focus on performance management. However, there is a much less punitive approach than in England (Timmins, 2013; Bevan et al, 2014).

Recent efforts to improve the health and social care system in Northern Ireland have been shaped by the Compton Review, *Transforming your care* (DHSSPS, 2011). This report outlined the case for change which included: a greater role for prevention; more patient-centred care; better arrangements for managing demand; renewed efforts to tackle health inequalities; stronger local commissioning; a shift to primary and community-based care; and rationalisation of the hospital sector. The report emphasised the need to focus on delivering high-quality services based on evidence and outcomes, while supporting the workforce in delivering change. The report also emphasised integrated care, choice and personalisation.

A further review, established in light of a series of service failures in Northern Ireland, reiterated the need for reform and urged speedier implementation of changes (Donaldson et al, 2014). Central to this was a recommendation to strengthen commissioning, which is much weaker and less developed than in England. As noted, the local commissioning bodies in Northern Ireland are committees of the health and social care board and primarily have an advisory role. There is no PBR system, and most services are delivered through block contracts. However, local commissioning groups are becoming become more engaged in seeking to shape local services in line with the priorities set out by ministers and the health and social care board.

The Donaldson report emphasised the need for clear system-wide targets and goals, better data and improved systems of measuring performance. It endorsed further rationalisation of the hospital sector, and expansion of primary care services (notably an extended role for pharmacists). The report also called for more support for self-management of chronic disease and a stronger patient voice (with greater independence for the Patient and Client Council). A stronger system of regulation was recommended, in particular, unannounced inspections. The report suggested that the role of the Regulation and Quality Improvement Authority be outsourced, and called for an improved system of incident reporting and the establishment of an institute for patient safety in Northern Ireland.

Differences in policy outcomes across the UK

In the initial period following devolution, some differences in policy outcomes were evident between the four countries of the UK (Connolly et al, 2010). Chiefly, these related to differences in NHS funding (with England being the least well-funded country), in efficiency (with England having higher levels of productivity), and in performance, especially with regard to access and, in particular, waiting times for hospital treatment (where England initially achieved the greatest reductions).

Although some of these differences have persisted, the overall picture has become less clear in recent years. This is partly due to changes in policy and performance. It is also due to greater acknowledgement of the difficulties of making comparisons, which led to a more cautious interpretation of the data (see NAO, 2012b; Bevan et al, 2014). As a result, there is now a more measured judgement about the impact of devolution on policy outcomes, namely, that policy and structural differences do not appear to have made much difference (Bevan et al, 2014).

This section summarises the main findings of the most recent research. It draws mainly on two comprehensive reviews: a report by the Health Foundation and Nuffield Trust (Bevan et al, 2014) and a National Audit Office review (NAO, 2012b). The policy outcomes are summarised under spending and efficiency; staffing and beds; access and quality; health outcomes; and public satisfaction.

Spending and efficiency

England still spends the lowest amount on healthcare per head of population. In 2012/13, this was £1,912 compared with £2,115 in Scotland, which is the most generous. NHS expenditure in Northern Ireland was £2,109 per head, and in Wales, £1,954 (Bevan et al, 2014). However, this does not tell the whole story, as the gap may be narrowing. The growth in NHS funding in England has risen faster than in the other countries of the UK (115 per cent between 2000/01 and 2012/13), much more than Scotland (99 per cent), Wales (98 per cent) and Northern Ireland (92 per cent). More recently, Wales has suffered the largest cuts to the NHS budget (10 per cent from 2010/11 to 2014/15), although it has protected social care spending more than in England (Timmins, 2013). It should be noted that the devolved governments receive the same health budget increase as England, but may choose not to pass this on to their NHS. In addition, it must be borne in mind that each country has different levels of health need, as indicated by mortality and illness rates. Overall, Northern Ireland has the highest health needs per person, followed by Wales, Scotland, and then England (although some parts of England have very high needs) (NAO, 2012b). Higher levels of spending on the NHS may therefore reflect higher needs rather than overgenerous funding.

Another approach is to examine the productivity as a measure of efficiency. The NAO (2012b) used a measure that weighted the costs of the inpatient, day case and outpatient activity per hospital medical staff member, and found that in 2008-09, England was the most productive, followed by Wales, Northern Ireland and Scotland. However, as the NAO and others have acknowledged, these findings are muddied by different data collection systems in the four countries and a lack of common definitions of basic terms such as admissions (Bevan et al, 2014). Also, these specific measures do not capture the productivity or efficiency of the whole NHS system, such as the contribution of primary care, community-based health services and public health.

Staffing and beds

There are also definitional and data collection differences when comparing human and physical resources. Nonetheless, it is quite clear that some countries have more healthcare professionals than others. Scotland has proportionally more GPs for its population, even allowing for the fact that its statistics are collected on a different basis from the other UK countries (Bevan et al, 2014). In 2009, Scotland had more (full-time equivalent) hospital medical staff and nurses/midwives/health visitors relative to its population size (NAO, 2012b). However, the ranking of the other UK countries on these indicators varies: for example, England comes second for GP staffing, but fourth for hospital medical staffing (and for nursing staff). Scotland also comes top for the number of beds in relation to population. In 2008/09, there were 500 beds per 100,000 population in Scotland, 440 in Wales, 430 in Northern Ireland and 310 in England (NAO, 2012b).

Access and quality

Waiting times have provided a key measure for the performance of the NHS across the four countries. However, difficulties of comparison also arise here from data collection differences and from the adoption of different measures (arising from the different targets adopted in each country). Furthermore, as already noted, the situation has been dynamic. England's success in reducing waiting times for treatment stimulated new performance regimes in other parts of the UK. England's early success was emulated by Scotland and followed, although to a lesser extent, in Wales and Northern Ireland (Bevan et al, 2014). In 2010, however, waiting times in Wales increased. In contrast, improvement continued in England and Scotland, although not as much as in the previous decade. The situation in Northern Ireland is more difficult to fathom as there is no comparable data from 2010 onwards. But as the financial squeeze on the NHS began, it became more difficult to meet the targets in all parts of the UK.

Access is only one dimension of quality, and perhaps the easiest to measure. Other aspects have been assessed, however. Researchers have concluded that, aside from waiting times, there is no systematic variation in quality between the UK countries (Sutherland and Coyle, 2009, cited in Bevan et al, 2014). One indicator of quality that is often used is reduced length of hospital stay. This is associated with greater patient satisfaction and recovery (although not always the case, for example, where there is an absence of community-based care). In general, lengths of stay in England and Northern Ireland are shorter than in Wales and Scotland, although there are variations between specialties (NAO, 2012b).

Other indicators relate to primary care. Analysis of practice performance in QOFs (see Chapter Seven) in 2010/11 found that GPs in Scotland and Northern Ireland appeared to perform better than in England and Wales, although the gap had narrowed (NAO, 2012b). Even so, the QOF has been criticised as a narrow assessment of quality and performance. Another indicator is immunisation rates, which again, shows Scotland and Northern Ireland in a better light than Wales and England (NAO, 2012b). Emergency admissions to hospital provide a further indicator of the effectiveness of primary care. In 2009/10, England had the second highest rate in the UK, Wales being the highest (partly, perhaps, due to its older population). But England endured a much faster growth in the rate of emergency admissions between 2000/01 and 2009/10 compared with Scotland and Wales. There was no comparable data for Northern Ireland for this period (NAO, 2012b).

Health outcomes

All countries of the UK have seen improvements in key health indicators in recent decades (Bevan et al, 2014). Rates of amenable mortality (defined as premature mortality in under-75s from causes that are amenable to timely and effective healthcare; see Nolte and McKee, 2004 cited in Bevan et al, 2014) have fallen dramatically. In 2010, England had the lowest rates, while Scotland had the highest. The gap between the countries has remained over time. All-cause mortality rates have also fallen (and again, Scotland has the highest rate and England the lowest), but this gap has widened (Bevan et al, 2014)

Similarly, life expectancy at birth varies across the countries of the UK. In 2010 England had the highest life expectancy and 'healthy life expectancy' in the UK for both men and women (NAO, 2012b). Scotland had the lowest life expectancy for women and men and the lowest healthy life expectancy for men. In contrast, Scotland had the biggest fall in infant mortality in the UK between 2002–10 (NAO, 2012b). During this period, infant mortality declined in England and Wales, but increased in Northern Ireland. In 2010, Northern Ireland and England had higher infant mortality rates than Scotland and Wales.

Public satisfaction

The best comparative data for public satisfaction is provided by the British Social Attitudes Survey. It asks the same questions to people across Britain, but does not include Northern Ireland. The 2011 data showed higher levels of satisfaction with the general running of the NHS in Wales than in Scotland and England (Park et al, 2012). Satisfaction with outpatient services was slightly higher in Scotland than England and Wales, and the same was true of inpatient services. More recent data (King's Fund, 2015) reveals that the highest overall level of satisfaction with the NHS is in Scotland (70 per cent very or quite satisfied), followed by England (65 per cent) and Wales (53 per cent). The high Scottish rating may, however, reflect the prominence of the NHS in independence referendum debates, which coincided with the survey. The poor level of satisfaction in Wales could be a reflection of patient experience and media coverage of its relatively longer waiting times. Periodic surveys in the UK have shown that public satisfaction is generally lower than levels of satisfaction expressed by recent patients. Both are influenced by media representation of health services and the prominence of the NHS in political debate (see Chapter Five).

Conclusion

Devolution has made a significant difference to health policy across the UK. Clear policy differences have arisen, partly as a consequence of devolved powers, and partly due to differences in political cultures and political systems, some features of which preceded the devolution settlement. There are major structural and organisational differences, although some occurred pre-devolution. Policy variation has resulted from policy innovation and by a refusal to pursue particular English policies. Yet factors promoting policy convergence remain, and have become stronger of late. Criticism of health policy and the state of the NHS has led devolved governments to adopt English approaches, notably waiting time targets. However, important differences remain both in policy style as well as outright rejection of certain policies.

There is clearly much scope for learning from different policies being pursued. Much can also be learned about the relative effectiveness of processes of policy-making and implementation, given the different policy styles that exist across the countries of the UK. However, there are concerns that the value of lesson drawing about both policy and processes is not being fully exploited (Connolly et al, 2010; Timmins, 2013; Bevan et al, 2014). More needs to be done to ensure this occurs, by, for example, providing consistent comparative data across the four countries and through independent evaluation of policy initiatives and processes (NAO, 2012b).

Summary

- Differences in health policy and NHS structures in different countries of the UK preceded devolution.
- Devolution has given the different countries of the UK new opportunities to develop distinctive health policies and to refashion NHS structures.
- Considerable variation has been evident. This has resulted from devolved governments introducing policies that differ from those in England. Divergence has also occurred as a result of refusing to pursue English policies.
- There are also forces that promote convergence, such as public opinion and the media, common health challenges, EU regulations and the reserved powers of the UK government.
- There is also an element of policy learning, with different parts of the UK learning from each other's experience and altering their policies. This is limited, however, by difficulties of comparison, poor quality data, shortcomings in evaluation and a reluctance to learn.
- The policy processes in other parts of the UK contrast with England. Lessons can be learned about the relative effectiveness of policy processes as well as policy impact.

Key questions

1. What are the main differences in health policy and NHS structures between the different countries of the UK today? What factors cause divergence?
2. How does the health policy process vary between the different countries of the UK?
3. What factors lead health policies to converge across the different countries of the UK?
4. Which country of the UK has the best NHS?

The international context of UK health policy

Overview

This chapter examines the global and international forces that impinge on UK health policies. It explores the impact of global trends and developments, and examines the activities of international institutions and organisations, such as UN bodies, NGOs and multinational corporations in the health policy arena. It also explores European influence on UK health policy, including EU institutions. In addition, it examines how the experiences of other countries have shaped health reforms.

Global influences on health policy

Global influences on UK health policy can be seen as part of a broader process of 'globalisation'. Although the precise meaning of globalisation is contested (see Lee and Collin, 2005; Koivusalo, 2006), it is often used as a convenient term for the growing interconnectedness of the world, and an increasing likelihood that decisions or events in one place will have a significant impact elsewhere (Giddens, 2002; Held et al, 1999; Labonte and Schrecker, 2004).

Health is affected by various global forces and trends from which individual countries cannot escape. The existence of such threats is not unprecedented, of course, as exemplified by the history of epidemics (Berlinguer, 1999). Rather, it is the combination of globalising forces in modern times that is unique, bringing new pressures for change across multiple policy arenas, including health. These forces are widely acknowledged (see Kickbusch

237

and de Leeuw, 1999; Lee and Collins, 2005; Kickbusch and Seck, 2007), and include:

- climate change, pollution and damage to ecological and agricultural systems;
- population displacement and migration (and health tourism);
- war and terrorism;
- increasing levels of chronic disease related to lifestyle and ageing populations;
- the threat of new and highly resistant strains of infectious disease, and the spread of infectious disease through increased trade and travel;
- concentration of capital and economic power;
- the spread of the Western consumer culture across the world;
- trade liberalisation, privatisation and deregulation;
- the global trade in legal and illegal recreational drugs;
- the movement of health professionals from poorer to richer countries;
- increasing inequalities, both within and between countries.

However, there are possible advantages from globalisation, in particular, from new communication technologies, including:

- pooling of expertise to tackle health problems;
- sharing of experiences about health reforms;
- improved transfer of health technologies;
- internationally coordinated action to combat the causes of ill health and to alleviate the consequences of illness.

Various international bodies are involved in the health policy process, including the World Health Organization (WHO), The World Bank and the World Trade Organization (WTO). Other players include nation states and their alliances, the most powerful of which is the 'G7/G8' group of countries. The health policy arena also includes NGOs, multinational corporations and trade organisations.

World Health Organization

The WHO was founded in 1948 as a specialist agency of the United Nations (UN) (K. Lee, 2009). Although not the first international body in this field, it heralded a more systematic and inclusive approach to improving cooperation on health policy and improving standards of health at the global level. All UN member states are eligible to join the WHO. They participate in decision-making through the World Health Assembly, while day-to-day decisions are in the hands of the WHO bureaucracy, headed by a director-general. Member states provide funding, which is supplemented by other sources (for example, from NGOs and the private sector).

The main functions of WHO are to provide scientific advice on health issues, to set international health standards, and to promote health and prevent disease. Its expertise is based on specialist staff and networks of external experts. Recommendations from WHO expert committees, task forces and commissions can provide momentum for action, both on specific health problems and on broader causes of illness. For example, the WHO Commission on the Social Determinants of Health (2008) provided a strong case for tackling the social, economic and environmental factors that influence health. The expertise and scientific advice provided by WHO and its associates has provided the basis for global strategies and programmes to improve health and to prevent disease.

WHO's early efforts focused mainly on the prevention of infectious diseases, and included the formulation of international health regulations that required notification of certain diseases (such as the plague, yellow fever and cholera). These regulations have since been extended to cover other potential international public health emergencies. WHO is also concerned with the prevention of non-communicable diseases (NCDs), such as most cancers and heart disease, which account for more deaths globally than infectious diseases.

During the 1970s, WHO began to formulate a global strategy, *Health for All by the year 2000*, to shift member states towards policies that prevented disease and promoted health (WHO and UNICEF, 1978; WHO, 1981). This emphasised the need to address health and social inequalities, the importance of primary healthcare, and the necessity for policies outside the health sector, for example, in trade, housing and welfare, to contribute to good health. *Health for All* was taken forward at international, regional and country level with a range of health improvement targets being set.

Health for All (and related initiatives, such as *Healthy Cities*, which coordinated local efforts to create healthier environments and communities) helped to place public health issues on the policy agenda. However, it could not compel governments to address such issues. In the UK, for example, governments were hostile to many elements of the strategy, especially targets on health inequalities; the strategy and its targets were later revised (WHO, 1999). Today WHO focuses on specific 'priority areas', such as tobacco, obesity and alcohol. Other priorities include malaria, TB, HIV/AIDS, mental health and maternal health. More recently, WHO has championed comprehensive intervention to address NCDs (diseases related to lifestyles such as smoking, obesity and alcohol misuse), which led to a UN strategy on NCDs, discussed further below. Another important strand of WHO's work is healthcare reform, which has involved comparative evaluations of different health systems.

WHO has attracted criticism from both friends and foes (K. Lee, 2009; Legge, 2012). It has been attacked by vested interests, such as the food, alcohol and tobacco industries, for policies that reduce their profitability. Governments that are heavily influenced by such interests (such as the US and UK) have also been critical of WHO. Others, however, believe that the WHO has been too cautious in its policies and unduly influenced by commercial interests. These critics point out that WHO's independence has been constrained by its funding, which is increasingly tied to specific projects. WHO is also dependent on major funders (including the UK, US and the Gates Foundation, see below), further reducing its autonomy (Sridhar et al, 2014). It has been criticised for lacking leadership, for being too bureaucratic and over-politicised. Many believe that WHO's leadership role in health has been ceded to other organisations (see below). It is also widely argued that it must do more to persuade other international bodies to acknowledge the health implications of their decisions (Prah Ruger and Yach, 2005; Horton, 2006; K. Lee, 2009).

WHO underwent various reforms from the late 1990s. The latest changes focused on improving health outcomes, promoting more coherence in global health strategies and interventions, and improving its organisation. WHO has sought to improve its reporting and accountability and information sharing, and has strengthened its commitment to leading and coordinating efforts to tackle global health issues. Nonetheless, much scepticism remains. This has been fuelled in particular by WHO's failings (acknowledged by its director-general) in tackling the Ebola crisis in 2014.

Other UN bodies

Other bodies have been involved in the health arena (Lee and Collin, 2005; Kickbusch and Seck, 2007; K. Lee, 2009). These include other UN agencies: the UN Children's Fund (UNICEF), the Food and Agriculture Organization (FAO) and the UN Educational, Scientific and Cultural Organisation (UNESCO). Other UN bodies also have an interest in health, such as the Joint Programme on HIV/AIDS (UNAIDS), the Population Fund, the UN Development Programme (UNDP), and the World Food Programme (WFP). Health is also on the agenda of others, including the International Labour Organization (ILO), the UN Office of Drugs and Crime (UNODC), the UN High Commission on Refugees (UNHCR) and the UN Conference on Trade and Development (UNCTAD). Health issues have been discussed by the UN Security Council. They are also extremely relevant to the work of the UN Environment Programme (UNEP), given the connections between health and the environment. The UNEP, along with its associated bodies, has been a key driver of efforts to combat climate change and to promote sustainable development. This had an impact through agreements and action plans, such as the 1997 Kyoto Protocol on climate change.

UN leadership and the General Assembly

The problems of coordinating the actions of these agencies, combined with a greater acknowledgement of the links between the key problems of world poverty, sustainable development, the environment and health, led the UN leadership to become more closely engaged with health and related issues. In 2000, the UN adopted the Millennium Development Goals (MDGs), which included reducing child mortality, improving maternal health, eradicating extreme poverty and hunger, combating HIV/AIDS, malaria, and other diseases, and ensuring environmental sustainability (see www. un.org/millenniumgoals/). This initiative specified key targets related to these objectives, to be achieved by 2015.

Recent developments have strengthened the links between sustainable development, environment and health objectives. The new approach is to replace the MDGs with integrated objectives across economic, social and environmental arenas. The targets cover a wider range of issues and are applicable to all countries, including industrialised states (UN Open Working Group on Sustainable Development, 2014).

Aside from this, the UN leadership and General Assembly have taken a much greater interest in health issues, including HIV/AIDs, women's health and NCDs. With regard to NCDs, the UN built on the work undertaken by the WHO to address the main causal factors. This led to a high level meeting of the General Assembly in 2011, which produced a political declaration (UN General Assembly, 2012). The declaration agreed a framework for action, including monitoring, indicators and targets, and a commitment to reduce premature mortality from NCDs by 25 per cent, by 2025.

Economic institutions: the World Bank and IMF

Another feature of recent decades has been the involvement of economic institutions in the health policy arena, such as The World Bank, the International Monetary Fund (IMF), the Organisation for Economic Co-operation and Development (OECD) and the WTO.

The World Bank is a key component in the financial system established after the Second World War (Lee and Collin, 2005; Prah Ruger, 2005). It is part of the UN system, but has considerable autonomy. Its original role was to help rebuild post-war economies by providing infrastructure loans.

Later, the World Bank's attention moved to developing countries and the implementation of structural adjustment programmes (SAPs) (Marshall, 2008). It increasingly pursued neoliberal policies that entailed reducing the public sector and liberalising markets in these countries, with adverse consequences for health and welfare (Lee and Collin, 2005). The World Bank has subsequently focused on the cost-effectiveness of health interventions, nutrition and poverty reduction, and building social capital through community development. It has supported partnership working between government, the private sector and NGOs to improve health (see below), and began to take a more enlightened approach on some key issues of health and trade, withdrawing support for the tobacco industry, for example. It also endorsed global action on NCDs, seeing these as a threat to the health standards and economies of lower and middle-income countries.

The IMF, like the World Bank, is an autonomous part of the UN system (Lee and Collin, 2005). It aims to expand international trade and lends to countries needing financial support (including industrialised countries). Like any 'banker' it imposes conditions, which usually involve reducing public spending, privatising public services and deregulation. It also issues reports on countries' economies and their economic policy, which can affect confidence and investment. These activities can affect health policy in a number of ways – health and other public service budgets may be curtailed due to IMF loan conditions, and privatisation and deregulation may be adopted in the health field to build IMF and investor confidence (Stuckler and Basu, 2009).

The Organisation for Economic Co-operation and Development

The OECD is an international economic organisation, although not a UN body. Its members, the main industrialised democracies, account for three-quarters of world trade (Koivausalo and Ollila, 1997). It was also established as part of the postwar reconstruction effort. Its current aims are to promote economic growth, improve standards of living and world trade through economic cooperation. It does this by promoting agreement between members on issues of common concern, undertaking research into economic and social issues, disseminating ideas about policy and reform, and comparing the performance of member states (Armingeon and Beyeler, 2004). It has taken a greater interest in healthcare reform issues since the 1990s, but is seen by critics (see, for example, de Vos et al, 2004) as promoting the same kind of neoliberal principles as the World Bank, IMF and WTO. Although regarded as less powerful than these bodies, it has a more subtle role, promoting reform through comparison, analysis and recommendations.

The World Trade Organization

The WTO was created in 1995 to monitor and enforce trade agreements. It is not a UN agency, but works closely with UN bodies. Its member states account for the vast majority of world trade. It aims to reduce barriers to trade by negotiating agreements and settling trade disputes. Its rules and decisions are binding on members and involve sanctions for those who do not comply. It is acknowledged that the richer industrialised countries exert most influence over WTO policies and decisions (Ostry, 2001).

Trade can improve health by raising levels of prosperity. However, liberalisation of trade is not necessarily good for health. It is argued that trade (rather than health) considerations are paramount in trade agreements (K. Lee et al, 2009; Smith et al, 2009), although trade agreements do allow for a degree of protection for health (Lee and Koivusalo, 2005; Waitzkin et al, 2005; Mitchell and Voon, 2011). While trade can be restricted 'to protect human, animal or plant life or health' (SPS, 1994), such restrictions must be based on clear scientific evidence, which is not always easy to provide, as risks are often difficult to quantify. Moreover, restrictions must not discriminate against particular countries or against foreign suppliers. Furthermore, measures to protect health must place the least possible restraint on trade. This implies that weaker forms of regulation (providing information to consumers, for example) will be chosen over stronger forms (such as taxes or bans on products).

WTO lacks in-house health expertise (Kimball, 2006), although this has been sought from other bodies. For example, international standards for food – labelling, content, additives, pesticides and drug residues – are set by the Codex Alimentarius Commission (or Codex), a body established by WHO and the FAO. Even so, there has long been concern that committees that advise WTO under-represent health and consumer interests (Millstone and van Zwanenberg, 2002). Indeed, critics argue that health standards have been compromised by WTO decisions (Lee and Koivusalo, 2005), pointing to the long-running dispute between the EU, US and Canada over the use of artificial growth hormones in cattle.

There is also concern that free trade rules may determine domestic policies on the organisation of health services. According to some, the extension of free trade rules to services raises the prospects of further privatisation of healthcare (Price, 2002; Lee and Koivusalo, 2005; Koivusalo, 2006). Although trade agreements exempt 'services supplied in the exercise of government authority' (Lee and Collin, 2005, p 93), they may be applied to public services where there is already private sector provision. While countries can exempt certain service areas, including health services, from the scope of trade agreements (Lipson, 2001), there are ways around this, notably where countries have health insurance-based funding systems or a system where a state body commissions healthcare from a range of public and private sector providers (as is now the case in the NHS). It is therefore possible that governments could be forced to open even more areas of healthcare to competition from private operators (Holden, 2005). All of these changes are seen as in the interests of global healthcare corporations, especially those based in the US, seeking to expand their businesses (Price, 2002; Tudor Hart, 2004; Holden, 2005).

A further consequence of the extension of trade rules to services is that trade restrictions now include government measures that incidentally affect the supply of services. This extends the remit of WTO to government regulation in areas such as health, environment and safety, thereby restricting public policy options (Price, 2002). This could benefit multinational corporations whose activities adversely affect health (such as the chemical, alcohol, tobacco and food industries). At the time of writing, concerns have been raised in connection with the negotiation of a bilateral agreement between the EU and US. The Transatlantic Trade and Investment Partnership (TTIP) seeks to reduce trade barriers and stimulate investment, but it may be bad for health. As it currently stands, US corporations will be able to claim compensation if they can prove that a government policy has disadvantaged them financially. This process, known as an investor–state dispute settlement, has been used in other trade agreements to inhibit governments from adopting public health policies that might adversely affect corporate interests (such as food, alcohol and tobacco businesses). If this process is included in TTIP without sufficient safeguards, it may lead to public health initiatives being blocked, and could force governments to open their healthcare systems to greater competition from the private sector.

Many commentators, especially those on the left, see institutions like the WTO, World Bank, IMF and OECD as acting in the interests of the richer countries of the world (although their activities can also adversely affect richer, industrialised countries as well as the less industrialised; see, for example, de Vos et al, 2004; Tudor Hart, 2006). The US is particularly powerful within these international organisations, and has a very strong pro-market, neoliberal ideology. This is counterbalanced to some extent by the EU, whose member states have a stronger tradition of social protection. However, neoliberalism has taken a stronger hold here in recent years with the creation of the single European market (discussed later in this chapter).

International fora

In addition to their weight within these global institutions, the rich countries also dominate other international fora. For example, the G7 and

G8 summits set the strategic context for policies across the globe. The G7 countries are France, the US, UK, Germany, Italy, Japan and Canada. The EU is also a member. The G7 plus Russia constitutes the G8 (although current international sanctions against Russia mean that the G8 is suspended).

The G7 and G8 have discussed a range of health-related issues including world poverty, food security, climate change, HIV/AIDS and illegal drugs (Labonte and Shrecker, 2004). This has led to decisions on poverty reduction, child and maternal health, and action on major diseases (notably, HIV/AIDS, TB and malaria). The G20 (which comprises the 20 largest economies, including the rapidly growing economies such as China and India) has also considered health issues, although its role in this field is less developed (Batniji and Woods, 2009).

Other players

The richer countries and commercial interests also dominate international networks that shape and reinforce opinion. One example is the World Economic Forum (WEF), a non-profit foundation, funded by big business, which builds partnerships between business, policy-makers and NGOs. It sees corporate expertise and resources and entrepreneurship as crucial to the solution of global economic and social problems. WEF analyses issues and produces reports. It provides networking opportunities, notably for high-level policy-makers and business people at its annual event in Davos, Switzerland (which also invites selected journalists and NGOs). WEF has been active on health issues, establishing a global health initiative in 2002. It has promoted partnership working in specific disease areas (HIV/AIDS, TB and malaria), focusing on certain regions and countries of the world (Africa, China and India). It is seen by critics as a pro-business and elitist organisation whose approach is strongly influenced by neoliberalism, corporate values and a Western industrialised nation perspective (Pigman, 2007).

The private sector is increasingly engaged in PPPs in the health field, for example, to extend vaccinations and to improve nutrition in poorer countries (Buse and Walt, 2000; Ollila, 2005). Although these initiatives have been broadly welcomed, they fall short of redistributive measures that many believe are needed to improve health in poorer countries (Fort et al, 2004; Labonte and Schrecker, 2004). There are concerns that the 'public' aims of PPPs are subverted by private profit motives (Nishtar, 2004). The private sector is also a key partner in worldwide efforts to promote health, especially in the context of reducing NCDs. Although portrayed as a sign that corporations are becoming more socially responsible, others are more sceptical. The participation of big businesses can be seen as a means by which they can block or dilute global efforts to prevent NCDs (by privately opposing effective policies from within), while at the same improving their public standing (see Fooks, 2011; Baggott, 2013).

It is generally acknowledged that multinational corporations are the dominant interests in global policy networks. However, on occasion they have been successfully challenged. An example was the tobacco control treaty (the Framework Convention on Tobacco Control) which entered into force in 2005. Another was the International Code of Marketing of Breast-milk Substitutes of 1981. Both resulted from successful campaigns by a range of organisations concerned about the health consequences of these products.

A range of other NGOs, including charities, foundations and think tanks, are involved in global health policy-making. Some are also engaged in funding or providing healthcare, such as the Bill & Melinda Gates Foundation, Oxfam and Médecins Sans Frontières. In addition, some international campaign groups focus on specific health issues (such as alcohol, tobacco or obesity). Health is also an issue for anti-globalisation, environmental and anti-poverty campaign groups, which oppose the current international order.

Health policy and Europe

A number of European institutions seek to influence UK health policy. These include the EU, the WHO Regional Office for Europe (WHO Europe) and the Council of Europe.

The European Union

Formally, the EU has limited powers over health in the member states (see Greer et al, 2014c; HM Government, 2013). The Treaty of Rome (1957) (see www.hri.org/docs/Rome57), which established the European Economic Community (EEC, a forerunner of the EU), did not provide a formal basis for action on health. Indeed, subsequent treaties made it clear that the definition of health policy, the management of health services and the allocation of resources were member state responsibilities. However, there was some scope for health-related initiatives under other Treaty provisions, concerning, in particular, the regulation of employment and trade. This enabled the introduction of measures on improving health and safety in the workplace, social protection arrangements for workers moving between countries (allowing them to use health services in other member states), and rules on product safety and labelling (including food and drugs).

The Single European Act 1987 increased the scope for such interventions. Although its principal aim was to stimulate competition and trade by harmonising regulation across member states, health protection was an important consideration. This meant that in a number of areas (including food, drugs, tobacco, motor vehicles and the workplace), European regulation was strengthened. The Act also strengthened EEC powers in environmental regulation, including water quality, waste control, chemicals and air pollution, areas that had important implications for health.

The key problem, however, was that these accumulated powers lacked a strategic framework. Although there were strong reasons for better coordination of public health matters, member states feared losing their autonomy. Nonetheless, in 1992, the Maastricht Treaty, which created the EU, contained a specific article on public health (Council of the European Communities and Commission of the European Communities, 1992). However, the new provision only enabled EU institutions to contribute towards protecting human health by encouraging cooperation and lending support to member states. Legislation was ruled out as a means of harmonisation, but research, information and incentives (such as funding for projects) were permitted.

Following the Maastricht Treaty, a framework for action was developed, including a network for the control and surveillance of communicable diseases. Specific programmes were formulated on cancer, HIV/AIDS, drug addiction, health monitoring, pollution-related disease, injury prevention and rare diseases (Randall, 2001). Following the BSE/Creutzfeld-Jakob disease (CJD) crisis, which exposed poor coordination between and within EU institutions as well as conflicts of interest between health and commerce, a new directorate for health and consumer protection was established within the European Commission (see **Box 10.1**). This body, later renamed the Directorate-General for Health and Consumers (DG SANCO), was given powers over food safety, including farm animal and plant health. In 2015, DG SANCO was retitled the Directorate-General for Health and Food Safety (DG SANTE), following the transfer of consumer responsibilities to another directorate.

The Amsterdam Treaty (European Union, 1997) further extended EU powers, stating that 'a high level of human health protection shall be ensured in the definition and implementation of all community policies and activities.' Actions could include measures to improve public health, to prevent illness and disease, and to address threats to public health. Member states agreed with greater cooperation in areas such as health monitoring and disease surveillance, but again, harmonisation of laws and regulations was not permitted. Nonetheless, there was now a sufficient foundation for a public health strategy. A programme of work was agreed for 2003-07, which had several aims: to improve health information and knowledge for the development of public health; to enhance capacity to respond to health threats; and to address health determinants (Decision of the European Parliament and of the Council, 2002). An evaluation of this programme

(European Court of Auditors, 2009) found that although it had achieved
some success in sharing experiences, facilitating learning and bringing
stakeholders together from different countries, there were significant
shortcomings. Its aims were too broad and ambitious, and too many diverse
topics were covered. The budget was insufficient and the programme lacked
strategic focus, and weaknesses were also found in monitoring projects and
their outcomes.

Box 10.1: European Union decision-making process

The EU decision-making process is complex, and a number of institutions
influence policy. The *European Commission* is the executive body of the EU. It
sets out priorities, develops policy and oversees implementation by specialist EU
agencies and the 28 member states. It has an important legislative role, drafting
proposals for consideration by other institutions. The Commission is organised into
departments known as directorate-generals, which have responsibility for an area
of policy (for example, DG SANTE). Each consists of permanent officials, overseen
by a commissioner. The commissioners are nominated by the member states, with
one commissioner drawn from each state. The president of the Commission is
responsible for allocating the commissioners' portfolios; they are also responsible
for strategic direction, central administrative functions and coordination, and
represent the Commission in its relations with other institutions, both within and
outside of the EU.

The *European Parliament* is directly elected by the member states in five-yearly
elections. It consists of 751 MEPs. The Parliament has a number of formal powers:
it elects the president of the Commission (following nomination by the European
Council), approves the appointment of the European Commission, and may block
appointments. It may censure the Commission, and has the power to remove the
entire Commission (although this has never been exercised, the potential threat
has put pressure on the Commission to make changes, and once pre-empted the
resignation of the entire Commission). The Parliament has budgetary powers
(which it shares with the Council of Ministers). Both must approve the medium-
term financial framework within which annual budgets are set. The Parliament and
Council of Ministers can also amend (and if necessary, reject) the annual budget
proposed by the Commission. The Parliament has used its powers in recent years
both to veto the budget and to freeze specific items of expenditure until certain
conditions are met.

Most legislation is now subject to a 'co-decision' procedure that involves Parliament.
Once the Commission has proposed a measure, the Parliament may amend it. The
Council of Ministers can also make changes. If there is disagreement between the

Council of Ministers and the Parliament, a conciliation process attempts to resolve the differences. Once agreement is reached, the measure can become law. The Parliament has established committees of MEPs that specialise in particular policy areas. These consider legislation, scrutinise EU health policy and produce reports and recommendations. The specialist committee for health is the Environment, Public Health and Food Safety Committee.

The *Council of Ministers* consists of ministers from each member state responsible for a particular area of policy. The composition of the Council therefore varies according to the issue being discussed (each particular arrangement is known as a configuration). Health matters fall within Employment, Social Policy, Health and Consumer Affairs (although other configurations also consider matters affecting health, such as the environment, for example). The Council of Ministers coordinates policy and, along with the European Parliament, legislates and approves budgets for EU programmes. Decisions in the Council are mostly made by a qualified majority, which makes it more difficult for countries (especially smaller states) to block proposals. It is led and coordinated by the presidency of the Council, a position held for six months by each member state on a rotating basis. The country in question chairs Council meetings, sets the agenda and is involved in seeking agreement on key issues.

The Council of Ministers is supported and coordinated by a body of civil servants and advisers drawn from the member states, known as COREPER (the Permanent Representatives Committee). COREPER prepares the agenda for discussions and decisions and helps to achieve compromise when there is disagreement. In addition, the heads of government meet four times a year as the *European Council*. This sets the strategic direction for the EU, deals with major concerns, and attempts to resolve major conflicts and tensions between governments. The European Council now has an elected president.

Finally, the *European Court of Justice* (since 2009 known as the Court of Justice of the European Union) considers cases brought before it under European law. Its case law judgments have affected health and healthcare issues, and include cross-border healthcare, tobacco advertising and alcohol regulation as well as judgments in employment law, competition and the regulation of goods and services.

EU strategy

The increasing political visibility of health problems such as obesity, alcohol and smoking, coupled with a growing awareness of the links between health, economic efficiency and competiveness (related to the EU's Lisbon Strategy, which linked social policy and competitiveness), and in light of threats to the health of European citizens from beyond its borders, led the EU to consider a more strategic approach (Byrne, 2004). In 2007, the European Commission launched a health strategy (European Commission, 2007a) that set out the fundamental principles of EU action in health: shared health values; health as a prerequisite for economic activity; the integration of Health in All Policies; and strengthening the voice of the EU in global health. Strategic aims included fostering good health in ageing populations, protecting citizens from health threats, and supporting health systems and new technologies. Proposed actions included the adoption of a statement on fundamental health values, a system of health indicators, action on reducing health inequities, health literacy programmes, studies of the relationship between health and economic growth, strengthening the integration of health across EU policies, and strengthening cooperation between the EU and global health policy actors.

The Council of Ministers (see **Box 10.1**) underlined its commitment to the strategy with a declaration on 'Health in All Policies' in Rome (EU Ministerial Conference, 2007). It also agreed that the EU should play a greater role in global public health. This highlighted the need to take action to improve health, reduce inequality and increase protection against global health threats, to recognise health as a key element in sustainable growth and development and poverty reduction, and for the increased leadership of WHO in global health.

A second health programme was agreed (Decision of the European Parliament and of the Council, 2007) covering the period 2008-13, with three objectives: to improve citizens' health security; to promote health for prosperity and solidarity (including the reduction of health inequities); and to generate and disseminate health information and knowledge. Examples of work funded by these programmes included information exchange on health threats and preparedness plans; promoting health impact assessment (HIA) of policies; healthy lifestyle campaigns; an overview of child obesity initiatives; exchange of good practice on nutrition and physical activity; the development of good practice on alcohol and the workplace; support for HIV/AIDS networks and groups; support for initiatives to build capacity in the field of tobacco control; prevention of illicit drug use; and the collection of data about health behaviours, diseases and conditions.

The funding for both the first and second programmes (€350 and €320 million respectively) was relatively small in comparison with the overall size of the EU budget (€123 billion in 2010). Most projects were small and specific. One might well question how they could produce the significant shifts in policy needed to make public health a top priority for the EU. However, it should be noted that the public health programme funding is dwarfed by other EU spending on health contained in other budgets (see

Greer et al, 2014c). In the period 2008–13, the EU spent around €12 billion on health, with the vast majority (around 98 per cent) from health research budgets and structural funds.

Health in All Policies and the third programme

EU interest in health has since extended, to some extent due to the environmental health agenda, particularly issues relating to pollution. There have also been greater efforts to address health inequalities and the social determinants of health. As a result, there has been a much stronger momentum towards 'Health in All Policies' and the promotion of intersectoral working on health. In addition, the Lisbon Treaty, which came into force in 2009, amended the EU's health responsibilities and powers in several ways. First, wellbeing was identified as a key aim of the EU. Second, the Treaty emphasised greater cooperation between member states to improve health services in cross-border areas. Third, it strengthened cooperation and coordination through guidelines, indicators, exchange of good practice, periodic monitoring and evaluation. Fourth, it confirmed that EU legislation would be permitted when setting high standards where there were common safety concerns (three areas were specified: blood products, organ transplants and other substances of human origin; medical products and devices; and measures in relation to animal or plant health with a direct objective of protecting public health). And fifth, EU competence in relation to cross-border health threats and the protection of public health from alcohol and tobacco was clarified, allowing incentives to be used but not legislation to harmonise laws.

A third programme for public health covering the period 2014–20 has since been launched with a larger budget (almost €450 million). It has four key objectives: to promote health, prevent disease and foster supportive environments for healthy lifestyles; to support public health capacity building and contribute to innovative, efficient and sustainable health systems; to protect citizens from serious cross-border health threats; and to facilitate access to better and safer healthcare (European Parliament and Council, 2014). The specific priorities of this programme include: addressing risk factors such as smoking, alcohol and obesity; ensuring effective responses to communicable disease, such as HIV/AIDS and TB; promoting action to address the health issues of an ageing society; and strengthening voluntary cooperation on a range of issues including e-health, health innovation, technology assessment and patient safety.

Healthcare services

The focus of EU health policy has shifted somewhat in recent years. In particular, there has been greater emphasis on the contribution of the health sector to economic growth (Greer et al, 2014c): it is increasingly acknowledged that financial investments in health generate significant economic activity; the health sector is both a user and a source of new technologies that can promote economic growth; and it is also a major employer, playing an important part in skills development and human capital. On the other hand, health services represent a major cost to the economies of the EU. In an era of austerity and the Eurozone crisis, this has produced further impetus to improve cost-effectiveness. EU financial institutions are increasingly concerned with public finances, and one of the biggest budgets is health and welfare systems. This has led to recommendations to member states on how to improve their health systems, for example, by hospital restructuring or primary care reform (Greer et al, 2014c). In light of the additional fiscal powers acquired in recent years, the EU now has greater scope to intervene in the fiscal policies of member states in ways that shape their health budgets and programmes (and although the UK has refused to concede its budgetary independence, it nonetheless receives advice on its economic management and fiscal policies).

As already mentioned, the responsibility for healthcare has been jealously guarded by member states. However, issues of cross-border care (where people resident in one country of the EU can obtain treatment in another) have allowed the EU to develop policies and legal instruments. Initially, rights to access health services were limited to EU migrant workers and temporary visitors (such as tourists and travellers). However, legal judgments in the European Court of Justice extended these rights to people in one EU country choosing treatment in another, paid for by their member state. This led to a new directive, which set out a framework for these cross-border flows of patients (Directive of the European Parliament and of the Council, 2011). Notably, it restricts cross-border flows in a number of ways (including prior authorisation by the patient's member state). Nonetheless, the potential for increased flows of patients between member states is considerable. This has generated further EU interest in ensuring that providers can compete on a level playing field, prompting efforts to promote greater collaboration between countries to manage patient flows and to improve the quality and safety of services provided.

Processes

As already indicated, the EU's formal powers in health matters, although expanded, are relatively limited. However, other policy tools and mechanisms have also been used to highlight priorities, to call for action, and to promote collaboration. The European Commission, the European Parliament (especially its specialist committee on health matters) and the Council of Ministers have all engaged with health issues and have issued declarations (in the form of Parliament opinions, Commission communications or Council conclusions) and other strategic statements. Examples include the health strategies adopted by the Commission and Council of Ministers, as already mentioned. In addition, there have been commitments on specific issues: for example, on the common values and principles in EU health systems (Council of the European Union, 2006); healthcare system reform (Council of the European Union, 2011); healthcare infections (Council of the European Union, 2009); health inequalities (European Parliament, 2011); alcohol (European Commission, 2006); obesity (European Commission, 2007b); and cancer screening (Council of the European Union, 2003).

Given the relative weakness of health legislation, there has been much effort to promote collaboration, coordination and cooperation between member states. The open method of coordination (OMC) enables member states to build consensus on issues where they retain a high degree of autonomy. In 2004, OMC was extended to health matters – under OMC, member states set out policy positions and plans, and share them, providing opportunities to learn from each other. In 2008, OMC was revamped to raise its profile, sharpen its focus and improve communication, coordination and mutual learning. It is believed that it has contributed to debates about the common issues facing health systems across the EU, and provided leverage for reform within member states. Even so, as the process is voluntary and there are no sanctions, its direct impact is limited (Greer et al, 2014c).

Working with stakeholders and external organisations

The EU system is open to pressure groups, business organisations and professional bodies seeking to influence policy. Increasingly they operate through pan-European lobby groups. Examples include the Standing Committee of European Doctors, the Association of European Cancer Leagues and the European Federation of Pharmaceutical Industries and Associations. The European Parliament is very accessible to interest groups, and its increased powers have attracted lobbyists' attention. The Commission is relatively open, partly because it lacks technical expertise and other information essential for policy development, and is therefore dependent on outside advice and information. The Commission also tends to proceed by consensus, and will usually canvas views before proceeding, giving outside bodies opportunities to comment.

Various stakeholder fora have been established. The Health Policy Forum, established in 2001, provides a vehicle for consultation. It consists of organisations representing trade unions, health professionals, health service providers and insurers, patients and consumers, and commercial interests. It identifies key areas of work within the context of an annual plan, examines specific issues and can adopt policy positions. Following criticism, however, new guiding principles on transparency were outlined for its members (EUHPF, 2007), including provisions on openness, conflicts of interest and governance, and the forum was subsequently reformed in 2009. Its mandate was renewed with the following aims: that the membership should concentrate on pan-European rather than national or regional associations, that preference should be given to umbrella bodies able to represent a wider constituency of organisations, and that membership should not exceed 50 groups.

Other consultative processes used by the European Commission to build collaboration and partnership with stakeholders include the Open Health Forum, which includes a wider range of organisations than the Health Policy Forum. In addition, a number of consultative 'platforms' have been created on specific issues. For example, the EU Platform for Action on Diet, Physical Activity and Health formed in 2005. The aim of such platforms is to create dialogue and to build consensus between different interests in these policy areas. Although they have provided the foundation for joint commitments, their impact on policy has been limited (see for example, Evaluation Partnership, 2010). They have tended to focus on areas of consensus, such as information and communication about risks and lifestyles, while thornier issues, such as regulation, tend to be avoided.

Achievements

As Greer et al (2014c) note, EU activities are rarely fully acknowledged because many lie outside its formal remit for public health. It is impossible to evaluate the EU's impact across the board, but some of the key achievements are listed below, in **Box 10.2** (see Greer et al, 2014c; HM Government, 2013).

> ## Box 10.2: Key EU achievements in health
>
> *Tobacco:* the EU has supported action on smoking and tobacco products. This includes measures to display health warnings on packs, ban advertising and sponsorship, reduce levels of toxins, and restrict smoking in the workplace and

in public places. EU action has been heavily based on health and safety at work legislation and internal market regulations. It has been challenged in the European Court of Justice, with occasional success. To counter this, and to address loopholes in the existing law, a comprehensive Tobacco Products Directive came into force in 2014.

Communicable diseases: the EU has promoted collaboration on communicable diseases. There has been monitoring and surveillance of communicable diseases across the EU since the 1980s, and these arrangements were formalised in the late 1990s. Subsequently, in 2004, a new agency, the European Centre for Disease Prevention and Control, was established to strengthen monitoring and to promote a coordinated response. There is also a Health Security Committee that addresses wider issues of preparedness for public health emergencies and helps to coordinate responses to such crises.

Rare diseases: the EU has done much to highlight the importance of responding to rare diseases. It has supported initiatives to increase access to expertise and information for rare diseases, and has also promoted the development of drugs for use in the treatment of rare conditions. The EU has also prompted member states to address this problem and to produce national plans.

Drugs and product safety: pharmaceuticals have been regulated by the EU for many years. There is a common system across the EU for licensing new drugs, consisting of two parts: a European-level system, where drugs are approved across the EU, and a national system, where approval in one member state is acknowledged by other national regulators. The European Medicines Agency oversees this system and operates the EU-level process. It also monitors any problems with drugs arising after their approval. Blood products, transplants and other healthcare products using human tissue are subject to separate legislative controls. There is also a separate system for regulating other medical and healthcare products, which involves national approval that enables them to be sold across the EU. This system has been found wanting (with a number of scandals involving inferior products, notably breast implants and hip replacements), and directives in this area are being revised.

While there are many examples of how the EU has contributed to better health across a whole range of policy issues, there has been criticism of its attempts to harmonise rules and regulations. Other criticisms have centred on a lack of priority given to health matters relative to other issues, and on the difficulty of coordinating various EU institutions. Another issue has been the problem of implementing EU policies and their variability of implementation across Europe. These and other issues are discussed in the next section.

Criticism of EU involvement in health

Health came late to the EU agenda, and has struggled to compete with established issues such as agriculture, industry, trade and competition, as well as welfare and environment issues. Notably, the European strategy for growth, Europe 2020, makes only a few brief references to health, despite its potential contribution to economic growth and social welfare (European Commission, 2010).

Commercial interests are very powerful within the EU, and highly skilled at opposing policies that threaten their profitability. They have strong links with the most powerful economic and trade directorates within the European Commission. Drugs companies, agricultural interests and food, drink, tobacco and alcohol corporations are particularly influential. Although the EU has developed policies, despite opposition from member states and business interests (for example, on tobacco), they have generally fallen far short of the demands of public health experts and campaigners (Rosenkötter et al, 2013). A major failure was the inability to ensure that the Common Agricultural Policy (CAP) meets health objectives (Elinder et al, 2003; Faculty of Public Health, 2007). There have been some gains (such as the phasing out of tobacco subsidies and the introduction of schemes to increase children's access to milk, fruit and vegetables), but generally, CAP remains geared to the economic interests of landowners and farmers.

Another area where commercial interests have been able to stifle policies is alcohol policy. Despite the scope for intervention at the European level, EU institutions have been reticent to address the major public health and social problems linked to alcohol, because of the power of multinational corporations in this sector and the vested interests of member states in alcohol production and trade (Anderson and Baumberg, 2006; Greer et al, 2014c).

In principle, health considerations are meant to be included in all EU decisions. Health was included in EU integrated impact assessment guidelines in 2002. Furthermore, it has encouraged the development of HIA tools (International Health Impact Assessment Consortium, 2004; Wismar et al, 2007). Nonetheless, the potential of HIA has not been realised (Lock and McKee, 2005; Salay and Lincoln, 2008; Rosenkötter et al, 2013; Greer et al, 2014c).

Furthermore, DG SANCO and its successor DG SANTE have been regarded as weak directorates within the Commission (Rosenkötter et al, 2013). This is because of the greater weight of the economic, agriculture and trade directorates, and because other functions affecting health, relating to environmental health, health and safety, and social policy, remain with other directorates and agencies. Despite growing EU interest in health issues, there are significant shortcomings in how health policy is developed and implemented. It is not a top priority. The EU's role in health remains restricted by the Treaties (HM Government, 2013; Greer et al, 2014c), and EU health programmes have been under-resourced. There has been, and still is, a diffusion of governance on health (Lear and Mossialos, 2008), with a lack of clear authority and accountability for health actions.

Fragmentation, coordination and leadership

The fragmentation of health responsibilities is exacerbated by poor coordination between the directorates and agencies whose activities impinge on health (Greer, 2009; Greer et al, 2014c). Although one can identify issues where great efforts have been made to promote a collaborative approach (such as communicable diseases, food safety and drug abuse, where specific EU bodies have been established), this is relatively unusual. For most directorates, health is not a priority (HM Government, 2013).

However, efforts have been made to strengthen coordination and leadership on health across EU institutions (Greer et al, 2014c). An inter-service group on public health was created in the 1990s to coordinate activities between different parts of the European Commission. Processes of consultation were established to exchange information and to strengthen coordination on the health aspects of policy and legislation. Specific subgroups were established to improve coordination on particular issues such as HIV/AIDS, global health and environmental health. Furthermore, in 2008 a working party on public health was established by the Council of Ministers as a forum for discussing major strategic issues and to consider issues arising for health systems and public health. This working party is supported by the Commission and reports to COREPER.

Other criticisms

There has been concern that the formation of EU policies does not take into account unintended consequences for member states (HM Government, 2013; Greer et al, 2014c). For example, the Working Time Directive (which aims to regulate hours of work and rest periods) has been opposed, particularly by the UK, for its potential adverse impact on the training of doctors (who traditionally spend long hours at work and on call). Another issue concerns the effect of the free movement of labour on health service quality. While this has benefits, allowing the NHS to attract staff from EU countries, there has been disquiet that EU rules prevent UK authorities from setting standards. This point has been made particularly about language competence, fuelled by cases where poor language skills have been identified as a factor in patient harm. Even so, it is fair to say that on some issues (notably regulation of clinical trials and on cross-border healthcare) the EU responded appropriately to concerns raised by member states to prevent potential problems (HM Government, 2013).

Unequal implementation of EU policies across member states has been a regular complaint (see HM Government, 2013) – some countries are better at implementing EU legislation than others. Those undertaking minimal implementation undermine the potential for harmonisation and undermine health and safety standards. This was evident in revelations about weak regulation of medical devices, mentioned earlier, where a failure of some national systems brought the EU process into disrepute. Another criticism of implementation is that the EU often reacts too slowly to impending problems, and its processes involve considerable delay (HM Government, 2013).

Some argue that EU policy is too often crisis-driven (Greer et al, 2014c). However, scandals such as BSE/CJD, contaminated blood products and faulty medical devices created a strong momentum for change. They led to stronger policies and institutional changes that benefit health. Even so, they also involved much human suffering, not to mention economic losses. In addition, policies forged in times of crisis may not be fully developed and thought through, which can store up problems for the future.

Finally, there is some criticism that the EU does not liaise as effectively as it might with other organisations in international and European health, for example, the WHO and the OECD (Rosenkötter et al, 2013). The net effect of this is that there is the potential for waste and duplication of initiatives.

WHO Europe

The WHO Regional Office for Europe (WHO Europe) has been a key exponent of action on public health and acts in collaboration with EU and other European bodies (Ziglio et al, 2005). Its membership is wider than that of the EU (53 member states), so it is valuable in building consensus and introducing initiatives across the continent. WHO Europe tailors global strategies and initiatives to the European setting. It also develops European initiatives, some of which are taken up by the WHO and other regions. An example is the *Healthy Cities* programme, mentioned earlier, which began in Europe and spread worldwide to over 600 municipalities.

WHO Europe has formulated broad regional strategies over a number of years. Its European *Health for All* strategy set specific aims and targets for the continent (WHO Regional Office for Europe, 1985, 1999). More recently, WHO developed Health 2020, a European policy framework for supporting action across government and society to improve health and wellbeing (WHO Regional Office for Europe, 2012a). In addition, it has promoted consensus across a range of issues enabling the formulation of specific resolutions, charters, strategies and action plans on topics such as alcohol, smoking, children's health, health systems, environmental health, NCDs, food and nutrition (see for example WHO Regional Office for Europe, 2006a, 2006b, 2010, 2011, 2012b). Other activities include specific programmes and projects such as Healthy Schools and Healthy Hospitals, which seek to promote health through the involvement of these sectors. Partnership and collaboration feature strongly in WHO Europe's work. This is embedded in specific plans and programmes. For example, Health 2020 refers to the importance of working across sectors, addressing the social and environmental determinants of health, and increasing the participation of all stakeholders, including citizens, in improving health. WHO Europe can play a subtle role in domestic health policy. By reporting on health issues it can raise their profile on national (and European) agendas. Also, by reviewing policies in individual countries, identifying good practice and evaluating the impact of policies and programmes, it can create opportunities for policy learning and transfer (see below).

Council of Europe

The Council of Europe is not an EU body (and is not to be confused with EU institutions, the European Council and the Council of Ministers; see **Box 10.1**). It was founded in 1949 to uphold democracy, human rights and the rule of law. Like WHO Europe, it has a larger membership than the EU (47 states), and it is similarly useful as a vehicle for securing agreement on issues across the continent. All member states have signed up to the European Convention on Human Rights (a Treaty to protect human rights, democracy and law). Signatories to this Convention (including the UK) are bound by its provisions. Individuals may pursue cases in the European Court of Human Rights (not the same as the European Court of Justice, discussed in **Box 10.1**) and (following the Human Rights Act 1998) in British courts (Montgomery, 2003). The Convention has been used to challenge healthcare practices, the actions of health authorities and decisions about access to care, on the grounds that they have breached an individual's human rights (such as the right to life, right to liberty, right to private and family life, prohibition of inhumane or degrading treatment, and discrimination on grounds of race or gender).

The UK is also signatory to a further Council of Europe convention, the *European Social Charter* (Council of Europe, 1996). This places a number of health responsibilities on states, which, if not undertaken, could provide a basis for legal challenges (Montgomery, 2003). These include the removal, as far as possible, of the causes of ill health, the provision of advisory and educational facilities for the promotion of health and encouragement of individual responsibility, and the prevention of infectious and other diseases, and accidents. The Charter requires states to ensure that people without resources can access care when sick, that such people should not suffer any loss of political or social rights, and that everyone may receive services such as advice and help to remove or alleviate personal or family want.

The principal focus of the Council of Europe's interest in health is on citizens' rights to health and healthcare, including access to services and participation in health matters. For example, it has promoted action on issues such as nutrition, HIV/AIDS, patient safety, the rights of minority ethnic groups to access healthcare, and the rights of elderly and disabled people, and people with chronic illness. It has also sought to improve systems of consultation and involvement in health, to enable citizens to have a say in matters affecting their health and health services. Its conventions have set a framework on important cross-border issues (for example, in 2011 it created a convention on counterfeit medical products). Its reports and projects often focus on neglected and controversial issues, raising their profile on domestic and European policy agendas. They also lay the foundations for policy formation by identifying key interventions and policies, on which individual states (and other EU-wide institutions) may draw. Examples include reports on the health dangers of Wi-Fi and mobile phones (2011), and a project to empower citizens in protecting health, to promote citizen participation and consultation, and to improve the protection of health by increased health literacy and health education (2012/13) (see www.coe.int/en/web/portal/home).

Over the years, the Council of Europe has cooperated with other European institutions such as EU bodies and WHO Europe on issues including school-based health promotion, drug dependence, hazardous chemicals and prison health, and has also facilitated cooperation on the safety of blood products and organs for transplant. For example, with regard to blood products, the Council of Europe is regarded as having played a key role in establishing an agreement on standards, paving the way for EU regulations on this issue (Greer et al, 2014c, p 62).

Learning lessons from elsewhere

Healthcare systems face similar challenges, such as ageing populations, changes in medical technology and rising public expectations and demands (OECD, 2004; Blank and Burau, 2010). In order to meet these challenges, most countries have undertaken healthcare system reform, and these have not occurred in isolation. Although each healthcare system is the product of a unique set of historical, cultural and political forces, changes have been influenced by the experience of other countries.

The UK is no exception – one can point to several key reforms imported from other healthcare systems. The creation of NHS foundation trusts was inspired by experiences from Spain, Sweden and Denmark, where health service providers were granted greater autonomy. The introduction of commissioning and the greater use of competition, both within the NHS and from the independent sector, were influenced by countries that adopted a market-led approach to healthcare, notably the US. They were also informed by the experiences of state insurance systems in continental Europe, which separate funding from provision, and which adopt a pluralist approach to the supply of health services (such as Germany and Holland, for example). Another example is the smoking ban, where UK policy-makers drew on the experiences of the early implementation of measures in California, New York and the Irish Republic.

It is often difficult to trace the genesis of a policy change. It may arise from an amalgamation of other countries' experiences rather than by simply drawing lessons from one country. Indeed, the spread of reform ideas across healthcare systems tends to happen multilaterally, rather than on a bilateral basis (for example, the development of competition and contracting across healthcare systems). Moreover, the legacy is often diluted. Other countries' experiences may provide the seeds of reform, but policy is then implanted differently once imported. For example, GP fundholding (see Chapter Seven) was loosely based on the experience of US health maintenance organisations (HMOs), but introduced in a way more suited to NHS values – expensive procedures were initially excluded (to avoid discrimination against 'high cost' patients), and the system was highly regulated to minimise the adverse effects of competition (Glennerster et al, 1994).

In practice, only minimal policy learning may actually occur (Ettelt et al, 2012). Developments elsewhere may be used to justify domestic policies rather than informing them. And there are questions about the quality of comparative data and evidence. Lessons based on poor information are unlikely to be worth learning. There are also issues of interpretation bias. Policy-makers may give insufficient consideration to the evidence about reforms being adapted from abroad, or select evidence to support their political inclinations. For example, it has been suggested that the NHS (in England at least) is learning the wrong lessons, by seeking to draw on the US experience of commissioning and competition in healthcare (Reynolds et al, 2012). Meanwhile, other lessons, from countries that made health gains by pursuing a more collaborative, primary care-led and public health-oriented approach, have been neglected. For example, Cuba's remarkable health record (see de Vos, 2005; Offredy, 2008) has been largely ignored by Western countries because of its relatively low level of economic development and because of its socialist approach to governance. But as Crisp (2010) notes, lessons can be learned from countries at lower levels of economic development, and there has been greater interest in such examples recently (see below).

Although the spread of reform ideas is complex, there are certain factors that appear to facilitate it (Ettelt et al, 2012). Academic research and other reports and investigations (commissions, committees of inquiry, health committee reports, think tanks) often identify potential reforms from other systems, and these may be taken up by policy actors. Notably the DH has an on-call facility from a group of academics, which it uses to acquire information about other healthcare systems. Overseas visits by policy actors can also generate new ideas for reform. An example was the visit in 2014 by a delegation of Northern Ireland Assembly members to Cuba to learn lessons about policies to reduce health inequalities. In addition, visiting academics and policy experts from overseas can generate new ideas. For example, Professor Alain Enthoven, a US academic who visited the UK in the mid-1980s, provided important intellectual arguments for using market forces in the NHS (Enthoven, 1985). Exchange schemes and fellowships can also be a means of transferring ideas between countries, such as the Commonwealth Fund's Harkness Fellowships (which enable researchers and practitioners from other countries including the UK to work in the US on research projects), identified as a channel through which US policy ideas have come to the UK (Reynolds et al, 2012).

In general, improvements in international travel and communication have expanded the scope for learning from other health policies and systems. The media can play a key role in highlighting what policies are being pursued in other countries, although its approach is highly selective and based on judgements of newsworthiness (see Chapter Five). Hence there has been considerable media interest in the decriminalisation of illicit drugs in some American and European countries, and on some other public health issues such as smoking bans.

There is now much more comparative information to enable the 'benchmarking' of health systems (see OECD, 2013; Davis et al, 2014). Variations in performance create pressures for reform, especially where highlighted by the media, and an impetus to learn lessons from 'high performing' countries. This also happens in specific policy and service areas. Comparisons on cancer survival produced by EUROCARE (2014) have pressured countries performing less well according to this data into exploring how they can become more successful in preventing and treating the disease.

Policy ideas are actively disseminated by global and international policy actors. These include institutions such as the OECD, WEF, World Bank, IMF, WHO (and its regional offices) and the EU as well as other organisations, such as multinational corporations and NGOs. Research bodies and think tanks also play a key role, not only in producing comparative data and evidence about the impact of reforms, but also by actively promoting particular reforms.

Conclusion

UK health policy cannot be examined in isolation from broader international and global forces. Indeed, many policies developed in the UK are connected to events, decisions, policies and ideas outside its borders. We have also seen that European institutions have an effect on individual health policies and health systems. The effects of global and European factors are often poorly understood, and frequently underestimated. Finally, domestic health policy is increasingly shaped by policy ideas from abroad. Policy learning and transfer can occur by individual countries picking up ideas from others, but international and supranational bodies can also play an important role in highlighting policies and identifying lessons.

Summary

- UK health policy must not be seen in isolation from international and global forces and institutions.
- International bodies influence health policy, including UN organisations, trade and financial bodies, international leadership fora, multinational corporations and NGOs.
- European institutions, including EU institutions, have taken a greater interest in health policy in recent years. They have influenced health policy in member states, despite having no direct control over their healthcare systems.
- Health policies in individual countries are influenced by developments in other health systems, and the UK is no exception.

Key questions

1. Which institutions and organisations are the most influential in shaping global health policies?
2. How, and to what extent, is UK health policy shaped by global institutions?

3. Give examples of UK health policies that have been derived, at least in part, from the experiences of other health systems.
4. How, and to what extent, has the EU increased its influence over health policy in the member states?
5. On balance, has UK membership of the EU been good or bad for the health of its people?

eleven

Conclusion

Overview

This chapter sets out the main conclusions of the book, and looks at possible future developments

Who makes health policy?

By exploring the role of key institutions and organisations and their involvement in various processes (such as agenda setting, consultation, policy advice and implementation), it has been possible to draw some broad conclusions, although a word of caution is perhaps needed. The analysis has been performed at a level of generality, albeit illustrated by particular cases. In any specific circumstance the balance of the institutions and forces described in this book will differ. The policy process is difficult to predict in advance, and one cannot simply 'read off' likely outputs or outcomes from a list of policy participants or the characteristics of a policy issue. What has been achieved here is a broad framework of analysis, which may be useful in investigating how specific policies have emerged and developed.

As shown in Chapter Two, party politics is important in setting the parameters and direction of health policy. However, there is considerable continuity between governments, irrespective of the party in power. There is also substantial policy change under governments of the same party. So party ideology does not automatically dictate what will happen in government. In practice, governments are more pragmatic than their rhetoric would suggest. Policy is shaped by party competition and the borrowing of ideas from other parties. Ideological policies may be discarded on grounds of ineffectiveness or impracticality, to be replaced by more pragmatic approaches. There is also a certain amount of path dependency in health, which limits the impact of new ideological policies. Political circumstances, internal party conflict and pressure group lobbying may also dilute parties' ideologically based policies. But this is not to say that ideology has not had any impact on policy. On the contrary, ideologies such as neoliberalism have been very influential. The parties have been vehicles for these ideologies, but they have also been expressed through other political and social institutions, such as international agencies, government bodies, the media, think tanks and pressure groups.

The party system is becoming more complex and unpredictable. New parties have emerged, and the public are less loyal to the established parties than was once the case. This makes it more difficult for parties to form majority governments, especially in those countries of the UK that use proportional representation. As coalitions (and minority governments) have to compromise to some extent on party policies in order to get their measures through, this makes it even more difficult to specify how party influences might have an impact on policy. Even when parties do have a working majority in Parliament (as is currently the case in Westminster and the Scottish Parliament), they still have to compromise, to minimise backbench rebellion and to ensure that they continue to appeal to the electorate by the time the next election is due.

Health policy-making is dominated by central government. Moreover, the core executive institutions (Prime Minister/Cabinet Office/Treasury) appear to have strengthened their grip on the policy-making process over the past few decades. In general, the health policy agenda has been driven more by the Prime Ministers and their advisers, who have played a key role in pushing particular policy ideas. The Treasury has acted as a counterweight to some of these ideas, as well as pursuing its own agenda. Under the coalition the centre's grip initially weakened, but was reinvigorated following the debacle surrounding the NHS reforms. Also, the DH was significantly weakened by these reforms.

Within central government key changes have taken place in the way in which policies are made. The most important developments have been the rise of special advisers and the decline of the traditional civil service role in policy formation. The genesis of most key health policies in recent years can be traced back to special advisers, with prime ministerial advisers particularly influential. In general, the influence of civil servants with a health professional background has waned, although some have exerted influence over key policies.

Parliament has only a marginal impact on health policy, largely because of its weakness in relation to central government, especially when the government has a large majority. Its influence over policy is limited by party discipline and by restrictions on its ability to initiate, amend and veto legislation. Parliament can play a valuable role in scrutinising central government and highlighting failures of public administration, but even these functions are hamstrung by limited powers. There are certain circumstances when Parliament can make a difference, however – on non-partisan issues, when the governing party is internally divided, or when the government cannot command a majority in the Commons. For example, under the 2010–15 coalition government, Parliament did exert considerable influence over the Health and Social Care Bill. Furthermore, MPs retain an important role in redressing grievances, and can bring cases to public attention, which may propel wider issues on to the political agenda. And in conjunction with others, such as the media and pressure groups, Parliament can shape agendas and contribute to policy change, particularly in the longer term.

The media has a very significant role in health policy. As has been shown, health issues attract media attention, and the reporting of health issues shapes perceptions of both the public and policy-makers. The media can influence the policy agenda in a positive way, by raising awareness about particular issues or policy options, although there is considerable media bias in the selection and coverage of issues. The media is mainly a negative force, limiting policy options and blocking policies. The importance of the media is borne out by the efforts of other policy actors to influence it (notably, government and external interests), and reflects the importance of agenda setting and symbolic politics in health policy. Media organisations also have their own agenda – many are now media businesses and their decisions are shaped by commercial considerations.

It is difficult to assess the role of policy networks in health policy. However, within these networks, the medical profession remains influential. Although organisations representing the profession have been challenged by non-medical groups and have faced a more difficult political environment, they still exert more influence than any other single interest. The health policy network, however, is more crowded than it once was. Some groups have become more influential, notably some private healthcare interests, think tanks and voluntary organisations, but there are considerable inequalities in influence within as well as between the various interests that seek to influence policy.

Access to key personnel within government is important for policy influence. External organisations and groups have responded to changes in policy processes within government (such as the rise of special advisers, czars and the involvement of the core executive institutions over health policy) by altering the focus of their lobbying. Although central government remains an important target for pressure groups, access does not guarantee influence. Groups are aware that they need to maintain good relationships with other political institutions (such as Parliament and the media) in order to influence policy, and influence often depends greatly on building alliances within and across the different interest groups (professional, commercial and the voluntary sector), and producing a coherent lobbying effort. These have increasingly coalesced around specific diseases and conditions (such as, for example, breast cancer, childbirth and mental health), which can be seen as competing with each other for resources and status.

Although most emphasis has been on the interaction between external organisations and policy-making institutions, one should not forget that influence is often exerted through the control of routine processes and practices, and the dominance of values and ideas within such systems. Indeed, it is acknowledged that the influence of the medical profession over policy has depended, to a large extent, on its hegemony within the healthcare system. This has enabled it to influence the agenda and 'non-decisions'. Commercial interests also exercise power in a similar way, as the neoliberal ethos is now firmly rooted in government. Meanwhile, challenging these dominant interests, other social forces, such as social movements, can exert influence over the health policy agenda in the longer term, by challenging dominant values and ideas in healthcare practice, as well as through the use of both direct action and conventional lobbying in the policy arena.

Turning to the implementation of health policy, it is clear that the political salience of health and healthcare has encouraged centralisation. Somewhat paradoxically, this has been accompanied by some decentralisation of functions and an attempt to shift responsibility on to local managers and professionals. The centralisation process has intensified in recent decades. New central regulatory bodies have been created, performance management has been strengthened, and centrally imposed priorities and targets have predominated. Even where autonomy is granted, this is only by compliance with central priorities. More recently, attempts to decentralise have gone beyond rhetoric and led to reforms that, if implemented fully, could lead to the devolution of power to local communities, managers and professionals. For the moment, such reforms remain controlled by central government regulatory frameworks.

Central intervention has often taken the form of reorganisations. Constant reorganisation can be counterproductive and costly, and has been increasingly discredited. The latest round of reforms is based on the idea that the NHS needs to be taken out of politics and moved from central control. But in reality, much scope for central intervention remains. Furthermore, as a key public service, many believe that the NHS should be a political issue.

Dissatisfaction with top-down models of decision-making, and concern that they are particularly inappropriate to complex policy areas such as health, has led to a growing interest in other approaches. These rely more on promoting cultural change, collaboration, networking and organisational learning than 'command and control' hierarchies. This may improve policy implementation, by engaging more closely with both clinicians and users, and offers the potential to develop better policies from the 'bottom up', by encouraging innovation and experimentation. Although several policy initiatives in recent years have sought to promote cultural change in the NHS, they do not sit easily with the dominant 'top down' style of policy-making.

It is now acknowledged that health policy implementation is contingent on other institutions outside the NHS. Increasingly, health policy and health services depend on a range of providers – statutory, voluntary and private sector. Indeed, the traditional problems of 'coordination' have multiplied partly as a result of government policy, which has encouraged competition, pluralism and privatisation in health and social care service provision. There are other challenges, too, such as the rising numbers of people with complex needs (for example, among elderly people), and the new public health agenda, which requires integrated care across a range of public and private sector organisations. In the past, the main emphasis has been on securing cooperation by financial incentives, planning arrangements, joint bodies, co-location and structural reorganisation. While these remain important, future efforts to improve collaboration should give greater weight to the cultural aspects of partnership, and in particular, the need to promote a common vision and commitment among partners. They must also involve a measure of decentralisation. Partnerships cannot be run effectively from Whitehall. The coalition government (and subsequently its Conservative successor) made some moves towards a more decentralised health and social care system with plans to devolve powers to cities and regions, but it remains to be seen whether or not these will come to fruition.

The devolution of powers to Scotland, Wales and Northern Ireland means that health policy in these parts of the UK is generated by different processes and contrasting political cultures compared to England. Consequently, policy differences have emerged between the four nations, in some cases resulting from a deliberate effort to set a new direction (such as free prescriptions and free personal care) or a refusal to follow England's lead (foundation trusts and competition in the NHS). Such variations offer the possibility of learning from different policy experiences, although, as noted, this is not fully exploited. In addition, there are factors that encourage convergence, not least the way in which healthcare systems in Northern Ireland, Wales and Scotland are judged with reference to the performance of the English NHS.

Significant reforms have taken place across the UK in relation to the voluntary sector and PPI. While these are broadly welcomed as a means of involving and perhaps empowering patients, there is much tokenism. Much more needs to be done to involve the public, patients and carers in public health and healthcare services. Care must be taken to ensure that the voluntary sector is not damaged by its involvement in publicly funded service provision, and in particular, its advocacy role on behalf of users must be protected.

Health policy is shaped by broader international and global forces. These include threats to health from communicable diseases and the health implications of economic pressures. Decisions made by international and supranational organisations, such as UN bodies and the EU, have a bearing on health. Health is therefore subject to multiple levels of governance. A process of 'hollowing out' has been identified, as international-level bodies have taken on a greater role in shaping domestic policies, while national government functions have been transferred to new agencies and to the independent sector (Rhodes, 1997). The reality is that a wide range of institutions at all levels, including central government, shape the formation and implementation of health policy.

Future directions

As has already been made clear, predicting the future direction of health policy is no easy task, but there are some clues. In 2014, the *NHS five year forward view* was published (NHS England et al, 2014). This document, authored by NHS England Chief Executive Simon Stevens and the leaders of five other national agencies (Health Education England, Monitor, CQC, NHSTDA and Public Health England) set out a future vision for health and care services in England. The highlights of this are set out in **Box 11.1** below. The other countries of the UK have either set out similar documents or are in the process of doing so (see Chapter Nine).

Box 11.1: A summary of the *NHS five year forward view*

The document set out the key issues facing the health and care system in England, including changing needs and new treatment options, variable quality of services, deep-rooted health inequalities and public health problems. In particular it called for:

- a radical upgrade in prevention and public health;
- a greater role for local authorities in leading public health;
- far greater control for patients of their care;
- greater engagement with communities and citizens in decisions about the future of health and care;
- more support for carers;
- steps to break down the division between family doctors and hospitals, physical and mental health, and health and social care;

- pioneering models of care to be developed at local levels, with a focus on establishing integrated care;
- redesign of urgent and emergency care services to meet needs;
- where supported by evidence, to reduce the number of specialist centres and improve quality;
- a new deal for GPs and primary care, with greater investment in these services;
- CCGs to acquire more control of the NHS budget;
- new options for midwife-led care;
- more NHS support for older people in care homes;
- better collaboration between regulators;
- an information revolution to support performance improvement, self-management of health, a paperless health record and online systems for prescriptions and appointments;
- acceleration of useful health innovation.

The document also made reference to the NHS budget, with £30 billion more needed per annum by 2020/21. It acknowledged that in order to address this gap, efficiency gains as well as additional funding from central government would be needed.

Source: NHS England et al (2014)

Despite party political rhetoric, and continuing controversy on issues such as the role of the private sector, a growing consensus was emerging about what must be done. This formed a basis for future policy development, now under a Conservative government (see Postscript below). It is likely that policy will shift to some extent with the departure of Lib Dem ministers. A greater emphasis on competition and the private sector seems inevitable. However, the early announcements of the Conservative government have so far exhibited a high degree of continuity with the coalition's policies (see Postscript). Other factors, not least the resources available to invest in the health and care system, will shape the response, whichever parties are in government. Furthermore, as before, other policy actors will exert influence on the direction and detail of policies.

Many of the issues identified in the *NHS five year forward view* are long-standing. They have been acknowledged in the past, but little has changed. In order for this vision to be achieved, a much stronger focus is needed on formulating workable policies that are accepted by professionals and the public, and which therefore have a greater chance of being fully implemented. In order for this to happen, a much more inclusive policy process is needed, more firmly based on evidence and research, and one that resists the need for simplistic initiatives and targets to placate media and public opinion.

Postscript

The Conservative Party's victory at the 2015 General Election enabled it to govern alone for the first time in almost 20 years. David Cameron continued as Prime Minister, while Secretary of State for Health, Jeremy Hunt, was also reappointed to his post. Although the government had won a working majority (12 seats more than the other parties together), the initial direction of policy changed little. The Conservatives promised to protect the NHS budget by providing a real-terms increase of £8 billion by 2020, coupled with £22 billion of planned efficiency gains. However, a cut to the public health budget (£200m in 2015/16) was also proposed. A new annual 1% pay increase limit was imposed on NHS staff until 2019/20. Some waiting time targets (those relating to inpatients and outpatients who had already been treated) were dropped. Changes to regulation were also announced. A new body, NHS Improvement, was proposed, to join up the provider regulation roles of Monitor and NHSTDA. It would also be responsible for patient safety (currently the responsibility of NHS England) and would host a new independent patient safety regulatory body. The government also called for all NHS services to be more widely available seven days a week, and indicated that if necessary it would impose this through contractual changes.

Key questions

1. What are the main features of the health policy process?
2. What is the likely future direction of health policy in the UK?

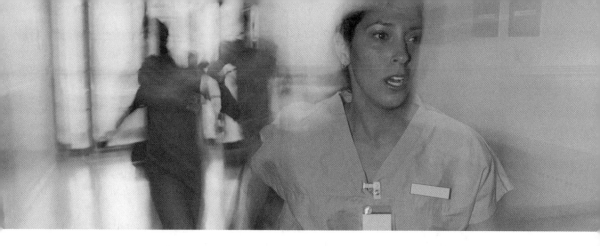

References

ABPI (Association of the British Pharmaceutical Industry) (2010) *The pharmaceutical industry's contribution to the UK economy and beyond*, London: ABPI.

Abraham, J. (2002) 'The pharmaceutical industry as a political player', *The Lancet*, vol 360, pp 1498-502.

ACEVO (Association of Chief Executives of Voluntary Organisations) (2010) *The organised efforts of society: The role of the voluntary sector in improving the health of the population*, London: ACEVO.

Adams, J. and Schmuecker, K. (eds) (2006) *Devolution in practice 2006: Public policy differences within the UK*, London: Institute for Public Policy Research.

Adams, J., Clark, M., Ezrow, L. and Glasgow, G. (2004) 'Understanding change and stability in party ideologies: do parties respond to public opinion or past election results?', *British Journal of Political Science*, vol 34, pp 589-610.

Addicott, R. (2011) *Social enterprise in health care*, London: King's Fund.

Addicott, R. (2013) *Working together to deliver the mandate*, London: King's Fund.

Addicott, R., McGivern, G. and Ferlie, E. (2006) 'Networks, organisational learning and knowledge management: NHS cancer networks', *Public Money & Management*, vol 26, no 2, pp 87-94.

Addison, P. (1975) *The road to 1945*, London: Cape.

Adonis, A. (2013) *Five days in May: The coalition and beyond*, London: Biteback.

ADPH (Association of Directors of Public Health) (2014) *English transition 2013 '6 months on' survey: Summary results*, London: ADPH.

Aggleton, P. (1990) *Health*, London: Routledge.

Alaszewski, A. and Brown, P. (2012) *Making health policy: A critical introduction*, Oxford: Polity Press.

Alcock, P. and Scott, D. (2002) 'Partnerships and the voluntary sector: can Compacts work?', in C. Glendinning, M. Powell and K. Rummery (eds) *Partnerships, New Labour and governance*, Bristol: Policy Press, pp 113-30.

Alford, R. (1975) *Health care politics*, Chicago, IL: University of Chicago Press.

Ali, N., Thoebe, L., Auvache, V. and White, P. (2001) 'Bad press for doctors: 21 year survey of three national newspapers', *British Medical Journal*, vol 323, pp 782-3.

Allen, P. (2013) 'An economic analysis of the limits of market-based reforms in the English NHS', *BMC Health Services Research*, vol 13, supp1, S1.

Allen, P. and Jones, L. (2011) 'Diversity of health care providers', in N. Mays. A. Dixon and L. Jones (eds) *Understanding New Labour's market reforms of the NHS*, London: King's Fund, pp 16-29.

Allen, P., Townsend, J., Dempster, P., Wright, J., Hutchings, A. and Keen, J. (2012) 'Organisational form as a mechanism to involve staff, public and users in public services: a study of NHS foundation trusts', *Social Policy & Administration*, vol 46, no 3, pp 239-57.

Allsop, J. and Saks, M. (eds) (2002) *Regulating the health professions*, London: Sage.

Alvarez-Rosete, A. and Mays N. (2008) 'Reconciling two conflicting tales of the English health policy process since 1997', *British Politics*, vol 3, pp 183-213.

Anderson, P. and Baumberg, B. (2006) *Alcohol in Europe: A public health perspective*, A Report for the European Commission, London: Institute of Alcohol Studies.

Appleby, J., Harrison, T., Hawkins, L. and Dixon, A. (2012) *Payment by results: How can payment systems deliver better care?*, London: King's Fund.

Appleby, J., Baird, B., Thompson, J. and Jabbal, J. (2015a) *The NHS under the coalition government: Part Two: NHS performance*, London: King's Fund.

Appleby, J., Thompson, J. and Jabbai, J. (2015b) *How is the NHS performing?* King's Fund Quarterly Monitoring Report, 16 July, London: King's Fund.

Armingeon, K. and Beyeler, M. (2004) *The OECD and European welfare states*, Cheltenham: Edward Elgar.

Armitage, G., Suter, E., Oelke, N. and Adair, C. (2009) 'Health systems and integration: state of the evidence', *International Journal of Integrated Care*, vol 9, no 17, pp 1-11.

Arora, S., Charlesworth, A., Kelly, E. and Stoye, G. (2013) *Public payment and private provision*, London: Nuffield Trust/Institute for Fiscal Studies.

Ashley, J. (1992) *Acts of defiance*, Harmondsworth: Penguin.

Ashworth, M., Medina, J. and Morgan, M. (2008) 'The effect of social deprivation on blood pressure monitoring and control in England', *British Medical Journal*, a2030.

Association of Medical Research Charities, Cancer Research UK and the Wellcome Trust (2012) *Leveson Inquiry: Culture, practice and ethics of the press (Evidence to the Leveson Inquiry)*, London: Association of Medical Research Charities.

Audit Commission (2003) *Targets in the public sector*, London: Audit Commission.

Audit Commission (2005) *Early lessons from payment by results*, London: Audit Commission.

Audit Commission (2009a) *Working better together: Managing local strategic partnerships*, London: The Stationery Office.

Audit Commission (2009b) *Means to an end: Joint financing across health and social care*, London: The Stationery Office.

Audit Commission and Healthcare Commission (2008) *Is the treatment working? Progress with the NHS system reform programme*, London: Audit Commission and Healthcare Commission.

Audit Scotland (2008) *Free personal and nursing care*, Edinburgh: Audit Scotland.

Audit Scotland (2011) *Review of community health partnerships*, Edinburgh: Audit Scotland.

Audit Scotland (2012) *Commissioning social care*, Edinburgh: Audit Scotland.

Audit Scotland (2013) *Improving community planning in Scotland*, Edinburgh: Audit Scotland.

Babor, T.F., Caetano, R., Casswell, S. et al (2003) *Alcohol: No ordinary commodity. Research and public policy*, Oxford: Oxford University Press.

Bachrach, P. and Baratz, M. (1962) 'Two faces of power', *American Political Science Review*, vol 56, no 4, pp 1947-52.

Baggott, R. (1990) *Alcohol, politics and social policy*, Aldershot: Avebury.

Baggott, R. (1995) *Pressure groups today*, Manchester: Manchester University Press.

Baggott, R. (2004) *Health and health care in Britain* (3rd edn), Basingstoke: Palgrave.

Baggott, R. (2007) *Understanding health policy*, Bristol: Policy Press.

Baggott, R. (2010a) *Public health: Policy and politics* (2nd edn), Basingstoke: Palgrave.

Baggott, R. (2010b) 'Alcohol policy and New Labour: a modern approach to an old problem', *Policy & Politics*, vol 38, no 1, pp 135-52.

Baggott, R. (2013) *Partnerships for public health and wellbeing*, Basingstoke: Palgrave.

Baggott, R. and Jones, K. (2014) 'The voluntary sector and health policy: the role of national level health consumer and patients' associations in the UK', *Social Science & Medicine*, vol 123, pp 202-9.

Baggott, R. and McGregor-Riley, V. (1999) 'Renewed consultation or continued exclusion? Organised interests and the Major governments', in P. Dorey (ed) *The Major premiership: Politics and policies under John Major 1990–97*, Basingstoke: Macmillan, pp 68-86.

Baggott, R., Allsop, J. and Jones, K. (2005) *Speaking for patients and carers*, Basingstoke: Palgrave.

Bale, T. (2010) *The Conservative Party from Thatcher to Cameron*, Cambridge: Polity.

Balloch, S. and Taylor, M. (2001) *Partnership working: Policy and practice*, Bristol: Policy Press.

Bara, J. and Budge, I. (2001) 'Party policy and ideology: still New Labour', *Parliamentary Affairs*, vol 54, no 4, pp 590-606.

Barber, M. (2008) *Instruction to deliver. Fighting to transform Britain's public services*, London: Methuen.

Bardsley, M., Steventon, A., Smith, J. and Dixon, J. (2013) *Evaluating integrated and community-based care: How do we know what works?*, London: Nuffield Trust.

Barker, A. and Peters, B.G. (1993) *The politics of expert advice: Creating, using and manipulating scientific knowledge for public policy*, Edinburgh: Edinburgh University Press.

Barnes, M., Harrison, S., Mort, M. and Shardlow, P. (1999) *Unequal partners: User groups and community care*, Bristol: Policy Press.

Barrett, S. (2004) 'Implementation studies: time for a revival? Personal reflections on 20 years of implementation studies', *Public Administration*, vol 82, no 2, pp 249-62.

Barrett, S. and Fudge, C. (eds) (1981) *Policy and action*, London: Methuen.

Bartlett, C., Sterne, J. and Egger, M. (2002) 'What is newsworthy? Longitudinal study of the reporting of medical research in two British newspapers', *British Medical Journal*, vol 325, pp 81-4.

Bate, P. (2000) 'Changing the culture of a hospital from hierarchy to networked community', *Public Administration*, vol 78, no 3, pp 485-512.

Batniji, R. and Woods, N. (2009) *Averting a crisis for global health: 3 actions for the G20*, Oxford: Global Economic Governance Programme.

Batty, D. (2001) 'The perils of celebrity endorsements', *The Guardian*, 3 August (www.theguardian.com/society/2001/aug/03/1).

Baumgartner, F. and Jones, B. (1993) *Agendas and instability in American politics*, Chicago, IL: University of Chicago Press.

BBC News (2007) 'Brown pledges hospital bug battle', 23 September (http://news.bbc.co.uk/1/hi/health/7008775.stm).

BBC News (2012) 'Tory blogger Tim Montgomerie questions coalition NHS plans', 10 February (http://www.bbc.co.uk/news/uk-politics-16984848).

Beer, S. (1965) *Modern British politics*, London: Faber & Faber.

Begg, N., Ramsay, M., White, J. and Bozoky, Z. (1998) 'Media dents confidence in MMR vaccine', *British Medical Journal*, vol 316, p 561.

Bell, D., Bowes, A. and Dawson, A. (2007) *Free personal care in Scotland: Recent developments*, York: Joseph Rowntree Foundation.

Bell, I. (1991) *The language of news media*, Oxford: Blackwell.

Bennett, C. (1991) 'What is policy convergence and what causes it?', *British Journal of Political Science*, vol 21, no 4, pp 215-33.

Benson, L., Boyd, A. and Walshe, K. (2004) *Learning from CHI: The impact of healthcare regulation*, Manchester: University of Manchester.

Bentley, A. (1967) *The process of government* (edited by P. Odegard), Cambridge, MA: Belknap.

Benton, M. and Russell, M. (2013) 'Assessing the impact of Parliamentary Oversight Committees in the British House of Commons', *Parliamentary Affairs*, vol 66, no 4, pp 772-97.

Berlinguer, G. (1999) 'Globalisation and global health', *International Journal of Health Services*, vol 29, no 3, pp 579-95.

Berman, S. (1998) 'Path dependency and political action: re-examining responses to the Depression', *Comparative Politics*, vol 20, no 4, pp 379-400.

Berridge, V. (1996) *AIDS in the UK: The making of policy 1981-1994*, Oxford: Oxford University Press.

Bevan, G. (2008) 'Changing paradigms of health governance and regulation of quality of healthcare in England', *Health, Risk & Society*, vol 10, no 1, pp 85-101.

Bevan, G. (2011) 'Regulation and system management', in N. Mays, A. Dixon and L. Jones (eds) *Understanding New Labour's market reforms of the English NHS*, London: King's Fund, pp 89-110.

Bevan, G. and Hood, C. (2006) 'Have targets improved performance in the English NHS?', *British Medical Journal*, vol 332, pp 419-22.

Bevan, G. and Skellern, M. (2011) 'Does competition between hospitals improve clinical quality? A review of evidence from two eras of competition in the English NHS', *British Medical Journal*, 343, d6740 (http://www.bmj.com/content/343/bmj.d6470).

Bevan, G., Karanikolos, M., Exley, J., Nolte, E., Connolly, S. and Mays, N. (2014) *The four health systems of the United Kingdom: How do they compare?*, London: Health Foundation/Nuffield Trust.

Birch, A.H. (1964) *Representative and responsible government*, London: George Allen & Unwin.

Black, D. (1987) *Recollections and reflections*, London: BMJ Books.

Blackstone, T. and Plowden, W. (1988) *Inside the think tank*, London: Heinemann.

Blair, T. (1997) *Speech to Trimdon Labour Club*, 30 April 1997.

Blair, T. (2010) *A journey*, London: Hutchinson.

Blake, R. (1985) *The Conservative Party from Peel to Thatcher*, London: Fontana.

Blank, R. and Burau, V. (2004) *Comparative health policy*, Basingstoke: Palgrave Macmillan.

Blaxter, M. (2004) *Health*, Oxford: Polity Press.

Bochel, C. and Bochel, H. (2004) *The UK social policy process*, Basingstoke: Palgrave.

Boero, N. (2013) 'Obesity in the media: social science weighs in', *Critical Public Health*, vol 23, no 3, pp 371-80.

Boffey, D. (2013) 'NHS chief admits to dismay at Jeremy Hunt's meddling', *The Observer*, 21 December (www.theguardian.com/society/2013/dec/21/nhs-service-jeremy-hunt-malcolm-grant).

Bogdanor, V. (2001) *Devolution in the United Kingdom*, Oxford: Oxford University Press.

Bojke, C., Castelle, A., Grasic, K. and Street, A. (2015) *Productivity of the English NHS 2012/13 update*, Research paper 110, York: Centre for Health Economics University of York.

Borkman, T. and Munn-Giddings, C. (2008) 'The contribution of self help groups and organisations to changing relations between patients/consumers and the health care system in the US and UK', in S. Chambre and M. Goldner (eds) *Patients, consumers and civil society: US and international perspectives, Vol 10, Advances in medical sociology*, Bingley: Emerald Publishing.

Bosanquet, N., de Zoete, H. and Haldenby, A. (2007) *NHS reform: The Empire strikes back*, London: Reform.

Bossert, T. (1998) 'Analysing the decentralisation of health systems in developing countries: decision, space, innovation and performance', *Social Science & Medicine*, vol 47, no 10, pp 1513-27.

Bovens, M. and t'Hart, P. (1996) *Understanding policy fiascoes*, New Brunswick, NJ: Transaction.

Bovens, M., t'Hart, P. and Peters, B.G. (eds) (2001) *Success and failure in public governance: A comparative analysis*, Cheltenham: Edward Elgar.

Boyd, A. and Coleman, A. (2011) 'Strategies used by health scrutiny committees to influence decision-makers', *Local Government Studies*, vol 37, no 3, pp 253-74.

Brainard, C. (2011) 'Mixed grades for medical coverage', *Columbia Journalism Review*, 22 April.

Brereton, L. and Vasoodaven, V. (2010) *The impact of the NHS market: An overview of the literature*, London: Civitas.

Brindle, D. (1999) 'Media coverage of social policy: a journalist's perspective', in B. Franklin (ed) *Social policy, the media and misrepresentation*, London: Routledge, pp 39-50.

Bristol Royal Infirmary Inquiry, The (2001) *The inquiry into the management of care of children receiving complex heart surgery at the Bristol Royal Infirmary – Final report*, London: The Stationery Office.

Britten, N. (2012) 'Doctor ran out of hours service for Londoners from his Norfolk home', *Daily Telegraph*, 26 January (http://www.telegraph. co.uk/news/health/news/9039195/Doctor-ran-out-of-hours-service-for-Londoners-from-his-Norfolk-home.html).

Brown, A. and Young, M. (2002) *NHS reform: Towards consensus?*, London: Adam Smith Institute.

Brown, P. and Zavestoski, S. (eds) (2004) 'Social movements in health: an introduction', *Sociology of Health & Illness*, vol 26, no 6, pp 679-94.

Brown, R. (1979) *Reorganising the NHS*, Oxford: Blackwell and Robertson.

Burch, M. and Holliday, I. (1996) *The British Cabinet system*, Hemel Hempstead: Prentice Hall.

Burch, M. and Holliday, I. (2004) 'The Blair government and the Core Executive', *Government and Opposition*, vol 39, no 1, pp 1-21.

Burns, H. (2004) 'Health tsars', *British Medical Journal*, vol 328, pp 117-18.

Bury, M. and Gabe, J. (1994) 'Television and medicine: medical dominance or trial by media?', in J. Gabe, D. Kelleher and G. Williams (eds) *Challenging medicine*, London: Routledge, pp 64-83.

Buse, K. and Walt, G. (2000) 'Global public-private health partnerships: part 2 – what are the issues for global governance', *Bulletin of the World Health Organisation*, vol 79, no 8, pp 699-79.

Buse, K., Mays, N. and Walt, G. (2005) *Making health policy*, Maidenhead: Open University Press.

Butler, J. (1992) *Patients, policies and politics: Before and after working for patients*, Buckingham: Open University Press.

Butler, I. and Drakeford, M. (2005) *Scandal, social policy and social welfare* (2nd edn), Bristol: Policy Press.

Byrne, D. (2004) *Partnerships for health in Europe*, Brussels: European Commission.

Byrne, P. (1997) *Social movements in Britain*, London: Routledge.

Cabinet Office (2007) *Capability review of the Department of Health*, London: Cabinet Office.

Cabinet Office (2009) *Department of Health: Progress and next steps*, London: Cabinet Office.

Cabinet Office (2010) *Building the big society*, London: Cabinet Office.

Cabinet Office (2014) *Special advisors in post*, November 2014, London: Cabinet Office.

Cairney, P. (2012) *Understanding public policy: Theories and issues*, Basingstoke: Palgrave.

Calkin, S. (2012) 'Commissioning board moves to halt NHS director exodus', *Health Service Journal*, 10 May.

Calkin, S. (2013) 'Bournemouth and Poole merger is blocked', *Health Service Journal*, 17 October.

Callaghan, K. and Schnell, F. (2001) 'Assessing the democratic debate: how the media frame elite policy discourse', *Political Communication*, vol 18, no 2, pp 182-213.

Cameron, D. (2009) *Our health priorities*, 2 November (www.conservatives. com/News/Speeches/200911/David_Cameron_Our_health _priorities. aspx).

Cameron, A. and Lart, R. (2003) 'Factors promoting and obstacles hindering joint working: systematic review of the research evidence', *Journal of Integrated Care*, vol 11, no 2, pp 9-17.

Cameron, A., Lart, R., Bostock, L. and Coomber, C. (2014) 'Factors that promote and hinder joint and integrated working between health and social care services: a review of research literature', *Health & Social Care in the Community*, vol 22, no 3, pp 225-33.

Campbell, A (2008) *The Blair years: Extracts from the Alastair Campbell diaries*, London: Hutchinson.

Campbell, D. (2013) 'Jeremy Hunt personally calls hospital bosses over A&E times', *The Guardian*, 22 November (www.theguardian.com/politics/2013/ nov/22/jeremy-hunt-hospital-personal-calls-times).

Cancer Research UK (2006) '"Kylie effect" can confuse women over breast cancer risk', Press Release, 23 October (www.cancerresearchuk. org/about-us/cancer-news/press-release/2006-10-23-kylie-effect-can-confuse-women-over-breast-cancer-risk).

Carers UK (2014) *Facts about carers*, London: Carers UK.

Carr, S. and Robins, D. (2009) *The implementation of individual budget schemes in adult social care*, London: Social Care Institute for Excellence.

Carvel, J. (2004) 'NHS Trusts bullied into private contracts', *The Guardian*, 1 June (www.theguardian.com/society/2004/jun/01/nhs2000.politics).

Carvel, J. (2008) 'NHS chief accused of eroding hospital's independence', *The Guardian*, 19 February (www.theguardian.com/society/2008/feb/19/ nhs.health).

Challis, L., Klein, R. and Webb, A. (1988) *Joint approaches to social policy: Rationality and practice*, Cambridge: Cambridge University Press.

Chambers, N., Pryce, A., Li., Y. and Poljsak, P (2011) 'The brilliant boards', *Health Service Journal*, 30 June, pp 19-22.

Chan, P., Dipper, A., Kelsey, P. and Harrison, J. (2010) 'Newspaper reporting of meticillin-resistant staphylococcus aureus and the "dirty hospital"', *Journal of Hospital Infection*, vol 75, pp 218-22.

Chapman, S. (2012) 'Does celebrity involvement in public health campaigns deliver long-term benefit? Yes', *British Medical Journal*, vol 345, e6364.

Chapman, S., Holding, S., Mcleod, K. and Wakefield, M. (2005) 'Impact of news of celebrity illness on breast cancer screening: Kylie Minogue's breast cancer diagnosis', *Medical Journal of Australia*, vol 183, no 5, pp 247-50.

Chard, J., Kuczawski, M., Black, N. and van der Meulen, J. (2011) 'Outcomes of elective surgery undertaken in independent sector treatment centres and NHS providers in England: audit of patient outcomes in surgery', *British Medical Journal*, 343, d6404.

Charleson, P., Lees, C. and Sikora, K. (2007) *Free at point of delivery – Reality or political mirage?*, London: Reform.

Checkland, K., Harrison, S., Snow, S., McDermott, I. and Coleman, A. (2012a) 'Commissioning in the English NHS: what's the problem?', *Journal of Social Policy*, vol 41, no 3, pp 553-50.

Checkland, K., Coleman, A., Segar, J., McDermott, I., Miller, R., Wallace, A., Petsoulas, C., Peckham, S. and Harrison, S. (2012b) *Exploring the early workings of emerging clinical commissioning groups: Final report*, Manchester: Manchester Policy Research Unit in Commissioning and the Healthcare System (https://www.escholar.manchester.ac.uk/uk-ac-man-scw:187083).

Childs, L. (2006) MRSA and the newspaper media', *Biologist*, vol 53, pp 252-5.

Clark, A. (2012) *Political parties in the UK*, Basingstoke: Palgrave.

Clark, G. and Kelly, S. (2004) 'Echoes of Butler? The Conservative Research Department and the making of Conservative policy', *Political Quarterly*, vol 75, no 4, pp 378-82.

Clarke, J. (1999) 'Breast cancer in mass circulating magazines in the USA and Canada 1974-1995', *Women and Health*, vol 8, no 4, pp 113-30.

Clarke, J. (2004) 'A comparison of breast, testicular and prostate cancer in mass print media (1996-2001)', *Social Science & Medicine*, vol 59, pp 541-51.

Clarke, J. and Everest, M. (2006) 'Cancer in the mass print media: fear, uncertainty and the medical model', *Social Science & Medicine*, vol 62, pp 591-600.

Clarke, J. and Newman, J. (1997) *The managerial state*, London: Sage.

Clwyd, A. and Hart, T. (2013) *Review of the NHS hospital complaints system: Putting patients back in the picture*, London: Department of Health.

Cobb, R. and Elder, C. (1972) *Participation in American politics: The dynamics of agenda-building*, Baltimore, MD: Johns Hopkins Press.

Cocker, P. and Jones, A. (2002) *Contemporary British politics and government* (3rd edn), Liverpool: Academic Press.

Coleman, A. and Glendinning, C. (2004) 'Local authority scrutiny of health: making the views of the community count?', *Health Expectations*, vol 7, pp 29-39.

Collier, J. (1989) *The health conspiracy – How doctors, the drug industry and government undermine our health*, London: Century Hutchinson.

Collingridge, D. and Reeve, C. (1986) *Science speaks to power: The role of experts in policy making*, London: Pinter.

Commission on Devolution in Wales (2014) *Empowerment and responsibility: Legislative powers to strengthen Wales*, Cardiff: Commission on Devolution in Wales.

Commission on the Future of Health and Social Care in England (2014) *A new settlement for health and social care – Final report*, London: King's Fund.

Commission to Strengthen Parliament (2000) *Report of the Commission*, London: Conservative Party.

Committee of Inquiry into the Cost of the NHS (1956) *Report (The Guillebaud report)*, Cmd 9663, London: HMSO.

Communities and Local Government Committee (2013) *The role of local authorities in health issues*, 8th report, 2012-13, London: The Stationery Office.

Comondore, V., Devereaux, P., Zhou, Q. et al (2009) 'Quality of care in for-profit and not-for-profit nursing homes: systematic review and meta-analysis', *British Medical Journal*, vol 339, b2732 (http://www.ncbi.nlm.nih.gov/pubmed/19654184).

Connolly, S., Bevan, G. and Mays, N. (2010) *Funding and performance of healthcare systems in the four countries of UK before and after devolution*, London: Nuffield Trust.

Conservative Party (2001) *Time for common sense: The Conservative manifesto*, London: Conservative Party.

Conservative Party (2003) *Setting patients free: A Conservative Party consultation*, London: Conservative Party.

Conservative Party (2005) *Action on health: Conservative manifesto*, Chapter 3, London: Conservative Party.

Conservative Party (2007a) *NHS autonomy and accountability: Proposals for legislation*, London: Conservative Party.

Conservative Party (2007b) *The patient will see you now doctor*, London: Conservative Party.

Conservative Party (2008) *Delivering some of the best health in Europe: Outcomes, not targets*, Responsibility Agenda Policy, Green Paper no 6, London: Conservative Party.

Conservative Party (2009) *Renewal plan for a better NHS: Plan for change*, London: Conservative Party.

Conservative Party (2010a) *A healthier nation*, Policy Green Paper no 12, London: Conservative Party.

Conservative Party (2010b) *Invitation to join the government of Britain: The Conservative manifesto 2010*, London: Conservative Party.

Conservative Research Department (2007) *Public health: Our priority*, London: Conservative Party.

Consumers' Association (2001) *The National Institute for Clinical Excellence: A patient-centred inquiry*, London: Which?

Cooper, Z., Gibbons, S., Jones, S. and McGuire, A. (2011) 'Does hospital competition save lives? Evidence from the English NHS patient choice reforms', *Economic Journal*, vol 121, F228-60.

Cope, J. (2002) 'Cause celebre', *The Guardian*, 4 April (www.theguardian.com/society/2002/apr/04/1).

Cottle, S. (2001) 'Television news and citizenship: packaging the public sphere', in M. Bromley (ed) *No news is bad news: Radio, television and the public*, London: Longman, pp 61-79.

Coulter, A. (2011) *Engaging patients in healthcare*, Maidenhead: Open University.

Coulter, A. and Collins, A. (2011) *Making shared decision-making a reality*, London: King's Fund.

Council of Europe (1996) *European Social Charter* (revised) (www.conventions.coe.int/treaty/en/Treaties/html/163.htm).

Council of the European Communities and Commission of the European Communities (1992) *Treaty on European Union*, (www.europa.eu).

Council of the European Union (2003) 'Recommendation of 2 December 2003 on cancer screening', *Official Journal*, L327/34.

Council of the European Union (2006) 'Council conclusions on common values and principles in EU health systems', *Official Journal*, vol 146, 22 June, p 1.

Council of the European Union (2009) 'Council recommendations on patient safety, including the prevention and control of healthcare associated infections', *Official Journal*, C151/1.

Council of the European Union (2011) *Council conclusions: Towards modern, responsive and sustainable health systems*, 3095th Employment, Social Policy, Health and Consumer Affairs Council Meeting: Health Issues, Luxembourg, 6 June.

Cox, J. (2001) 'Appointed czars, elected presidents and windows of opportunity', *British Journal of Psychiatry*, vol 178, pp 292-3.

Coxall, W. (2001) *Pressure groups in British politics*, London: Longman.

CQC (Care Quality Commission) (2011) *Review of compliance: Castlebeck Care (Teesdale) Ltd: Summary of our findings*, London: Care Quality Commission.

Craig, F.W.S. (1975) *British general election manifestos 1900-74*, Basingstoke: Macmillan.

Craig, G. and Taylor, M. (2002) 'Dangerous liaisons: local government and the voluntary and community sectors', in C. Glendinning, M. Powell and K. Rummery (eds) *Partnerships, New Labour and governance*, Bristol: Policy Press, pp 131-48.

Craig, G., Taylor, M. and Parkes, T. (2004) 'Protest or partnership? The voluntary and community sectors in the policy process', *Social Policy & Administration*, vol 38, no 3, pp 221-39.

Crayford, T., Hooper, R. and Evans, S. (1997) 'Death rates of characters in soap operas on British television: is a government health warning required?', *British Medical Journal*, vol 315, pp 1649-52.

Crinson, I. (2005) 'The direction of health policy in New Labour's third term', *Critical Social Policy*, vol 25, no 4, pp 507-16.

Crinson, I. (2009) *Health policy: A critical perspective*, London: Sage.

Crisp, N. (2010) *Turning the world upside down: The search for global health in the 21st century*, London: Royal Society of Medicine Press.

Crisp, N. (2011) *24 hours to save the NHS: The Chief Executive's account of reform 2000-2006*, Oxford: Oxford University Press.

Crossley, N. (2006) 'The field of psychiatric contention in the UK, 1960-2000', *Social Science & Medicine*, vol 62, pp 552-63.

Crossman, R. (1972) *Inside view: Three lectures on prime ministerial government*, London: Jonathan Cape.

Curry, N., Goodwin, N., Naylor, C. and Robertson, R. (2008) *Practice-based commissioning: Reinvigorate, replace, abandon?*, London: King's Fund.

Curry, N., Mundle, C., Sheil, F. and Weaks, L. (2011) *The voluntary and community sector in health: Implications of the proposed NHS reforms*, London: King's Fund.

D'Ancona, M. (2013) *In it together*, London: Viking.

Darjee, R. and Crichton, J. (2004) 'New mental health legislation', *British Medical Journal*, vol 329, pp 634-35.

David, P. (1985) 'Clio and the economics of qwerty', *American Economic Review*, vol 75, no 2, pp 332-7.

Davies, A. (2000) 'Don't trust me, I'm a doctor – medical regulation and the 1999 NHS reforms', *Oxford Journal of Legal Studies*, vol 20, pp 437-56.

Davies, P. (2012) 'Behind closed doors: how much power does McKinsey wield?', *British Medical Journal*, vol 344, e2905.

Davis, K., Stremekis, K., Squires, D. and Schoen, C. (2014) *Mirror, mirror on the wall: How the performance of the US health care system compares internationally*, Washington, DC: Commonwealth Fund.

Davis, S. (2005) 'Public medicine: the reception of a medical drama', in M. King and K. Watson (2005) *Representing health: Discourses of health and illness in the media*, Basingstoke: Palgrave, pp 27-46.

Day, P. and Klein, R. (1989) 'Interpreting the unexpected: the case of AIDS policy making in Britain', *Journal of Public Policy*, vol 9, no 3, pp 337-53.

Day, P. and Klein, R. (1992) 'Constitutional and distributional conflict in British medical politics: the case of general practice, 1911-1991', *Political Studies*, vol 40, pp 462-78.

Day, P. and Klein, R. (1997) *Steering but not rowing: The transformation of the Department of Health*, Bristol: Policy Press.

Day, P. and Klein, R. (2004) *The NHS improvers: A study of the Commission for Health Improvement*, London: King's Fund.

Deacon, D. (1999) 'The construction of voluntary sector news', in B. Franklin (ed) *Social policy, the media and misrepresentation*, London: Routledge, pp 51-68.

Deakin, N. and Parry, R. (2000) *The Treasury and social policy*, London: Macmillan.

Dean, M. (2013) *Democracy under attack*, Bristol: Policy Press.

Decision of the European Parliament and of the Council (2002) *Adopting a programme of community action in the field of public health (2003-08)*, Decision 1786/2002, *Official Journal*, L271, 9 October.

Decision of the European Parliament and of the Council (2007) *Establishing a second programme of community action in the field of health (2008-13)*, Decision 1350/2007, *Official Journal*, L30, 20 November.

Declerq, E. (1998) 'Changing childbirth in the United Kingdom: lessons for US health policy', *Journal of Health Politics, Policy and Law*, vol 23, no 5, pp 833-59.

Deeming, C. (2004) 'Decentring the NHS: a case study of resource allocation decisions within a health district', *Social Policy & Administration*, vol 38, no 1, pp 57-72.

Deer, B. (2011) 'How the case against the MMR vaccine was fixed', *British Medical Journal*, vol 342, c5347.

Della Porta, D. and Diani, M. (2005) *Social Movements: An introduction*, 2nd edition, London: Wiley Blackwell.

Denham, A. and Garnett, M. (2006) 'What works? British think tanks and the end of ideology', *Political Quarterly*, vol 77, no 2, pp 156-65.

Department for Communities and Local Government (2006) *Strong and prosperous communities: The Local Government White Paper*, Cm 6939, London: The Stationery Office.

Devereux, E. (2007) *Understanding the Media*, London: Sage.

Devereaux, P., Choi, P., Lachetti, C. et al (2002) 'A systematic review and meta analysis of studies comparing mortality rates of private for-profit and private not-for-profit hospitals', *Canadian Medical Association Journal*, vol 166, no 11, pp 1399-406.

de Vos, P. (2005) 'No one left abandoned: Cuba's national health system since the 1959 revolution', *International Journal of Health Services*, vol 35, pp 189-207.

de Vos, P., Dewitte, H. and van der Stuyft, P. (2004) 'Unhealthy European policy', *International Journal of Health Services*, vol 34, no 2, pp 255-69.

DH (Department of Health) (1987) *Promoting better health*, Cm 249, London; HMSO.

DH (1989) *Working for patients*, Cm 555, London: HMSO.

DH (1991) *The patient's charter*, London: DH.

DH (1992) *The health of the nation: A strategy for health in England*, Cm 1986, London: The Stationery Office.

DH (1997) *The NHS: Modern, dependable*, Cm 3807, London: The Stationery Office.

DH (1998a) *Independent Inquiry into Inequalities in Health*, London: The Stationery Office.

DH (1998b) *Partnership in action: New opportunities for joint working between health and social services: A discussion document*, London: DH.

DH (1998c) *Modernising health and social services: National priorities guidance 1999-2000/2001-2*, London: DH.

DH (1999a) *With respect to old age. Long-term care – Rights and responsibilities. A report by the Royal Commission on Long-Term Care*, Cm 4192, London: The Stationery Office.

DH (1999b) *Saving lives*, Cm 4386, London: The Stationery Office.

DH (2000) *The NHS Plan: A plan for investment – A plan for reform*, Cm 4818, London: The Stationery Office.

DH (2001) *Shifting the balance of power within the NHS: Securing delivery*, London: DH.

DH (2002) *Delivering the NHS Plan: Next steps on investment, next steps on reform*, Cm 5503, London: The Stationery Office.

DH (2003) *Building on the best: Choice, responsiveness and equity in the NHS*, Cm 6079, London: The Stationery Office.

DH (2004a) *The NHS Improvement Plan*, Cm 6268, London: The Stationery Office.

DH (2004b) *Choosing health*, Cm 6374, London: The Stationery Office.

DH (2004c) *Making partnership work for patients, carers and service users: A strategic agreement between the Department of Health, the NHS and the voluntary and community sector*, London: DH.

DH (2004d) 'Government and industry launch joint report encouraging innovations in NHS and healthcare', DH press release, 2004/0412.

DH (2005) *Creating a patient-led NHS: Delivering the NHS Improvement Plan*, London: DH.

DH (2006a) *Our health, our care, our say: A new direction for community services*, Cm 6737, London: The Stationery Office.

DH (2006b) *Good doctors, safer patients: A report by the Chief Medical Officer*, London: DH.

DH (2008) *High quality healthcare for all* (Darzi Review), Cm 7432, London: The Stationery Office.

DH (2010a) *Equity and excellence: Liberating the NHS*, Cm 7881, London: The Stationery Office.

DH (2010b) *Healthy lives: Healthy people*, Cm 7985, London: The Stationery Office.

DH (2010c) *Liberating the NHS: Report of the arm's length bodies review*, London: DH.

DH (2012) *Transforming care: A national response to Winterbourne View hospital – Final report*, London: DH.

DH (2013a) *The Mandate: A mandate from the government to the NHS Commissioning Board April 2013–March 2015*, London: DH.

DH (2013b) *Annual report and accounts 2012–13*, London: DH.

DH (2014) *The Mandate: A mandate from the government to NHS England, April 2014–March 2015*, London: DH.

DH (2015) *The NHS constitution for England*, London: DH.

DH/Cabinet Office (2012) *Department of Health Capability Action Plan 2011-12*, London: Cabinet Office.

DH, ADASS (Association of Directors of Adult Social Services), CQC (Care Quality Commission), LGA (Local Government Association) et al (2013) *Integrated care and support: Our shared commitment*, London: DH.

DHSS (Department of Health and Social Security) (1976) *Priorities for health and personal social services in England: A consultative document*, London: HMSO.

DHSS (1981) *Care in action*, London: DHSS.

DHSS (1983) *NHS management inquiry* (Griffiths Management Report), London: DHSS.

DHSSPS (Department of Health, Social Services and Public Safety) (2002) *Investing for health*, Belfast: DHSSPS.

DHSSPS (2010) *Investing for health strategy: Final report*, Report prepared by RSM International, Belfast: DHSSPS.

DHSSPS (2011) *Transforming your care: A review of health and social care in Northern Ireland* (Compton Review), Belfast: DHSSPS.

DHSSPS (2014) *Making life better: A whole system framework for public health 2013-23*, Belfast: DHSSPS.

Dickinson, H., Ham, C., Snelling, I. and Spurgeon, P. (2013a) *Are we there yet? Models of medical leadership and their effectiveness*, Southampton: National Institute for Health Research.

Dickinson, H., Glasby, J., Nicholds, A., Jeffares, S., Robinson, S. and Sullivan, H. (2013b) *Joint commissioning in health and social care: An exploration of processes, services and outcomes- final report*, NIHR Service Delivery and Organisation Programme, Southampton: National Institute for Health Research.

Dimbleby, H. and Vincent, J. (2013) *The school food plan* (www.schoolfoodplan.com/wp-content/uploads/2013/07/School_Food_Plan_2013.pdf).

Directive of the European Parliament and of the Council (2011) 'On the application of patients' rights in cross-border healthcare', 9 March, 2011/24/EU, *Official Journal*, 4.4.2011 L88/45-65.

Dixon, A. and Alvarez-Rosete, A. (2008) *Governing the NHS: Alternatives to an independent board*, London; King's Fund.

Dixon, A. and Jones, L. (2011) 'Local implementation of market reforms', in N. Mays, A. Dixon and L. Jones (eds) *Understanding New Labour's market reforms of the NHS*, London: King's Fund, pp 124-42.

Dixon, A. and Robertson, R. (2011) 'Patient choice of hospital', in N. Mays, A. Dixon and L. Jones (2011) *Understanding New Labour's market reforms of the English NHS*, London: King's Fund, pp 52-65.

Dixon, A., Appleby, J., Robertson, R., Burge, P., Devlin, N. and Magee, H. (2010) *Patient choice*, London: King's Fund.

Dixon, A., Khachatryan, A., Wallace, A., Peckham, S., Boyce, T. and Gillam, S. (2011) *Impact of quality and outcomes framework on health inequalities*, London: King's Fund.

Dolowitz, D. (2012) 'Policy transfer: what have we learned and where should we go?', *Regional and Federal Studies*, vol 22, no 3, pp 341-51.

Dolowitz, D. and Marsh, D. (1996) 'Who learns what from whom: a review of the policy transfer literature', *Political Studies*, vol 44, no 2, pp 343-57.

Donaldson, L., Rutter, P. and Henderson, M. (2014) *The right time, the right place*, Belfast: Department of Health, Social Services and Public Safety.

Dopson, S. and Fitzgerald, L. (2006) *Knowledge to action? Evidence-based healthcare in context*, Oxford: Oxford University Press.

Dopson, S., Locock, L. and Stewart, R. (1999) 'Regional offices in the new NHS: an analysis of the effects and significance of recent changes', *Public Administration*, vol 77, no 1, pp 91-110.

Doran, T., Fullwood, C., Kontopantelis, E. and Reeves, D. (2008) 'Effect of financial incentives on inequalities in the delivery of primary clinical care in England: analysis of clinical indicators for the quality and outcomes framework', *The Lancet*, vol 372, no 9640, pp 728-36.

Doran, T., Kontopantelis, K., Reeves, D., Sutton, M. and Ryan, A. (2014) 'Setting performance targets in pay for performance programmes: what can we learn from QOF?', *British Medical Journal*, vol 348, g1595.

Dorey, P. (2005) *Policy making in Britain: An introduction*, London: Sage.

Dorey, P. (2007) 'A new direction or another false dawn? David Cameron and the crisis of British Conservatism', *British Politics*, vol 2, pp 137-66.

Dowler, C. (2013a) 'Mandate update will impose additional burden on NHS', *Health Service Journal*, 15 July.

Dowler, C. (2013b) 'NHS England warning: Monitor's proposals could put services at risk', *Health Service Journal*, 9 September.

Dowling, B. (1997) 'Effect of fundholding on waiting times: a database study', *British Medical Journal*, vol 315, pp 290-2.

Dowling, B., Powell, M. and Glendinning, C. (2004) 'Conceptualising successful partnerships', *Health & Social Care in the Community*, vol 12, no 4, pp 309-17.

Downs, A. (1957) *An economic theory of democracy*, New York: Harper & Row.

Downs, A. (1972) 'Up and down with ecology: the issue attention cycle', *Public Interest*, vol 28, no 1, pp 38-50.

Doyal, L. (1979) *The political economy of health*, London: Pluto.

Doyle, H. (2000) 'Health scares, media hype, policy making', in A. Hann (ed) *Analysing health policy*, Aldershot: Ashgate, pp 147-64.

Drakeford, M. (2006) 'Health policy in Wales: making a difference in conditions of difficulty', *Critical Social Policy*, vol 26, no 3, pp 543-61.

Driver, S. and Martell, L. (2002) *Blair's Britain*, Cambridge: Polity Press.

Drummond, C. (2004) 'An alcohol strategy for England: the good, the bad and the ugly', *Alcohol and Alcoholism*, vol 39, no 5, pp 377-9.

Dunlop, C. and Radaelli, C. (2013) 'Systematising policy learning: from monoliths to dimensions', *Political Studies*, vol 31, no 3, pp 599-619.

Dunsire, A. (1978) *Implementation in a bureaucracy*, Oxford: Martin Robinson.

Eckstein, H. (1960) *Pressure group politics: The case of the BMA*, London: George Allen & Unwin.

Edelman, M. (1964) *The symbolic uses of politics*, Urbana, IL: University of Illinois Press.

Edelman, M. (1971) *Politics as symbolic action*, New York: Academic Press.

Edelman, M. (1977) *Political language: Words that succeed and policies that fail*, New York: Institute for the Study of Poverty.

Edelman, M. (1985) *The symbolic uses of politics*, Urbana, IL: University of Illinois Press.

Edwards, B. (1993) *The National Health Service: A manager's tale 1946-92*, London: Nuffield Provincial Hospitals Trust.

Edwards, B. (2007) *An independent NHS: A review of the options*, London: Nuffield Trust.

Edwards, B. and Fall, M. (2005) *The executive years of the NHS: The England account 1985-2003*, Oxford: Radcliffe.

Edwards, N. (2010) *Triumph of hope over experience*, London: NHS Confederation.

Edwards, N. (2014) *Community services: How they can transform care*, London: King's Fund.

Egglestone, K. Shen,Y.-C., Lau, J., Schmid, C. and Chan, J. (2006) 'Hospital ownership and quality of care: what explains the different results?', Working Paper 12241, Cambridge, MA: National Bureau of Economic Research.

Eldridge, J., Kitzinger, J. and Williams, K. (1999) *The mass media and power in modern Britain*, Oxford: Oxford University Press, pp 160-80.

Elinder, L., Joosens, L. and Raw, M. (2003) *Public health aspects of the Common Agricultural Policy*, Ostersund: Swedish National Institute of Public Health.

Elliot, F. (2009) 'Short, hard life of Ivan Cameron, whose suffering could change Britain', *The Times*, 26 February.

Ellmore, R. (1980) 'Backward mapping: implementation research and policy decisions', *Political Science Quarterly*, vol 94, no 4, pp 601-16.

Ennew, C.,Whynes, D., Jolleys, J. and Robinson, P. (1998) 'Entrepreneurship and innovation among GP fundholders', *Public Money & Management*, vol 18, no 1, pp 59-68.

Enthoven, A. (1985) *Reflections on the management of the NHS*, London: Nuffield Provincial Hospitals Trust.

Entwhistle,V. (1995) 'Reporting research in medical journals and newspapers', *British Medical Journal*, vol 310, pp 920-3.

Entwhistle, V. and Beaulieu–Hancock, M. (1992) 'Health and medical coverage in the UK national press', *Public Understanding of Science*, vol 1, no 4, pp 367-82.

Entwhistle,V. and Sheldon,T. (1999) 'The picture of health? Media coverage of the health service', in B. Franklin (ed) *Social policy, the media and misrepresentation*, London: Routledge, pp 118-34.

Entwhistle,V., Watt, I., Bradbury, R. and Pehl, L. (1996) 'Media coverage of the Child B Case', *British Medical Journal*, vol 312, pp 1587-91.

Ettelt, S., Mays, N. and Nolte, E. (2012) 'Policy learning from abroad: why it is more difficult than it seems', *Policy & Politics*, vol 40, no 4, pp 491-504.

Etzioni, A. (1993) *The spirit of community*, New York: Random House.

EU (European Union) (1997) *Treaty of Amsterdam* (www.eurotreaties.com/amsterdamtext.html).

EUHPF (European Union Health Policy Forum) (2007) *Guiding principles with regard to transparency*, Brussels: EUHPF.

EU Ministerial Conference (2007) *Rome Declaration: Health in all policies – achievements and challenges*, 18 December, Rome.

EUROCARE (2014) *Survival of cancer patients in Europe*, EUROCARE-5 (www.eurocare.it).

European Commission (2006) *An EU strategy to support member states in reducing alcohol related harm*, COM (2006) 625, Brussels: European Commission.

European Commission (2007a) *Together for health: A strategic approach for the EU*, COM 2007/630, Brussels: European Commission.

European Commission (2007b) *A strategy for Europe on nutrition, overweight and obesity-related health issues*, COM 2007/279 final, Brussels: European Commission.

European Commission (2010) *Communication from the Commission: Europe 2020: A strategy for smart, sustainable and inclusive growth*, COM (2010) 2020 final, Brussels: European Commission.

European Court of Auditors (2009) *Special Report 2/2009: The European Union's Public Health Programme (2003-2007): An effective way to improve health?*, Luxembourg: European Court of Auditors.

European Parliament (2011) *Report on reducing health inequalities in the EU*, 2010/2089 NI, European Parliament Plenary sitting A7-0032/2011.

European Parliament and Council (2014) Regulation 282/2014 11.3.14, Establishment of a Third Programme for the Union's actions in the field of health 2014-20, *Official Journal*, 21.3.14 L86/1.

Evaluation Partnership (2010) *Evaluation of the European platform for action on diet, physical activity and health*, Brussels: European Commission.

Evans, M. and Davies, J. (1999) 'Understanding policy transfer: a multi-level, multi-disciplinary perspective', *Public Administration*, vol 77, no 1, pp 361-85.

Evans, R. (2008) 'Brown unveils vision for 21st century', *Health Service Journal*, 10 January, pp 45.

Evans, S. and Williams, S. (2002) *The wrong prescription? A critique of Labour's management of the NHS*, London: Conservative Policy Unit.

Exworthy, M. and Frosini, F. (2008) 'Room for manoeuvre? Explaining local autonomy in the English National Health Service', *Health Policy*, vol 86, pp 204-12.

Exworthy, M. and Hunter, D. (2012) 'The challenge of joined up government in tackling health inequalities', *International Journal of Public Administration*, vol 34, no 4, pp 201-12.

Exworthy, M., Peckham, S., Powell, M. and Hann, A. (eds) (2011) *Shaping health policy: Case studies methods and analysis*, Bristol: Policy Press.

Faculty of Public Health (2007) *The impact of the EU Common Agricultural Policy on public health*, London: Faculty of Public Health.

Fairclough, N. (2000) *New Labour, new language?*, London: Routledge.

Farrar, S., Yi, D., Sutton, M., Chalkley, M., Sussex, J. and Scott, A. (2009) 'Has payment by results affected the way that English hospitals provide care?' *British Medical Journal*, vol 339, b3407 (http://www.bmj.com/content/339/bmj.b3047).

Fawcett, H. (2004) 'The making of social justice in Scotland: devolution and social exclusion' in A. Trench and A. Hazell (eds) *Has devolution made a difference? The state of the nations*, Exeter: Imprint, pp 237-54.

Ferlie, E., Ashburner, L., Fitzgerald, L. and Pettigrew, A. (1996) *The new public management*, Oxford: Oxford University Press.

Ferner, R. (2005) 'The influence of big pharma', *British Medical Journal*, vol 330, pp 857-8.

Ferner, R. and McDowell, S. (2006) 'How NICE may be outflanked', *British Medical Journal*, vol 332, pp 1268-71.

File on 4 (2012) 'NHS queues', BBC Radio 4, 17 June.

File on 4 (2013) 'A healthy market?', BBC Radio 4, 12 November.

File on 4 (2014) 'NHS: testing the market', BBC Radio 4, 19 October.

Fischer, F. (1990) *Technocracy and the politics of expertise*, Newbury Park, CA: Sage.

Fitzgerald, L. and Dufour, Y. (1997) 'Clinical management as boundary management: comparative analysis of Canadian and UK health institutions', *International Journal of Public Sector Management*, vol 10, no 1/2, pp 5-10.

Fooks, G. (2011) 'Corporate social responsibility and access to policy elites: an analysis of tobacco industry documents', *PLoS Medicine*, vol 8, no 8, e10001076.

Foot, C., Gilburt, H., Dunn, P., Jabbai, J., Seale, B., Goodrich, J., Buck, D. and Taylor, J. (2014) *People in control of their own health and care: The state of involvement*, London: King's Fund.

Foot, M. (1975) *Aneurin Bevan: A biography, Vol 2, 1945-60*, London: Paladin.

Forder, J., Jones, K., Glendinning, C., Caeils, J., Welch, E., Baxter, K., Davison, J., Windle, K., Irvine, A. King, D. and Dolan, P. (2012) *Evaluation of the personal health budget pilot programme*, Canterbury: Personal Social Services Research Unit, University of Kent.

Fort, M., Mercer, M. and Gish, O. (eds) (2004) *Sickness and wealth: The corporate assault on global health*, Cambridge, MA: South End Press.

Fotaki, M., Ruane, S. and Leys, C. (2013) *The future of the NHS? Lessons from the market in social care in England*, London: Centre for Health and the Public Interest.

Fowler, N. (1991) *Ministers decide: A personal memoir of the Thatcher years*, London: Chapman.

Fox, M.J. (2002) *Lucky man: A memoir*, London: Ebury Press.

Franklin, B. (ed) (1999) *Social policy, the media and misrepresentation*, London: Routledge.

Friedman, M. (1962) *Capitalism and freedom*, Chicago, IL: University of Chicago Press.

Fulop, N., Mowlem, A. and Edwards, N. (2005) *Building integrated care*, London: NHS Confederation.

Furness, D. and Gough, B. (2009) *From feast to famine: Reforming the NHS for an age of austerity*, London: Social Market Foundation.

Gainsbury, S. (2009) '"Organic" reduction in PCTs under Tories', *Health Service Journal*, vol 27, 4 August.

Gamble, A. (1994) *The free economy and the strong state: The politics of Thatcherism* (2nd edn), London: Macmillan.

Garcia, J., Redshaw, M., Fitzsimmons, B. and Keene, J. (1998) *First class delivery: A national survey of women's views of maternity care*, London: Audit Commission/NPEU (National Perinatal Epidemiology Unit).

Gard, M. and Wright, J. (2005) *The obesity epidemic: Science, morality and ideology*, London: Routledge.

Gaynor, M., Moreno-Serra, R. and Propper, C. (2011) 'Death by market power: reform, competition and patient outcomes in the National Health Service', CMPO Working Paper 10/242, Bristol: University of Bristol.

Gerrard, M. (2009) *A stifled voice?*, Brighton: Pen Press.

Giddens, A. (1998) *The Third Way: The renewal of social democracy*, Cambridge: Polity Press.

Giddens, A. (2002) *Runaway world: How globalisation is reshaping our lives*, London: Profile.

Gilbert, B. (1970) *British social policy 1914–1939*, London: Batsford.

Glasby, J. (2012) *Understanding health and social care* (2nd edn), Bristol: Policy Press.

Glasby, J. and Dickinson, H. (2014) *Partnership working in health and social care*, Bristol: Policy Press.

Glasby, J. and Peck, E. (2003) *Care trusts: Partnership working in action*, Abingdon: Radcliffe Medical Press.

Glasby, J., Martin, G. and Regen, E. (2008) 'Older people and the relationship between hospital services and intermediate care: results from a national evaluation', *Journal of Interprofessional Care*, vol 22, no 6, pp 639-49.

Glasby, J., Smith, J. and Dickinson, H. (2006) *Creating NHS Local: A new relationship between PCTs and local government*, Birmingham: Health Services Management Centre.

Glendinning, C., Coleman, A. and Rummery, K. (2003) 'Looking outwards: primary care organisations and local partnerships', in B. Dowling and C. Glendinning (eds) *The new primary care*, Maidenhead: Open University Press, pp 196-216.

Glendinning, C., Hudson, B. and Means, R. (2005) 'Under strain? Exploring the troubled relationship between health and social care', *Public Money & Management*, vol 25, no 4, August, pp 245-51.

Glendinning, C., Challis, D., Fernandez, J., Jacobs, S., Jones, K., Knapp, M., Manthorpe, J., Moran, N., Netten, A., Stevens, M. and Wilberforce, M. (2008) *Evaluation of individual budgets pilot programme*, York: Social Policy Research Unit, University of York.

Glennerster, H., Owens, P. and Matsaganis, M. (1994) *Implementing GP fundholding: Wild card or winning hand?*, Buckingham: Open University Press.

GMC (General Medical Council) (2013) *Good medical practice* (www.gmc-uk.org/guidance).

Goldacre, B. (2008) *Bad science*, London: Fourth Estate.

Goldacre, B. (2013) *Bad pharma*, London: Fourth Estate.

Goodchild, S. (2015) 'Soaps, mental health and cancer: how TV is shaping our attitudes', *The Guardian*, 22 January (www.theguardian.com/healthcare-network/2015/jan/22/soaps-mental-health-cancer-hollyoaks-eastenders-coronation-street).

Goodwin, N. (2013) 'Understanding integrated care', *International Journal of Integrated Care*, vol 13, URN:NBN:NL: UI: 10.1.114416.

Gornall, J. (2014) 'Under the influence', *British Medical Journal*, vol 348, f7646.

Grant, W. (2000) *Pressure groups and British politics*, Basingstoke: Macmillan.

Grant, W. (2005) 'Pressure politics: a politics of collective consumption?', *Parliamentary Affairs*, vol 58, no 2, pp 366-79.

Gray, A. and Harrison, S. (2004) *Governing medicine*, Maidenhead: Open University Press.

Gray, A.M. and Birrell, D. (2013) 'The structures of the NHS in Northern Ireland: divergence, policy copying and policy deficiency', *Public Policy and Administration*, vol 28, no 3, pp 274-89.

Green, D.S. (1987) *The new right: The counter-revolution in political, economic and social thought*, Brighton: Wheatsheaf.

Green, J. (2007) 'When voters and parties agree: valence issues and party competition', *Political Studies*, vol 55, pp 629-55.

Green, J. and Thorogood, N. (1998) *Analysing health policy*, London: Longman.

Green-Pedersen, C. (2007) 'The growing importance of issue competition: the changing nature of party competition in Western Europe', *Political Studies*, vol 55, pp 607-28.

Greenaway, J. (2003) *Drink and British politics since 1830: A study in policy-making*, Basingstoke: Palgrave.

Greener, I. (2004a) 'Three moments of Labour's health policy discourse', *Policy & Politics*, vol 32, no 3, pp 303-16.

Greener, I. (2004b) 'The political economy of health service organisation', *Public Administration*, vol 82, no 3, pp 657-76.

Greener, I. (2006) 'Path dependency, realism and the NHS', *British Politics*, vol 1, no 3, pp 319-43.

Greener, I., Harrington, B., Hunter, D., Mannion, R. and Powell, M. (2014) *Reforming healthcare: What's the evidence?*, Bristol: Policy Press.

Greer, S. (2004) *Territorial politics and health policy: UK health policy in comparative perspective*, Manchester: Manchester University Press.

Greer, S. (2005) 'The territorial bases of health policy making in the UK after devolution', *Regional and Federal Studies*, vol 15, no 4, pp 501-18.

Greer, S. (2009) *Territorial politics and health policy*, Manchester: Manchester University Press.

Greer, S. and Trench, A. (2010) 'Intergovernmental relations and health in Great Britain after devolution', *Policy & Politics*, vol 38, no 4, pp 509-29.

Greer, S., Jarman, H. and Azorsky, A. (2014a) *A reorganisation you can see from space: The architecture of power in the new NHS*, London: Centre for Health and the Public Interest.

Greer, S., Wilson, I., Stewart, E. and Donnelly, P. (2014b) 'Democratising the public sector? Representation and elections in the Scottish NHS', *Public Administration*, vol 92, no 4, pp 1090-105.

Greer, S., Fahey, N., Elliott, H., Wismar, M., Jarman, H. and Palm, W. (2014c) *Everything you always wanted to know about European Union Health Policies but were afraid to ask?*, European Observatory on Health Systems and Policies, Copenhagen: World Health Organization.

Gregory, S., Dixon, A. and Ham, C. (2012) *Health policy under the coalition: A mid-term assessment*, London: King's Fund.

Guthrie, B., Inkster, M. and Fahey, T. (2007) 'Tackling therapeutic inertia: role of treatment data in quality indicators', *British Medical Journal*, vol 335, pp 542-44.

Gwyn, R. (1999) 'Killer bugs, silly buggers, politically correct pals, competing discourses in health care reporting', *Health*, vol 3, no 3, pp 335-45.

Habermas, J. (1987) *The theory of communicative action*, vol 2, Cambridge: Polity Press.

Ham, C. (2000) *The politics of the NHS reform 1988-97: Metaphor or reality?*, London: King's Fund.

Ham, C. (2004) *Health policy in Britain* (5th edn), Basingstoke: Palgrave Macmillan.

Ham, C. and Walsh, N. (2013) *Making integrated care happen at scale and pace*, London: King's Fund.

Ham, C., Heenan, D., Longley, M. and Steel, D. (2013) *Integrated care in Northern Ireland, Scotland and Wales: Lessons for England*, London: King's Fund.

Ham, C., Baird, B., Gregory, S., Jabbal, J. and Alderwick, H. (2015) *The NHS under the coalition government: Part one: NHS reform*, London: King's Fund.

Hamblin, R. and Gamesh, J. (2007) *Measure for measure: Using outcome measures to raise standards in the NHS*, London: Policy Exchange.

Hammond, P. (2009) *Trust Me, I'm (Still) a Doctor*, Edinburgh: Black and White Publishing.

Hansard Society (2012) *What next for E-petitions?*, London: Hansard Society.

Hansard Society Commission on Parliamentary Scrutiny (2001) *The challenge for Parliament: Making government accountable*, London: Vacher Dod Publishing.

Harrabin, R., Coote, A. and Allen, J. (2003) *Health in the news: Risk reporting and media influence*, London: King's Fund.

Harrison, S. (1988) *Managing the National Health Service: Shifting the frontier?*, London: Chapman and Hall.

Harrison, S. (2001) 'Reforming the medical profession in the United Kingdom 1989-97: structural interests in health care', in M. Bovens, B.G. Peters and P. t'Hart (eds) *Success and failure in public governance*, Aldershot: Edward Elgar, pp 277-92.

Harrison, S. and Pollitt, C. (1994) *Controlling health professionals*, Buckingham: Open University Press.

Harrison, S. and Wood, B. (1998) 'Designing health service organisation in the UK, 1968 to 1998: from blueprint to bright idea and manipulated emergence', *Public Administration*, vol 77, no 4, pp 751-68.

Harrison, S., Hunter, D., Marnoch, G. and Pollitt, C. (1992) *Just managing: Culture and power in the National Health Service*, Basingstoke: Macmillan.

Hart, C. (2004) *Nurses and politics: The impact of power and practice*, Basingstoke: Palgrave.

Hawkes, N. (2014) 'The Better Care Fund: a disaster in waiting?', *British Medical Journal*, vol 348, g3345.

Hawkins, B. and Holden, C. (2012) 'Water dripping on stone? Industry lobbying and UK alcohol policy', *Policy & Politics*, vol 42, no 1, pp 55-70.

Hayek, F. (1976) *The road to serfdom*, London: Routledge & Kegan Paul.

Health and Social Care Committee (2013) *Inquiry into measles outbreak*, Cardiff: Welsh Assembly.

HCIO (House of Commons Information Office) (2010) *Private Member's Bill procedure*, London: HCIO.

Health Committee (2001) *The National Institute for Clinical Excellence*, 2nd report, 2001-2, London: The Stationery Office.

Health Committee (2005a) *Smoking in public places*, 1st report, 2005-6, London: The Stationery Office.

Health Committee (2005b) *The influence of the pharmaceutical industry*, 4th report, 2004-5, London: The Stationery Office.

Health Committee (2006a) *Changes to primary care trusts*, 2nd report 2005-6, London: The Stationery Office.

Health Committee (2006b) *Independent sector treatment centres*, 4th report, 2005-6, London: The Stationery Office.

Health Committee (2009) *Health inequalities*, 3rd report, 2008-9, London: The Stationery Office.

Health Committee (2010) *Commissioning*, 4th report, 2009-10, London: The Stationery Office.

Health Committee (2011a) *Public health*, 12th report, 2010-12, London: The Stationery Office.

Health Committee (2011b) *Commissioning*, 3rd report, 2010-11, London: The Stationery Office.

Health Committee (2011c) *Commissioning: Further issues*, 5th report, 2010-12, London: The Stationery Office.

Health Committee (2012) *Social care*, 14th report, 2010-12, London: The Stationery Office.

Health Committee (2014) *Public expenditure on health and social care*, 7th report, 2013-14, London: The Stationery Office.

Healthcare Commission and Audit Commission (2008) *Are we choosing health? The impact of policy on the delivery of health improvement programmes and services*, London: Healthcare Commission.

Healthwatch (2014) *Suffering in silence, Listening to consumer experiences of the health and social care complaints system*, London: Healthwatch England.

Heenan, D. (2013) 'Northern Ireland', in C. Ham, D. Heenan, M. Longley and D. Steel (eds) *Integrated care in Northern Ireland, Scotland and Wales: Lessons for England*, London: King's Fund, pp 2-24.

Heenan, D. and Birrell, D. (2006) 'The integration of health and social care: the lessons from Northern Ireland', *Social Policy & Administration*, vol 40, no 1, pp 47-66.

Heinz, J., Laumann, E., Nelson, R. and Salisbury, R. (1993) *The hollow core: Private interests in national policy making*, Cambridge, MA: Harvard University Press.

Held, D., McGrew, A., Goldblatt, D. and Perraton, J. (1999) *Global transformations: Politics, economics and culture*, Palo Alto, CA: Stanford University Press.

Helm, T. and Syal, R. (2009) 'Key Tory MPs backed call to dismantle NHS', *The Observer*, 16 August (www.theguardian.com/politics/2009/aug/16/tory-mps-back-nhs-dismantling).

Henderson, L. (1999) 'Producing serious soaps', in G. Philo (ed), *Messages received, Glasgow Media Group Research 1993-98*, London: Longman, pp 62-81.

Henderson, L. and Kitzinger, J. (1999) 'The human drama of genetics: "hard" and "soft" media representations of inherited breast cancer', *Sociology of Health & Illness*, vol 21, no 5, pp 560-78.

Heywood, A. (1994) *Political ideas and concepts: An introduction*, Basingstoke: Macmillan.

Hilder, P. (2005) 'Open parties? A map of 21st century democracy', Open Democracy, 19 January (www.opendemocracy.net/democracy-open_politics/article_2312.jsp).

Hill, M. (1997) 'Implementation theory: yesterday's issue?', *Policy & Politics*, vol 25, no 4, pp 375-85.

Hill, M. and Hupe, P. (2002) *Implementing public policy*, London: Sage.

Himmelstein, D., Woolhandler, S., Hellander, I. and Wolfe, S. (1999) 'Quality of care in investor-owned vs not for profit HMOs', *Journal of the American Medical Association*, vol 282, no 2, pp 159-63.

HM Government (1999a) *Caring about carers: A national strategy for carers*, London: Cabinet Office.

HM Government (1999b) *Modernising government*, Cm 4310, London: The Stationery Office.

HM Government (2008) *Carers at the heart of 21st century families and communities*, London: Cabinet Office.

HM Government (2010a) *The coalition: Our programme for government*, London: Cabinet Office.

HM Government (2010b) *Recognised, valued and supported: Next steps for the carers strategy*, London: Department of Health.

HM Government (2013) *Review of the balance of competences between the United Kingdom and the European Union: Health*, London: HM Government.

HM Government (2014) *Carers strategy: Second national action plan 2014–2016*, London: Department of Health.

Hobolt, S. and Klemmemson, R. (2005) 'Responsive government? Public opinion and government policy preferences in Britain and Denmark', *Political Studies*, vol 53, pp 379-402.

Hogg, C. (1999) *Patients, power and politics*, London: Sage.

Hogg, C. (2002) *National service frameworks: Involving patients and the public*, London: The Patients Forum.

Hogg, C. (2009) *Citizens, consumers and the NHS: Capturing voices*, Basingstoke: Palgrave.

Hogwood, B. and Gunn, L. (1984) *Policy analysis for the real world*, Oxford: Oxford University Press.

Hogwood, B. and Peters, B.G. (1983) *Policy dynamics*, Brighton: Wheatsheaf.

Holden, C. (2005) 'Privatisation and trade in health services: a review of the evidence', *International Journal of Health Services*, vol 35, no 4, pp 675-89.

Holder, H. (2013) *The role of the voluntary sector in providing commissioning support*, London: Nuffield Trust.

Home Office (1998) *Compact on Relations with the Voluntary and Community Sector in England*, Cm 4100, London: The Stationery Office.

Honigsbaum, F. (1970) *The struggle for the Ministry of Health*, London: Social Administration Research Trust.

Hood, C. (1976) *The limits of administration*, London: John Wiley.

Hopkins, J. (2000) 'Celebrity illnesses raise awareness but can give the wrong message', *British Medical Journal*, vol 321, p 1099.

Hoque, K., Davis, S. and Humphreys, M. (2004) 'Freedom to do what you are told: senior management autonomy in an NHS acute trust', *Public Administration*, vol 82, no 2, pp 355-75.

Horton, R. (2004) *MMR: Science and fiction*, London: Granta.

Horton, R. (2006) 'WHO: strengthening the road to renewal', *The Lancet*, vol 367, pp 1793-5.

House of Commons (2014) *Register of Member's financial interests* (www. publications.parliament.uk/pa/cm/cmregmem/130507/130507.pdf).

House of Lords Select Committee on Public Service and Demographic Change (2013) *Ready for ageing?*, Report of 2012-13, London: The Stationery Office.

House of Lords and House of Commons (2013) *Draft Care and Support Bill*, Session 2012-13, London: The Stationery Office.

House of Lords Select Committee on the Constitution (2011a) *Health and Social Care Bill*, 18th report, 2010-12, London: The Stationery Office.

House of Lords Select Committee on the Constitution (2011b) *Health and Social Care Bill: Follow-up report*, 22nd report, 2010-12, London: The Stationery Office.

Hudson, B. (2002) 'Interprofessionality in health and social care: the Achilles' heel of partnership?', *Journal of Interprofessional Care*, vol 6, no 1, pp 7-15.

Hudson, B. (2011) 'Big society: a concept in pursuit of a definition', *Journal of Integrated Care*, vol 19, no 5, pp 17-24.

Hudson, B. (2015) 'Devo Manc: five early lessons for the NHS', *The Guardian*, 24 March (www.theguardian.com/healthcare-network/2015/mar/24/devo-manc-five-early-lessons-for-the-nhs).

Hudson, B. and Hardy, B. (2002) 'What is a successful partnership and how can it be measured?', in C. Glendinning, M. Powell and K. Rummery (eds) *Partnerships, New Labour and governance*, Bristol: Policy Press, pp 51-66.

Hudson, B. and Henwood, M. (2002) 'The NHS and social care: the final countdown', *Policy & Politics*, vol 30, no 2, pp 153-66.

Hudson, J. and Lowe, S. (2004) *Understanding the policy process*, Bristol: Policy Press.

Hughes, D. and Griffiths, L. (1999) 'On penalties and the Patient's Charter: centralism v decentralised governance in the NHS', *Sociology of Health & Illness*, vol 2, no 1, pp 71-94.

Hultberg, E.-L., Glendinning, C., Allebeck, P. and Lönnroth, K. (2005) 'Using pooled budgets to integrate health and welfare services: a comparison of experiments in England and Sweden', *Health & Social Care in the Community*, vol 13, no 6, pp 531-41.

Humphries, R. (2013) *Paying for social care: Beyond Dilnot*, London: King's Fund.

Humphries, R. and Galea, A. (2013) *Health and wellbeing boards: One year on*, London: King's Fund.

Humphries, R., Galea, A., Sonola, L. and Mundle, C. (2012) *Health and wellbeing boards: Systems leaders or talking shops?*, London: King's Fund.

Hunter, D. and Perkins, N. (2014) *Partnership working in public health*, Bristol: Policy Press.

Hunter, D., Wilkinson, J. and Coyle, E. (2005) 'Would regional government have been good for your health?', *British Medical Journal*, vol 330, pp 159-60.

Hunter, D., Perkins, N., Bambra, C., Marks, L., Hopkins, T. and Blackman, T. (2011) *Partnership working and the implications for governance: Issues affecting public health partnerships*, Southampton: NIHR Service Delivery and Organisation Programme/HMSO.

Iacobucci, G. (2013) 'More than a third of GPs on commissioning groups have conflicts of interest', *British Medical Journal*, 346: f1569 accessed 2.7.15.

Iacobucci, G. (2014) 'Raiding the public health budget', *British Medical Journal*, 27 March, 348:g2274 accessed 2.7.15.

IHA (Independent Healthcare Association) and DH (Department of Health) (2000) *For the benefit of patients: A concordat with the private and voluntary health provider sector*, London: IHA and DH.

Immergut, E. (1992) *Health politics, interests and institutions in Western Europe*, Cambridge: Cambridge University Press.

Independent Commission on Whole Person Care (2014) *One person, one team, one system: Report of the Independent Commission on Whole Person Care for the Labour Party*, (chairman, Sir John Oldham) (www.yourbritain.org.uk/uploads/editor/files/One_Person_One_Team_One_System.pdf).

Independent Review of Free Personal and Nursing Care in Scotland (2008) *A report by Lord Sutherland*, Edinburgh: Scottish Government.

Ingle, S. and Tether, P. (1981) *Parliament and health policy: The role of MPs 1970-5*, Farnborough: Gower.

International Health Impact Assessment Consortium (2004) *European Policy Health Impact Assessment: a guide*, Brussels: European Commission.

Ipsos MORI (2012) *Department of Health 2012 stakeholder research*, London: Ipsos MORI.

Ipsos MORI (2013) *Department of Health 2013 stakeholder research*, London: Ipsos MORI.

Irvine, D. (2003) *The doctor's tale: Professionalism and public trust*, Oxford: Radcliffe Medical Press.

Jarman, H. and Greer, S. (2010) 'In the eye of the storm: civil servants and managers in the UK Department of Health', *Social Policy & Administration*, vol 44, no 2, pp 172-92.

Jeffrey, C. (2005) 'Devolution and the European Union: trajectories and futures', in A. Trench (ed) *The dynamics of devolution: The state of nations 2005*, Exeter: Imprint Academic, pp 179-99.

Jeffrey, C. (2006) 'Devolution and the lopsided state', in P. Dunleavy, R. Heffernan, P. Cowley and C. Hay (eds) *Developments in British politics*, Basingstoke: Palgrave, pp 138-58.

Jenkins-Smith, H. and Sabatier, P. (1994) 'Evaluating the advocacy coalition framework', *Journal of Public Policy*, vol 14, no 2, pp 175-203.

Jennings, M.K. (1999) 'Political responses to pain and loss: presidential address, American Political Science Association, 1998', *American Political Science Review*, vol 93, no 1, pp 1-15.

Jervis, P. and Plowden, W. (2003) *The impact of political devolution on the UK's health services*, London: Nuffield Trust.

John, P. (2012) *Analysing public policy* (2nd edn), London: Pinter.

Johnson, C., Coleman, A., Boyd, A., Bradshaw, D., Gains, F., Shacklady-Smith, A. and Smith, L. (2007) *Scrutinising for health*, Manchester: University of Manchester.

Jones, J. (1990) 'Party committees and all party groups', in M. Rush (ed) *Parliament and pressure politics*, Oxford: Clarendon, pp 112-36.

Jones, K. (2008) 'In whose interest? Relationships between health consumer groups and the pharmaceutical industry in the UK', *Sociology of Health & Illness*, vol 30, no 6, pp 929-43.

Jones, L., Exworthy, M. and Frosini, F. (2013) 'Implementing market-based reforms in the English NHS: bureaucratic coping strategies and social embeddedness', *Health Policy*, vol 111, pp 52-9.

Jones, N. (2002) *The control freaks: How New Labour gets its own way*, London; Politico's.

Jones, T. (1996) *Remaking the Labour Party*, London: Routledge.

Jordan, G. (1990) 'Policy community realism v "new" institutionalist ambiguity', *Political Studies*, vol 38, pp 470-84.

Jordan, G. and Maloney, W. (1997) *The protest business: Mobilising campaign groups*, Manchester: Manchester University Press.

Judge, K. and Bauld, L. (2007) 'Learning from policy failure? Health Action Zones in England', *European Journal of Public Health*, vol 16, no 4, pp 341-4.

Kammerling, R. and Kinnear, A. (1996) 'The extent of the two tier service for fundholders', *British Medical Journal*, vol 312, pp 1399-401.

Kane, D. and Allen, J. (2011) *Counting the cuts: The impact of spending cuts on the UK voluntary and community sector*, London: NCVO.

Karpf, A. (1988) *Doctoring the media: The reporting of health and medicine*, London: Routledge.

Kavanagh, D. and Seldon, A. (2000) 'Support for the Prime Minister: the hidden influence of No 10', in R. Rhodes (ed) *Transforming British government, Vol 2, Changing roles and relationships*, Basingstoke: Macmillan, pp 63-78.

Keane, J. (1991) *The media and democracy*, Cambridge: Polity Press.

Keating, M. (2005) 'Policy making and policy divergence in Scotland after devolution', *Regional Studies*, vol 39, pp 453-63.

Keefe, R., Lane, S. and Swarts, H. (2006) 'From the bottom up: tracing the impact of four health-based social movements on health and social policies', *Journal of Health and Social Policy*, vol 21, no 3, pp 55-69.

Kelaher, M., Cawson, J., Miller, J., Kavanagh, A., Dunt, D. and Studdert, D. (2008) 'Use of breast cancer screening and treatment services by Australian women aged 25-44 years following Kylie Minogue's breast cancer diagnosis', *International Journal of Epidemiology*, vol 37, no 6, pp 1326-32.

Keogh. B. (2013) *Report into the quality of care and treatment provided by 14 hospital trusts in England: Overview report*, London: Department of Health.

Keynes, S. and Tetlow, G. (2014) *Survey of public spending in the UK*, London, Institute for Fiscal Studies.

Kerr, D. (2005) *Building a health service fit for the future: A national framework for service change in the NHS in Scotland*, Edinburgh: Scottish Executive.

Kickbusch, I. and de Leeuw, E. (1999) 'Global public health: revisiting healthy public policy at the global level', *Health Promotion International*, vol 14, no 4, pp 285-88.

Kickbusch, I. and Seck, B. (2007) 'Global public health', in J. Douglas, S. Earle, S. Handsley, C. Lloyd and S. Spurr (eds) *A reader in promoting public health: Challenge and controversy*, London: Sage/Open University, pp 159-68.

Kimball, A. (2006) 'The health of nations: Happy Birthday WTO', *The Lancet*, vol 367, pp 188-9.

King, D., Ramirez-Cano, D., Greaves, F., Vlaev, I., Beales, S. and Darzi, A. (2013) 'Twitter and the health reforms in the English National Health Service', *Health Policy*, vol 110, pp 291-7.

King, M. and Street, C. (2005) 'Mad cows and mad scientists', in M. King and K. Watson (eds) *Representing health: Discourses of health and illness in the media*, Basingstoke: Palgrave, pp 115-32.

King's Fund (2002) *The future of the NHS: A framework for debate*, London: King's Fund.

King's Fund (2011) *The future of leadership and management in the NHS: No more heroes*, Commission on Leadership and Management in the NHS, London: King's Fund.

King's Fund (2012) *Leadership and engagement for improvement in the NHS: Together we can*, London: King's Fund.

King's Fund (2013) *Patient-centred leadership: Rediscovering our purpose*, London: King's Fund.

King's Fund (2015) *Public satisfaction with the NHS in 2014*, London: King's Fund.

Kingdon, J. (1984) *Agendas, alternatives and public policy*, Boston, MA: Little Brown.

Kingsley, H. (1993) *Casualty: The inside story*, London: BBC.

Kirby, I. (2010) 'Tories paid an unhealthy sum', *News of the World*, 24 January, p 18.

Kitzinger, J. (2000) 'Media templates: patterns of association and the (re) construction of meaning over time', *Media, Culture & Society*, vol 22, no 1, pp 61-84.

Klein, R. (1990) 'The state and the profession: the politics of the double-bed', *British Medical Journal*, vol 301, pp 700-2.

Klein, R. (1995) *The new politics of the NHS* (3rd edn), London: Longman.

Klein, R. (2000) *The new politics of the NHS* (4th edn), London: Prentice Hall.

Klein, R. (2001) 'First past the post', *Health Service Journal*, 12 April, pp 26-7.

Klingemann, H.-D., Hofferbert, R. and Budge, I. (1994) *Parties, policies and democracy*, Boulder, CO: Westview Press.

Kmietowicz, Z. (2013) 'Peer publishes bill to reinstate legal duty of health secretary to provide NHS', *British Medical Journal*, vol 346, p 1605.

Koivusalo, M. (2005) 'The future of European health policies', *International Journal of Health Services*, vol 35, no 2, pp 325-42.

Koivusalo, M. (2006) 'The impact of economic globalisation on health', *Theoretical Medicine and Bioethics*, vol 27, no 1, pp 1-34.

Koivusalo, M. and Ollila, E. (1997) *Making a healthy world*, London: Zed Books.

Koteyko, N., Nerlich, B., Crawford, P. and Wright, N. (2008) '"Not rocket science" or "no silver bullet"? Media and government discourses about MRSA and cleanliness', *Applied Linguistics*, vol 29, no 2, pp 223-43.

Kuznetsova, D. (2012) *Healthy places: Councils leading on public health*, London: New Local Government Network.

Labonte, R. and Schrecker, T. (2004) 'Committed to health for all? How the G7/G8 rate', *Social Science & Medicine*, vol 59, pp 1661-76.

Labour Party (1990) *A fresh start for health*, London: Labour Party.

Labour Party (1992) *Your good health: A White Paper for a Labour government*, London: Labour Party.

Labour Party (1994) *Health 2000: The health and wealth of the nation in the 21st century*, London: Labour Party.

Labour Party (1995) *Renewing the NHS*, London: Labour Party.

Larson, R., Woloshin, S., Schwartz, L. and Welsh, H. (2005) 'Celebrity endorsements of cancer screening', *Journal of the National Cancer Institute*, vol 97, no 9, pp 693-5.

Laver, M. and Budge, I. (1992) *Party policy and government coalitions*, Basingstoke: Macmillan.

Laver, M. and Schofield, N. (1998) *Multiparty government: The politics of coalition in Europe*, Ann Arbor, MI: University of Michigan Press.

Lawrie, S. (2000) 'Newspaper coverage of psychiatric and physical illness', *Psychiatric Bulletin*, vol 24, pp 104-6.

Lear, J. and Mossialos, E. (2008) 'EU law and health policy in Europe', *Euro Observer*, vol 10, no 3, pp 1–3.

Leatherman, S. and Sutherland, K. (2003) *The quest for quality in the NHS*, London: Nuffield Trust.

Lee, K. (2009) *The World Health Organization*, London: Routledge.

Lee, K. and Collin, J. (eds) (2005) *Global change and health*, Maidenhead: Open University Press.

Lee, K. and Koivusalo, M. (2005) 'Trade and health: is the community ready for action?', *PLoS Medicine*, vol 2, no 1, p 8.

Lee, K., Sridhar, D. and Patel, M. (2009) 'Bridging the divide: global governance of trade and health', *Lancet*, vol 371, no 9661, pp 416–22.

Lee, S. (2009) 'David Cameron and the renewal of policy', in S. Lee and M. Beech (eds) *The Conservatives under David Cameron: Built to last?*, Basingstoke: Palgrave, pp 44–59.

Legge, D. (2012) 'The future of WHO hangs in the balance', *British Medical Journal*, vol 345, e6877.

Le Grand, J., Mays, N. and Mulligan, J. (eds) (1998) *Learning from the NHS internal market: A review of evidence*, London: King's Fund.

Leveson, Lord (2012) *Report of an inquiry into the culture, practices and ethics of the press*, London: The Stationery Office.

Levitt, R. and Wall, A. (1984) *The reorganised National Health Service* (3rd edn), London: Croom Helm.

Leys, C. and Player, S. (2011) *The plot against the NHS*, Pontypool: Merlin Press.

LGA (Local Government Association) Health Commission (2008) *Report of the LGA Commission on Health*, London: LGA.

LGIU (Local Government Information Unit) (2010) *All's well that end's well? Local government leading on health improvement*, London: LGIU.

Liaison Committee (2012) *Select Committee effectiveness, resources and powers*, 2nd report, 2012-13, London: The Stationery Office.

Liberal Democrats (1992) *Restoring the nation's health*, London: Liberal Democrats.

Liberal Democrats (2008) *Empowerment, fairness and quality in healthcare*, London: Liberal Democrats.

Liberal Democrats (2010) *Manifesto 2010*, London: Liberal Democrats.

Lindblom, C. (1959) 'The science of muddling through', *Public Administration Review*, vol 19, no 2, pp 78–88.

Lindblom, C. (1965) *The intelligence of democracy*, New York: Free Press.

Lipsky, M. (1979) *Street-level bureaucracy*, New York: Russell Sage.

Lipson, D. (2001) 'The World Trade Organization's health agenda', *British Medical Journal*, vol 329, pp 1139–40.

Lister, J. (2006) 'Simons Stevens and his amazing dancing balance sheet', *Red Pepper*, March, p 10.

Lock, S., and McKee, M. (2005) 'Health impact assessment: assessing opportunities and barriers to intersectoral health improvement in an expenaded European Union', *Journal of Epidemiology and Public Health*, vol 59, pp 356-60.

Longley, M. (2013) 'Wales', in C. Ham, D. Heenan, M. Longley and D. Steel (eds) *Integrated care in Northern Ireland, Scotland and Wales*, London: King's Fund, pp 57-77.

Longley, M., Riley, N., Davies, P. and Hernandez-Quevedo, C. (2012) 'United Kingdom (Wales) health system review', *Health Systems in Transition*, vol 14, no 11, pp 1-84.

Lowe, R. (1993) *The welfare state in Britain since 1945*, London: Macmillan.

Lukes, S. (1974) *Power: A radical view*, London: Macmillan.

Lupton, D. (1994) 'Femininity, responsibility and the technological imperative: discourses on breast care in the Australian press', *International Journal of Health Services*, vol 24, no 1, pp 73-89.

McBride, D. (2013) *Power trip: A decade of policy, plots and spin*, London: Biteback.

McConnell, A. (2010) *Understanding policy success: Rethinking public policy*, Basingstoke: Palgrave.

McDonald, R. et al (2013) *Evaluation of the CQUIN framework*, London: Department of Health.

McGregor-Riley, V. (1997) 'The politics of medical representation: the case of the BMA from 1979-1995', Unpublished PhD thesis, Leicester: De Montfort University.

McKee, M., Dubois, C.-A. and Sibbald, B. (2006) 'Changing "professional boundaries"', in C.-A. Dubois, M. McKee and E. Nolte (eds) *Human resources for health in Europe*, Maidenhead: Open University Press, pp 63-78.

McLachlan, G. (1990) *What price quality? The NHS in review*, London: Nuffield Provincial Hospitals Trust.

McLelland, S. (2002) 'Health policy in Wales: distinctive or derivative?', *Social Policy & Society*, vol 1, no 4, pp 325-33.

McNulty, T. and Ferlie, E. (2002) *Re-engineering health care*, Oxford: Oxford University Press.

McQuail, D. (2005) *Mass communication theory* (5th edn), London: Sage.

McSmith, A. (2010) 'Jamie Oliver health approach "doesn't work" says Health Secretary', *The Independent*, 30 October (www.independent.co.uk/news/uk/politics/jamie-oliver-health-approach-doesnt-work-says-health-secretary-2014780.html).

Maloney, W., Jordan, A.G. and McLaughlin, A. (1994) 'Interest groups and the policy process: the insider/outsider model revisited', *Journal of Public Policy*, vol 14, no 1, pp 17-38.

Mandelson, P. (2011) *The third man*, London: Harper Press.

Mandelstam, M. (2006) *Betraying the NHS: Health abandoned*, London: Jessica Kingsley Publishers.

Maniadakis, M., Hollingsworth, B. and Thanassoulis, E. (1999) 'The impact of the internal market on hospitals efficiency, productivity and service quality', *Health Care Management Science*, vol 2, no 2, pp 75-85.

Mannion, R., Davies, H. and Marshall, M. (2005a) 'Impact of star performance ratings in English acute hospital trusts', *Journal of Health Service Research & Policy*, vol 10, no 1, pp 18-24.

Mannion, R., Davies, H. and Marshall, M. (2005b) *Cultures for performance in health care*, Maidenhead: Open University Press.

Mannion, R., Marini, G. and Street, A. (2006) 'Demand management and administrative costs under payment by results', *Health Policy Matters*, vol 12, pp 1-8.

March, J.G. and Olsen, J. (1984) 'The new institutionalism: organisational factors in political life', *American Political Science Review*, vol 78, no 3, pp 734-48.

Marks, L. and Hunter, D. (2007) *Social enterprises and the NHS*, London: Unison.

Marsh, D. and Rhodes, R. (eds) (1992a) *Implementing Thatcherite policies*, Buckingham: Open University Press.

Marsh, D. and Rhodes, R. (eds) (1992b) *Policy networks in British government*, Oxford: Clarendon.

Marsh, D. and Smith, M. (2000) 'Understanding policy networks: towards a dialectic approach', *Political Studies*, vol 48, no 4, pp 4-21.

Marshall, K. (2008) *The World Bank*, London: Routledge.

Marshall, L., Charlesworth, A. and Hurst, J. (2014) *The NHS payment system: evolving policy and emerging evidence*, London: Nuffield Trust.

Mason, A., Goddard, M. and Weatherley, H. (2014) *Financial mechanisms for integrating funds for health and social care: An evidence review*, CHE Research Paper 97, York: Centre for Health Economics, University of York.

Mason, W. and Maxwell, L. (2008) *Freedom for public services*, London: Centre for Policy Studies.

May, J. and Wildavsky, A. (eds) (1978) *The policy cycle*, Beverly Hills, CA: Sage.

Mays, N., Dixon, A. and Jones, L. (2011) *Understanding New Labour's market reforms of the English NHS*, London: King's Fund.

Mays, N., Mulligan, J. and Goodwin, N. (2000) 'The British quasi market in health care: a balance sheet of the evidence', *Journal of Health Services Research & Policy*, vol 5, pp 49-58.

Melucci, A. (1989) *The nomads of the present*, London: Radius.

Mid Staffordshire Inquiry (2013) *The Mid Staffordshire NHS Foundation Trust Public Inquiry – Final report* (Francis Report), London: The Stationery Office.

Milburn, A. (2001) *Reforming public services: Reconciling equity with choice*, London: Fabian Society.

Miliband, R. (1982) *Capitalist democracy in Britain*, Oxford: Oxford University Press.

Miller, D. and Reilly, J. (1994) *Food scares in the media*, London: Routledge.

Miller, D., Kitzinger, J., Williams, K. and Beharrell, P. (1998) *The circuit of mass communication. Media strategies, representation and audience reception in the AIDS crisis*, London: Sage.

Miller, R., Dickinson, H. and Glasby, J. (2011) 'The Care Trust pilgrims', *Journal of Integrated Care*, vol 19, no 4, pp 14-21.

Millstone, E. and van Zwanenberg, P. (2002) 'The evolution of food safety policy making institutions in the UK, EU and Codex Alimentarius', *Social Policy & Administration*, vol 36, no 6, pp 593-609.

Millward Brown (2004) *National media coverage of public health issues and the NHS*, London: Department of Health.

Ministry of Health (1962) *A Hospital Plan for England and Wales*, Cmnd. 1604, London: HMSO.

Ministry of Health (1963) *Health and Welfare: The Development of Community Care. Plans for the health and welfare services of the local authorities in England and Wales*, Cmnd. 1973, London: HMSO.

Mitchell, A. and Voon, T. (2011) 'Implications of the World Trade Organization in combatting non-communicable diseases', *Public Health*, vol 125, pp 832-9.

Mitchell, J. and Mitchell, A. (2011) *Devolution in the UK*, Manchester: Manchester University Press.

Modernisation of the House of Commons (2006) *The legislative process*, 1st report, 2005-6, London: The Stationery Office.

Mohan, J. (1995) *A national health service?*, Basingstoke: Macmillan.

Mohan, J. (2002) *Planning, markets and hospitals*, London: Routledge.

Molloy, C. (2013) 'Paying for private failure in England's NHS – again!', *openDemocracy* (https://www.opendemocracy.net/ournhs/caroline-molloy/paying-for-private-failure-in-englands-nhs-again).

Monitor (2013) *Walk in centre review: Preliminary report*, London: Monitor.

Monitor (2014) *Enabling integrated care in the NHS*, London: Monitor.

Montero, J. and Gunther, R. (2003) *The literature on political parties: A critical reassessment*, Barcelona: Institut de Ciencies Politiques i Socials.

Montgomery, J. (2003) *Health care law* (2nd edn), Oxford: Oxford University Press.

Moore, A. (2014) 'A new angle on public involvement', *Health Service Journal*, 22 August, pp 16-19.

Moran, M. (1999) *Governing the health care state: A comparative study of the United Kingdom, the United States and Germany*, Manchester: Manchester University Press.

Moran, M. (2000) 'Understanding the welfare state: the case of health', *British Journal of Politics and International Relations*, vol 92, pp 135-60.

Morgan, R. (2003) 'Clear red water', *Agenda*, Spring, Cardiff: Institute of Welsh Affairs.

Morrell, K. and Hewison, A., (2013) 'Rhetoric in policy texts: the role of enthymeme in Darzi's review of the NHS', *Policy & Politics*, vol 41, no 1, pp 59-79.

Mosca, I. (2006) 'Is decentralisation the real solution? A three country study', *Health Policy*, vol 77, no 1, pp 113-20.

Moynihan, D., Doran, E. and Henry, D. (2008) 'Disease mongering is now part of the global health debate', *PLoS Medicine*, vol 5, no 5, e106.

Moynihan, R. (1998) *Too much medicine: The business of health and its risks for you*, Sydney: ABC Books.

Moynihan, R. and Cassels, A. (2006) *Selling sickness*, New York: Nation Books.

Moynihan, R., Heath, I. and Henry, D. (2002) 'Selling sickness: the pharmaceutical industry and disease-mongering', *British Medical Journal*, vol 324, pp 886-91.

Nairne, P. (1984) 'Parliamentary control and accountability', in R. Maxwell and N. Weaver (eds) *Public participation in health*, London: King Edward's Fund for London, pp 33-51.

NAO (National Audit Office) (2003) *Achieving improvement through clinical governance: A progress report*, London: The Stationery Office.

NAO (2009) *Reducing healthcare associated infections in hospitals in England*, London: The Stationery Office.

NAO (2011) *The Care Quality Commission: Regulating the quality and safety of health and adult social care 2010-12*, London: The Stationery Office.

NAO (2012a) *Progress in making NHS efficiency savings*, London: The Stationery Office.

NAO (2012b) *Healthcare across the UK: A comparison of the NHS in England, Scotland, Wales and Northern Ireland*, London: The Stationery Office.

NAO (2013a) *NHS reorganisation: Making the transition to the reformed health system*, London: The Stationery Office.

NAO (2013b) *Managing NHS consultants: Room for improvement in managing the NHS contract*, London: The Stationery Office.

NAO (2013c) *Memoranda on provision of out of hours GP services in Cornwall*, London: The Stationery Office.

NAO (2014a) *Adult social care in England: Overview*, London: The Stationery Office.

NAO (2014b) *Waiting times for elective care in England*, London:The Stationery Office.

National Advisory Group on the Safety of Patients in England (2013) *A promise to learn:A commitment to act: Improving the safety of patients in England* (Berwick Review), London: Department of Health.

National Audit of Intermediate Care (2013) *Report* (http://www.nhsbenchmarking.nhs.uk/CubeCore/.uploads/icsurvey/NAIC%202013/NAICNationalReport2013.pdf).

National Statistics (2014) *Free personal and nursing care, Scotland 2012-13*, Edinburgh: Scottish Government.

Navarro, V. (1978) *Class struggle, the state and medicine*, Oxford: Martin Robertson.

NAVCA (National Association for Voluntary and Community Action) (2015) *Voluntary sector annual survey: Findings from the health and care voluntary sector strategic partnership 2014 survey*, London: NAVCA.

NEF (New Economics Foundation) (2010) *Cutting it*, London: NEF.

Negrine, R. (1994) *Politics of the mass media in Britain*, London: Routledge.

Nerlich, B. and Halliday, C. (2007) 'Avian flu: the creation of expectations in the interplay between science and the media', *Sociology of Health & Illness*, vol 29, no 1, pp 45-65.

Newman, J. (2001) *Modernising governance: New Labour policy and society*, London: Sage.

Newton, K. (2001) 'The transformation of governance?', in B. Axford and R. Huggins (eds) *New media and politics*, London: Sage, pp 151-71.

NHS Alliance (2002) *The vision in practice*, Retford: NHS Alliance.

NHS Benchmarking Network (2013) *National audit of intermediate care report 2013*, (http://www.nhsbenchmarking.nhs.uk/CubeCore/.uploads/icsurvey/NAIC%202013/NAICNationalReport2013.pdf).

NHS Confederation (2012) *Making integrated out of hospital care a reality*, London: NHS Confederation.

NHS Confederation (2013) *Ambition, challenge, transition: Reflections on a decade of NHS commissioning*, London: NHS Confederation.

NHS England (2014) *NHS England's commitment to carers*, London: NHS England.

NHS England, CQC (Care Quality Commission), Health Education England, Public Health England, Monitor and NHSTDA (NHS Trust Development Authority) (2014) *NHS five year forward view*, London: NHS England.

NHS Future Forum (2011) *Summary report on proposed changes to the NHS*, London: Department of Health.

NHS Future Forum (2012) *Summary report: Second phase*, London: Department of Health.

NHSIII (National Health Service Institute for Innovation and Improvement) (2011) *Leading large scale change: A practical guide*, London: NHSIII.

Nishtar, S. (2004) 'Public–private partnerships in health: a global call to action', *Health Research Policy and Systems*, vol 2, no 5 (http://www.health-policy-systems.com/content/2/1/5).

NLIAH (National Leadership and Innovation Agency for Healthcare) (2009) *Getting collaboration to work in Wales*, Llanharan: NLIAH.

Nolte, E. and McKee, M. (2004) *Does healthcare save lives? Avoidable mortality revisited*, London: Nuffield Trust.

Nolte, E and Pitchforth, E. (2014) *What is the evidence on the economic impacts of integrated care?*, Copenhagen: WHO Europe.

Nuffield Trust (2013) *Rating providers for quality: A policy worth pursuing?*, London: Nuffield Trust.

Nunes, V., Neilson, J., O'Flynn, N. et al (2009) *Medicines adherence: involving patients in decisions about prescribed medicines and supporting adherence. Full Guideline*, London: National Collaborating Centre for Primary Care and Royal College of GPs.

O'Connor, J. (1973) *The fiscal crisis of the state*, New York: St Martin's Press.

O'Donovan, O. and Glavanis-Grantham, K. (2003) 'Researching the political and cultural influence of the transnational pharmaceutical industry in Ireland', *Administration*, vol 52, no 3, pp 21-42.

O'Neill, C., McGregor, P. and Merkur, S. (2012) 'UK: Northern Ireland health system review', *Health Systems in Transition*, vol 14, no 10, London: European Observatory on Health Systems and Policies.

Oborne, P. and Walters, S. (2004) *Alistair Campbell*, London: Aurum.

OECD (Organisation for Economic Co-operation and Development) (2004) *Towards high performing health systems*, Paris: OECD.

OECD (2013) *Health at a Glance 2013: OECD indicators*, Paris: OECD (www.oced.org/health/healthataglance).

Offe, C. (1984) *The contradictions of the welfare state*, London: Hutchinson.

Offredy, M. (2008) 'The health of a nation: perspectives from Cuba's national health system', *Quality in Primary Care*, vol 16, no 4, pp 269-77.

Oliver, J. (2011) 'This obesity strategy is a cop out', *The Guardian*, 13 October (www.theguardian.com/commentisfree/2011/oct/13/obesity-strategy-jamie-oliver).

Ollila, E. (2005) 'Global health priorities: priorities of the wealthy?', *Globalisation and Health*, vol 1, no 6, pp 1-6.

Olson, M. (1965) *The logic of collective action*, Cambridge, MA: Harvard University Press.

ONS (Office for National Statistics) (2013) *Expenditure on healthcare in the UK*, London: ONS.

ONS (2015) *Expenditure on healthcare in the UK*, London: ONS.

Ostry, A. (2001) 'International trade regulation and publicly funded health care in Canada', *International Journal of Health Services*, vol 31, no 3, pp 475-80.

PAC (Public Accounts Committee) (2002) *Inappropriate adjustments to NHS waiting lists*, HC 517, 46th report, 2001/2, London: The Stationery Office.

PAC (2012) *Learning the lessons from PFI and other projects*, 44th report, Session 2010-12, London: The Stationery Office.

PAC (2014a) *Monitor: Regulating NHS foundation trusts*, 4th report, Session 2014-15, London: The Stationery Office.

PAC (2014b) *Adult social care in England*, 6th report, Session 2014-15, London: The Stationery Office.

PAC (2015) *Planning for the Better Care Fund*, 37th report, Session 2014-15, London: The Stationery Office.

Paine, D. (2014) 'One in six councils without a director of public health', *Health Service Journal*, 22 May.

Park, A., Clery, E., Curtice, J., Phillips, M. and Utting, D (eds) (2012) *British Social Attitudes Survey: The 29th report*, London: National Centre for Social Research.

Parliament First (2003) *Parliament's last chance*, London: Parliament First.

Parsons, W. (1995) *Public policy*, Aldershot: Edward Elgar.

PASC (Public Administration Select Committee) (2010) *Goats and Tsars: Ministerial and other appointments from outside Parliament*, 8th Report 2009-10 HC 330, London: The Stationery Office.

PASC (Public Administration Select Committee) (2012) *Special advisors*, 6th report, 2012-13 HC 134, London: The Stationery Office.

Paton, C. (2014) *At what cost? Paying the price for the market in the NHS*, London: Centre for Health and the Public Interest.

PCRC (Political and Constitutional Reform Committee) (2013a) *Revisiting 'Rebuilding the house': The impact of the Wright reforms*, 3rd report, 2013-14, London: The Stationery Office.

PCRC (2013b) *Ensuring the standards of quality in legislation*, 1st report, Session 2013-14, London: The Stationery Office.

Peck, E., Gulliver, P. and Towell, D. (2002) *Modernising partnerships: Evaluation of Somerset's innovations in the commissioning and organisation of mental health services – final report*, London: Institute for Applied Social Policy, King's College London.

Peckham, S., Exworthy, M., Powell, M. and Greener, I. (2005) *Decentralisation as an organisational model for health care in England*, London: NHS Coordinating Centre for Service Delivery and Organisation.

Peckham, S., Exworthy, M., Powell, M. and Greener, I. (2008) 'Decentralising health services in the UK: a new conceptual framework', *Public Administration*, vol 86, no 2, pp 559-80.

Petch, A., Cook, A. and Miller, E. (2013) 'Partnership working and outcomes: do health and social care partnerships deliver for users and carers?', *Health & Social Care in the Community*, vol 21, no 6, pp 623-33.

Pharmaceutical Industry Competitiveness Task Force (2001) *Final report*, London: Department of Health and Association of the British Pharmaceutical Industry.

Pharoah, F., Mari, J., Rathbone, J. and Wong, W. (2006) 'Family intervention for schizophrenia', *Cochrane Review, Cochrane Database of Systematic Reviews*, Issue 4, CD000088.

Phelps, K. and Regen, E. (2008) *To what extent does the use of Health Act flexibilities promote effective partnership working with positive outcomes for frail older people?, Final report*, Leicester: University of Leicester.

Philo, G. (ed) (1996) *Media and mental distress*, London: Longman.

Philo, G. (1999) 'Media and mental illness', in G. Philo (ed) *Message received, Glasgow Media Group Research 1993-98*, London: Longman, pp 54-61.

Picker Institute Europe (2014) *Policy briefing: The friends and family test*, Oxford: Picker Institute Europe.

Pigman, G. (2007) *The World Economic Forum: A multi-stakeholder approach to global governance*, Oxford: Routledge.

Platt, S. (1998) *Government by task force*, London: Catalyst.

PMSU (Prime Minister's Strategy Unit) (2004) *Alcohol harm reduction strategy for England*, London: Cabinet Office.

Pollitt, C. (2008) *Time, policy, management: Governing with the past*, Oxford: Oxford University Press.

Pollitt, C., Birchall, J. and Putman, K. (1998) *Decentralising public service management*, Basingstoke: Macmillan.

Pollock, A. (2004) *NHS Plc: The privatisation of our health care*, London: Verso.

Pollock, A., Price, D. and Liebe, M. (2011a) 'Private finance initiatives during NHS austerity', *British Medical Journal*, vol 342, d324.

Pollock, A., Macfarlane, A., Kirkwood, G., Majeed, F., Greener, I., Morelli, C., Boyle, S., Mellett, H., Godden, S., Price, D. and Brhlikova, P. (2011b) 'No evidence that patient choice saves lives', *The Lancet*, vol 378, no 9809, pp 2057-60.

Powell, M. (1997) *Evaluating the NHS*, Buckingham: Open University Press.

Powell, M. and Glendinning, C. (2002) 'Introduction', in C. Glendinning, M. Powell and K. Rummery (eds) *Partnerships, New Labour and governance*, Bristol: Policy Press, pp 1-15.

Powell, M., Millar, R., Mulla, A., Brown, H., Fewtrell, C., McLeod, H., Goodwin, N., Dixon, A. and Naylor, C. (2011) *Comparative case studies of health reform in England*, London: Department of Health, Policy Research Programme.

Prah Ruger, J. (2005) 'The changing role of the World Bank in global public health', *Journal of Public Health*, vol 95, no 1, pp 65-70.

Prah Ruger, J. and Yach, D. (2005) 'Global functions at the World Health Organization', *British Medical Journal*, vol 330, pp 1099-100.

Pressman, J. and Wildavsky, A. (1973) *Implementation*, Berkeley, CA: University of California Press.

Price, D. (2002) 'How the WTO extends the rights of private property', *Critical Public Health*, vol 12, no 1, pp 55-63.

Price, L. (2011) *Where power lies: Prime ministers v the media*, London: Simon & Schuster.

Procedure Committee (2012) *Debates on Government e-Petitions*, 7th Report 2010-12, HC 1706, London: The Stationery Office.

Procedure Committee (2013a) *Debates on Government e-Petitions in Westminster Hall*, 6th Report 2012-13, HC 1094, London: The Stationery Office.

Procedure Committee (2013b) *Early Day Motions Report*, 1st Report 2013-14, HC 189, London: The Stationery Office.

Propper, C., Burgess, S. and Gossage, D. (2008) 'Competition and quality: evidence from the NHS internal market 1991-9', *The Economic Journal*, vol 118, no 525, pp 138-70.

Propper, C., Croxson, B. and Shearer, A. (2002) 'Waiting times for hospital admissions: the impact of GP fundholding', *Journal of Health Economics*, vol 21, no 2, pp 227-52.

Propper, C., Sutton, M., Whitnall, C. and Windmeijer, F. (2010) 'Incentives and targets in hospital care: evidence from a natural experiment', *Journal of Public Economics*, vol 94, no 3-4, pp 318-35.

Public Health for the NHS (2012) 'Health and Social Care Bill will leave public health compromised, weaker and less safe', Press release, 5 March.

Public Services Improvement Policy Group (2007) *Restoring pride in our public services*, Submission to the Shadow Cabinet, London: Conservative Party.

Raftery, J. (2006) 'Review of NICE's recommendations 1999-2005', *British Medical Journal*, vol 332, pp 1266-8.

RAND Europe/Ernst & Young LLP (2012) *National evaluation of the Department of Health's integrated care pilots, Final report*, London: Department of Health.

Randall, E. (2001) *The European Union and health policy*, Basingstoke: Palgrave.

Rawnsley, A. (2001) *Servants of the people: The inside story of New Labour*, Harmondsworth: Penguin.

Rawnsley, A. (2010) *The end of the party*, Harmondsworth: Penguin.

Rayner, G. (2012) 'Does celebrity involvement in public health campaigns deliver long term benefit? No', *British Medical Journal*, vol 345, e6362.

Register of All Party Groups (2015) As at 30 March 2015 www.publications. parliament.uk/pa/cm/csmallparty/memi01.htm accessed 26.6.15.

Reynolds, L. and McKee, M. (2012) 'Any qualified provider in NHS reforms: but who will qualify?', *Lancet*, vol 379, no 9821, pp 1083-4.

Reynolds, L., Gerada, C. and McKee, M. (2012) 'Ditching the single payer system in the National Health Service: how the English Department of Health is learning the wrong lessons from the United States', *International Journal of Health Services*, vol 42, no 3, pp 539-47.

Rhodes, R. (1997) *Understanding governance: Policy networks, governance, reflexivity and accountability*, Buckingham: Open University Press.

Richards, D. and Smith, M. (2002) *Governance and public policy in the UK*, Oxford: Oxford University Press.

Richards, P. (1972) *The backbenchers*, London: Faber.

Richards, S. (2013) 'Making news', Radio 4, 2nd, 9th, 16th April.

Richardson, J. (2000) 'Governments, interest groups and policy change', *Political Studies*, vol 48, pp 1006-25.

Richardson, J. and Jordan, G. (1979) *Governing under pressure*, Oxford: Martin Robertson.

Richardson, J. and Moon, J. (1984) 'The politics of unemployment in Britain', *Political Quarterly*, vol 55, pp 29-37.

Riddell, P. (2000) *Parliament under Blair*, London: Politico's.

Ridley, F. and Jordan, G. (1998) *Protest politics: Cause groups and campaigns*, Oxford: Oxford University Press.

Ridley, J., McKeown, M., Machin, K. et al (2014) *Exploring family carer involvement in forensic mental health services*, Edinburgh: Support in Mind Scotland.

Ries, N., Rachul, S. and Caulfied, T. (2011) 'Newspaper reporting on legislative policy interventions to address obesity: United States, Canada, and the United Kingdom', *Journal of Public Health Policy*, vol 32, no 1, pp 73-90.

Riker, W. (1962) *The theory of political coalitions*, New Haven, CT: Yale University Press.

Rivett, G. (1998) *From cradle to grave: Fifty years of the NHS*, London: King's Fund.

Robb, B. (1967) *Sans everything*, London: Nelson.

Robbins, M. (2012) 'The lay scientist', *The Guardian*, 1 March (www.theguardian.com/science/the-lay-scientist/2012/mar/01/1).

Robertson, D. (1976) *A theory of party competition*, London: Wiley.

Robinson, A., Coutinho, A., Bryden, A. and McKee, M. (2013) 'Analysis of health stories in daily newspapers in the UK', *Public Health*, vol 127, pp 39-45.

Rogers, A. and Pilgrim, D. (1991) 'Pulling down churches: accounting for the British mental health users movement', *Sociology of Health & Illness*, vol 13, no 2, pp 129-48.

Rogers A. and Pilgrim, D. (2001) *Mental health policy in Britain* (2nd edn), Basingstoke: Palgrave.

Rondinelli, D. (1981) 'Government decentralisation in comparative perspective: theory and practice in developing countries', *International Review of Administrative Science*, vol 47, pp 137-45.

Room, R. (2004) 'Disabling the public interest: alcohol strategies and policies for England', *Addiction*, vol 99, no 9, pp 1083-99.

Rose, D. (1998) 'Television, madness and community care', *Journal of Community & Applied Social Psychology*, vol 8, pp 213-28.

Rose, R. (1973) 'Comparing public policy: an overview', *European Journal of Political Research*, vol 1, pp 67-94.

Rose, R. (1984) *Do parties make a difference?* (2nd edn), London: Macmillan.

Rose, R. (1991) 'What is lesson drawing?', *Journal of Public Policy*, vol 11, no 1, pp 3-30.

Rose, R. and Davies, P. (1994) *Inheritance in public policy: Change without choice in Britain*, New Haven, CT: Yale University Press.

Rosenau, P. (2003) 'Performance evaluations of for-profit and non-profit US hospitals since 1980', *Nonprofit Management & Leadership*, vol 13, no 4, pp 401-23.

Rosenkötter, N., Clemens, T., Sorensen, K. and Brand, H. (2013) 'Twentieth anniversary of the European Union health mandate: taking stock of perceived achievements, failures, and missed opportunities – a qualitative study', *BMC Public Health*, vol 13, p 1074.

Ross, W. and Tomaney, J. (2001) 'Devolution and health policy in England', *Regional Studies*, vol 35, no 3, pp 265-70.

Roy, M., Donaldson, C., Baker, R. and Kerr, S. (2014) 'The potential of social enterprise to enhance health and well-being: a model and systematic review', *Social Science and Medicine*, DOI: 10.1016/j.socscimed.2014.o7.031.

Royal Commission on Local Government in England (1969a) *Volume 1: Report* (The Redcliffe-Maud report), Cmnd 4040, London: HMSO.

Royal Commission on Local Government in England (1969b) *Volume II: Memorandum of dissent by Mr Derek Senior*, Cmnd 4040, London: HMSO.

Royal Commission on the NHS (1979) *Report* (The Merrison Report), Cmnd 7615, London: HMSO.

Royal Liverpool Children's Inquiry (2001) *The report of the Royal Liverpool Children's Inquiry*, London: The Stationery Office.

Ruane, S. (2002) 'Public–private partnerships: the case of the PFI', in C. Glendinning, M. Powell and K. Rummery (eds) *Partnerships, New Labour and the governance of welfare*, Bristol: Policy Press, pp 199-212.

Ruane, S. (2005) 'The future of healthcare in the UK: think tanks and their policy prescriptions', in M. Powell, L. Bauld and K. Clarke (eds) *Social Policy Review 17*, Bristol: Policy Press, pp 147-66.

Rush, M. (2005) *Parliament today*, Manchester: Manchester University Press.

Russell, M. (2013) *The Contemporary House of Lords: Westminster bicameralism revived*, Oxford: Oxford University Press.

Russell, M. and Benton, M (2011) *Selective influence: The policy influence of House of Commons Select Committees*, London: UCL Constitution Unit.

Russell, M., Morris, B. and Larkin, P. (2013) *Fitting the Bill: Bringing the Commons legislation committees into line with best practice*, London: UCL Constitution Unit.

Sabatier, P. (1987) 'Knowledge, policy-orientated learning and policy change', *Knowledge: Creation, Diffusion, Utilisation*, vol 8, no 4, pp 649-92.

Sabatier, P. (ed) (1999) *Theories of the policy process*, Boulder, CO: Westview Press.

Salay, R and Lincoln, P. (2008) 'Health impact assessments in the European Union', *The Lancet*, vol 372, pp 860-1.

Salter, B. (1998) *The politics of change in the health service*, Basingstoke: Macmillan.

Salter, B. (2003) 'Patients and doctors: reformulating the UK health policy community?', *Social Science & Medicine*, vol 57, no 5, pp 927-36.

Salter, B. (2004) *The new politics of medicine*, Basingstoke: Palgrave Macmillan.

Saltman, R., Bankhauskaite, V. and Vrangback, K. (eds) (2007) *Decentralisation in healthcare*, Maidenhead: McGraw-Hill.

Sampson, A. (2004) *Who runs this place? The anatomy of Britain in the 21st century*, London: John Murray.

Sanderson, I. (2002) 'Evaluation, policy learning and evidence-based policy making', *Public Administration*, vol 80, no 1, pp 1-22.

Saywell, C., Beattie, L. and Henderson, L. (2000) 'Sexualised illness: the newsworthy body in media representations of breast cancer', in L. Potts (ed) *Ideologies of breast cancer: Feminist perspectives*, Basingstoke: Macmillan, pp 37-62.

Scally, G. (2013) 'Chief medical officers: the need for public health at the heart of government', *British Medical Journal*, vol 346, f688.

Schattschneider, E. (1960) *The semi-sovereign people*, New York: Holt, Rinehart & Winston.

Schwitzer, G. (2008) 'How do journalists cover treatment, tests, products, and procedures? An evaluation of 500 stories', *PLoS Medicine*, vol 5, no 5, e95.

Science Media Centre (2011) *Evidence from the Science Media Centre to the Leveson Inquiry*, London: Science Media Centre.

Science Media Centre (2012) *10 best practice guidelines for reporting science and health stories*, London: Science Media Centre.

Scott, A. (1990) *Ideology and the new social movements*, London: Unwin Hyman.

Scottish Executive (2000) *Our national health: A plan for action, a plan for change*, Edinburgh: Scottish Executive.

Scottish Executive (2003a) *Improving health in Scotland: The challenge*, Edinburgh: Scottish Office.

Scottish Executive (2003b) *Partnership for care: Scotland's Health White Paper*, Edinburgh: Scottish Office.

Scottish Executive (2004) *Fair to all, personal to each: The next steps for NHS Scotland*, Edinburgh: Scottish Executive.

Scottish Government (2007a) *Better health, better care: A discussion document*, Edinburgh: Scottish Government.

Scottish Government (2007b) *Better health, better care: Action plan*, Edinburgh: Scottish Government.

Scottish Government (2015) *Scottish government: Strategic objectives* (www.gov.scot).

Scottish Office (1991) *Health education in Scotland: A national policy statement*, Edinburgh: Scottish Office.

Scottish Office (1992) *Scotland's health: A challenge to us all*, Edinburgh; Scottish Office.

Scottish Office (1999) *Towards a healthier Scotland*, Cm 4269, Edinburgh: Scotland.

Seale, C. (2001) 'Sporting cancer: struggle language in news reports of people with cancer', *Sociology of Health & Illness*, vol 23, no 3, pp 308-29.

Seale, C. (2002) *Media and health*, London: Sage.

Seale, C. (2003) 'Health and the media: an overview', *Sociology of Health & Illness*, vol 25, no 6, pp 513-31.

Seale, C. (2005) 'Threatened children: media representations of childhood cancer', in M. King and K. Watson (eds) *Representing health: Discourses of health and illness in the media*, Basingstoke: Palgrave, pp 94-114.

Seldon, A. (1994) 'Policy making and Cabinet', in D. Kavanagh and A. Seldon (eds) *The Major effect*, London: Macmillan, pp 154-66.

Seldon, A. (2004) *Blair*, London: Free Press.

Select Committee on Public Administration (2002) *Ministerial accountability and parliamentary questions*, 9th report, 2001-2, London: The Stationery Office.

Select Committee on Public Administration (2003) *On target? Government by measurement*, 5th report, 2002-3, London: The Stationery Office.

Shaw, E. (2004) 'What matters is what works: the Third Way and the case of the private finance initiative', in W. Leggett, S. Hale and L. Martell (eds) *The Third Way and beyond: Criticisms, futures and alternatives*, Manchester: Manchester University Press, pp 64-82.

Shaw, S., Rosen, R. and Rumbold, B. (2011) *What is integrated care?*, London: Nuffield Trust.

Shaw, S., Russell, J., Greenhalgh, T. and Korica, M. (2014) 'Thinking about think tanks in health care: a call for a new research agenda', *Sociology of Health & Illness*, vol 36, no 3, pp 447-61.

Sheard, S. (2010) 'Quacks and clerks: historical and contemporary perspectives on the structure and function of the British medical civil service', *Social Policy & Administration*, vol 44, no 2, pp 193-207.

Sheard, S. and Donaldson, L. (2006) *The nation's doctor: The role of the Chief Medical Officer 1855-1998*, Oxford: Radcliffe.

Sheldon, T., Cullum, N., Dawson, D., Lankshear, A., Lowson, K., Watt, I., West, P., Wright, D. and Wright, J. (2004) 'What's the evidence that NICE guidance has been implemented? Results from a national evaluation using time series analysis, audit of patients' notes and interviews', *British Medical Journal*, vol 329, p 999.

Shipman Inquiry, The (2001) *First report*, London: The Stationery Office.

Shipman Inquiry, The (2004) *Fifth report: Safeguarding patients. Lessons from the past – Proposals for the future*, London: The Stationery Office.

Short, C. (2005) *An honourable deception: New Labour, Iraq and the misuse of power*, London: Free Press.

Shugart, H. (2011) 'Heavy viewing: emergent frames in contemporary news coverage of obesity', *Health Communication*, vol 26, pp 635-48.

Sibbald, B., Shen, J. and McBride, A. (2004) 'Changing the skill mix of the healthcare workforce', *Journal of Health Services Research & Policy*, vol 9, no 1, Supplement, S1-28.

Silk, P. and Walters, R. (1998) *How Parliament works* (4th edn), London: Longman.

Simon, H. (1945) *Administrative behaviour*, Glencoe, IL: Free Press.

Simon, H. (1960) *The new science of management decision*, Englewood Cliffs, NJ: Prentice Hall.

Sky News (2009) 'Tory Party of NHS claims in tatters again', 23 August (http://news.sky.com/story/718845/tories-party-of-nhs-claims-in-tatters-again).

Slater, E. and Beckford, M. (2011) '£500m wasted in private treatment centres for NHS', *Daily Telegraph*, 20 May (www.telegraph.co.uk/news/health/news/8526111/500m-wasted-in-private-treatment-centres-for-NHS.html).

Smith, J., Walshe, K. and Hunter, D. (2001) 'The redisorganisation of the NHS', *British Medical Journal*, vol 323, pp 1262-3.

Smith, K. and Hellowell, M. (2012) 'Beyond rhetorical differences: a cohesive account of post devolution developments in UK health policy', *Social Policy & Administration*, vol 46, no 2, pp 178-98.

Smith, M. (1993) *Pressure, power and policy*, Brighton: Harvester Wheatsheaf.

Smith, M. (1999) *The core executive in Britain*, Basingstoke: Macmillan.

Smith, M., Richards, D. and Marsh, D. (2000) 'The changing role of central government departments', in R. Rhodes (ed) *Transforming British government, Vol 2: Changing roles and relationships*, Basingstoke: Macmillan, pp 146-63.

Smith, P. (2005) 'Performance measurement in healthcare: history, challenges and prospects', *Public Money & Management*, vol 25, no 4, pp 213-20.

Smith, R., Chanda, R. and Tancharoensathien, V. et al (2009) 'Trade in health-related services', *The Lancet*, vol 373, pp 593-601.

Snape, S. (2003) 'Health and local government partnerships: the local government context', *Local Government Studies*, vol 29, no 3, pp 73-98.

Social Justice Policy Group (2007) *Breakthrough Britain: Policy recommendations to the Conservative Party*, London: Conservative Party.

Society Guardian (2000) 'The 15 most powerful people in health', 14 November (www.theguardian.com/society/2000/nov/14/longtermcare. socialcare).

Söderlund, N., Csaba, I., Gray, A., Milne, R. and Raftery, J. (1997) 'Impact of the NHS reforms on English hospital productivity: an analysis of the first three years', *British Medical Journal*, vol 315, pp 1126-9.

Sontag, S. (1991) *Illness as metaphor: AIDS and its metaphors*, London: Penguin.

Speers, T. and Lewis, J. (2004) 'Journalists and jabs: media coverage of the MMR vaccine', *Communication & Medicine*, vol 1, no 2, pp 171-82.

SPS (Sanitary and Phytosanitary Measures) (1994) *Agreement on the application of sanitary and phytosanitary measures*, Uruguay Round Agreement, World Trade Organization (www.wto.org/english/docs_e/legal_e/15sps_01_e. htm).

Sridhar, D., Frenk, J., Gostin, L. and Moon, S. (2014) 'Global rules for global health: why we need an independent, impartial WHO', *British Medical Journal*, vol 348, g3841.

Steel, D. (2013) 'Scotland', in C. Ham, D. Heenan, M. Longley and D. Steel (eds) *Integrated care in Northern Ireland, Scotland and Wales: Lessons for England*, London: King's Fund, pp 25-56.

Stevens, P., Stokes, L. and O'Mahony, M. (2006) 'Metrics, targets and performance', *National Institute Economic Review*, vol 197, no 1, pp 80-92.

Stewart, J. (1958) *British pressure groups: Their role in relation to the House of Commons*, London: Greenwood.

Stewart, J. (2004) *Taking stock: Scottish welfare after devolution*, Bristol: Policy Press.

Stoker, G. (2004) 'New localism, progressive politics and democracy', in A. Gamble and T. Wright (eds) *Restating the state*, Oxford: Blackwell, pp 117-29.

Storey, J., Bullivant, J. and Corbett-Nolan, A. (2011) *Governing the new NHS: Issues and tensions in health service management*, London: Routledge.

Storey, J., Holti, R., Winchester, N., Green, R., Salaman, G. and Bate, P. (2010) *The intended and unintended outcomes of new governance arrangements within the NHS: Project report*, NIHR Research programme project 08/1618/129 (www.nets.nihr.ac.uk).

Strom, K. (1990) 'A behavioural theory of competitive political parties', *American Journal of Political Science*, vol 34, no 2, pp 565-98.

Summers, D. and Glendinning, L. (2009) 'Cameron rebukes Tory MEP who rubbished NHS in America', *The Guardian*, 14 August (www.theguardian.com/politics/2009/aug/14/health-nhs).

Stuckler, D. and Basu, S. (2009) 'The International Monetary Fund's effects on global health: before and after the 2008 financial crisis', *International Journal of Health Services*, vol 39, no 4, pp 771-81.

Sullivan, H. and Skelcher, C. (2002) *Working across boundaries: Collaboration in public services*, Basingstoke: Palgrave.

Sumner, P., Vivian-Richards, S., Boivin, J. et al (2014) 'The association between exaggeration in health related science news and academic press releases: retrospective observational study', *British Medical Journal*, vol 349, g7015.

Sutherland, K. and Coyle, N. (2009) *Quality healthcare in England, Wales, Scotland and Northern Ireland: An intra-UK chartbook*, London: Health Foundation

Sylvester, R. (2012) 'Is Lansley the exception to the no sacking policy?', *The Times*, 7 February.

Tallis, R. (2004) *Hippocratic oaths: Medicine and its discontents*, London: Atlantic Books.

Tam, H. (1998) *Communitarianism: A new agenda for politics and citizenship*, Basingstoke: Macmillan.

Tarrow, S. (1998) *Power in movement*, Cambridge: Cambridge University Press.

Taylor, D. and Balloch, S. (2005) *The politics of evaluation: Participation and policy evaluation*, Bristol: Policy Press.

Taylor, M. (2006) 'Communities in partnership: developing a strategic voice', *Social Policy and Society*, vol 5, no 2, pp 269-79.

Terkildsen, N., Schnell, F. and Ling, C. (1998) 'Interest groups, the media and policy debate formation: an analysis of message structure, rhetoric and source cues', *Political Communication*, vol 15, pp 45-61.

Tew, M. (1998) *Safer childbirth? A critical history of maternity care* (3rd edn), London: Free Association Books.

Thatcher, M. (1982) Speech to the Conservative Party Conference, Brighton, 8 October.

Thatcher, M. (1993) *The Downing Street years*, London: HarperCollins.

The BSE Inquiry (2000) *The Report (The Phillips Report)*, London: The Stationery Office.

Thistlethwaite, P. (2011) *Integrating health and social care in Torbay*, London: King's Fund.

Thompson, L. (2013) '"More of the same or a period of change": the impact of bill committees in the twenty-first century House of Commons', *Parliamentary Affairs*, vol 66, pp 459-79

Thorlby, R. and Maybin, J. (2010) *A high performing NHS: A review of progress 1997-2010*, London: King's Fund.

Time to Change (2015) *Making a drama out of a crisis*, London: Time to Change.

Timmins, N. (1995) *The five giants: A biography of the welfare state*, London: Fontana.

Timmins, N. (2012) *Never again: The story of the Health and Social Care Act 2012: A study in coalition government and policy making*, London: King's Fund and Institute for Government.

Timmins, N. (2013) *The four UK health systems: Learning from each other*, London: King's Fund.

Torfing, J. (1999) *New theories of discourse: Laclau, Mouffe, and Zizek*, Oxford: Blackwell.

Toynbee, P. and Walker, D. (2001) *Did things get better?*, London: Penguin.

Treasury Committee (2011) *Private finance initiative*, 17th report, session 2010-12, London: The Stationery Office.

Tudor Hart, J. (2004) 'Health care or health trade? A historic moment of choice', *International Journal of Health Services*, vol 34, no 2, pp 245-54.

Tudor Hart, J. (2006) *The political economy of health care: A clinical perspective*, Bristol: Policy Press.

Tudor Jones, G. (2013) *Assessing the transition to a more localist health system – The first step towards a marriage between the NHS and local government?*, London: Localis.

Turner, S., Allen, P., Bartlett, W. and Perotin, V. (2011) 'Innovation and the English national health service: a qualitative study of the independent sector treatment centre programme', *British Medical Journal*, vol 73, no 4, pp 522-9..

Ungoed-Thomas, J. and Summers, H. (2012) 'Overcrowded A&Es force patients to wait in ambulances', *Sunday Times*, 14 October.

UN (United Nations) General Assembly (2012) Resolution adopted by the General Assembly, 66th Session, 19 September, *Political declaration of the High-level Meeting of the General Assembly on the prevention and control of non-communicable diseases*, A/RES/66/2.

UN Open Working Group on Sustainable Development (2014) *Introduction and proposed goals and targets on sustainable development for the post 2015 development agenda*, 2 June.

Verzulli, R., Jacobs, R. and Goddard, M. (2011) *Do hospitals respond to greater autonomy? Evidence from the English*, Research Paper 64, York: NHS Centre for Health Economics, University of York.

Vizard, P. and Obolenskaya, P. (2015) *The coalition's record on health: Policy, spending and outcomes 2010-15*, Social Policy in a Cold Climate, Summary Working Paper 16, London: Centre for Analysis of Social Exclusion, London School of Economics and Political Science.

Vize, R. (2013) 'Goodbye (and good riddance?) to PCTs', *British Medical Journal*, vol 246, f2039.

Wait, S. and Nolte, E. (2006) 'Public involvement policies in health: explaining their conceptual basis', *Health Economics, Policy and Law*, vol 1, pp 149-62.

Waitzkin, H., Jasso-Aguilar, R., Landwehr, A. and Mountain, C. (2005) 'Global trade, public health, and health services: stakeholders' constructions of the key issues', *Social Science & Medicine*, vol 61, pp 893-906.

Wales Audit Office (2006) *NHS waiting times: Follow-up report*, Cardiff: Wales Audit Office.

Walker, D. (2002) *In praise of centralism: A critique of the new localism*, London: Catalyst.

Walshe, K. (2003) *Regulating healthcare: A prescription for improvement*, Buckingham: Open University Press.

Walshe, K. (2010) 'Reorganisation of the NHS in England', *British Medical Journal*, vol 341, c3843.

Walt, G. (1994) *Health policy: An introduction to process and power*, London: Zed Books.

Wanless, D. (2007) *Our future health secured? A review of NHS funding and performance*, London: King's Fund.

Washer, P. (2004) 'Representation of SARS in the British newspapers', *Social Science & Medicine*, vol 59, pp 2561-71.

Watt, E., Ibe, O. and McLelland, N. (2010) *Study of community health partnerships*, Edinburgh: Scottish Government Social Research.

Webb, P. (2000) *The Modern British party system*, London: Sage.

Webster, C. (1988) *The health services since the war, Vol 1, Problems of health care. The National Health Service before 1957*, London: HMSO.

Webster, C. (1996) *Government and health care, Vol 2, The National Health Service 1958-79*, London: HMSO.

Webster, C. (1998) 'The BMA and the NHS', *British Medical Journal*, vol 317, pp 45-7.

Webster, C. (2002) *The National Health Service: A political history* (2nd edn), Oxford: Oxford University Press.

Welikala, J. and West, D. (2015) 'CCGs' fear of competition rules grows', *Health Service Journal*, 24 April, p 5.

Welsh Assembly Government (2002) *Wellbeing in Wales*, Cardiff: Welsh Assembly Government.

Welsh Assembly Government (2003) *Wales: A better country*, Cardiff: Welsh Assembly Government.

Welsh Assembly Government (2005) *Designed for life*, Cardiff: National Assembly for Wales.

Welsh Assembly Government (2009) *Our healthy future*, Cardiff: Welsh Assembly Government.

Welsh Office (1989) *Welsh Health Planning Forum: Strategic intent and direction for the NHS in Wales*, Cardiff: Welsh Office.

Welsh Office (1998) *Strategic Framework: Better health, better Wales*, Cardiff: Welsh Office.

Welsh Government (2014) *Listening to you – Your health matters*, Cardiff: Welsh Government.

West, D. (2013) 'Reform deputy director moves to Number 10', *Health Service Journal*, 8 May.

West, D. (2014) 'CCGs open services to competition out of fear of rules', *Health Service Journal*, 4 April.

Whiteley, P. and Winyard, S. (1987) *Pressure for the poor: The poverty lobby and policy making*, London: Methuen.

WHO (World Health Organization) (1946) *Preamble to the Constitution of the World Health Organization as adopted by the International Conference*, New York, 19 June-22 July, Official Records of the World Health Organization, no 2.

WHO (1981) *Global health strategy for Health for All by the year 2000*, Geneva: WHO.

WHO (1998) *Health for All for the 21st century*, Geneva: WHO.

WHO Commission on the Social Determinants of Health (2008) *Closing the gap in a generation*, Geneva: WHO.

WHO Regional Office for Europe (1985) *Targets for Health for All: Targets in support of the European regional strategy for health for all*, Copenhagen: WHO Europe.

WHO Regional Office for Europe (1999) *Health 21: The Health for All policy framework for the 21st century*, Copenhagen: WHO Europe.

WHO Regional Office for Europe (2006a) *European Charter on Counteracting Obesity*, Copenhagen: WHO Europe.

WHO Regional Office for Europe (2006b) *Framework for Alcohol Policy in the WHO European Region*, Copenhagen: WHO Europe.

WHO Regional Office for Europe (2010) *Parma Declaration on Environment and Health*, Copenhagen: WHO Europe.

WHO Regional Office for Europe (2011) *Action Plan for the Implementation of the European Strategy for the Prevention and Control of Non-communicable Diseases 2012-16*, Copenhagen: WHO Europe.

WHO Regional Office for Europe (2012a) *Health 2020*, Copenhagen: WHO Europe.

WHO Regional Office for Europe (2012b) *Addressing the Social Determinants of Health: the urban dimension and the role of local government*, Copenhagen: WHO Europe.

WHO and UNICEF (United Nations Children's Fund) (1978) *Declaration of Alma Ata*, Report of the International Conference on Primary Health Care, Geneva: WHO and UNICEF.

Williams, K. (1999) '"Dying of ignorance?" Journalists, news sources and media reporting of HIV/AIDS', in B. Franklin (ed) *Social policy, the media and misrepresentation*, London: Routledge, pp 69-85.

Williams, S. (2002) *Alternative prescriptions: A survey of international healthcare systems*, London: Conservative Policy Unit.

Wilsford, D. (1994) 'Path dependency, or why history makes it difficult but not impossible to reform health care systems in a big way', *Journal of Public Policy*, vol 13, no 3, pp 251-83.

Wismar, M., Blau, J., Ernst, K. and Figueras, J. (2007) *The effectiveness of health impact assessment: Scope and limitations of supporting decision making in Europe*, Copenhagen: WHO/European Observatory on Health Systems and Policies.

Wistow, G. (2013) 'Still a fine mess? Local government and the NHS 1962 to 2012', *Journal of Integrated Care*, vol 20, no 2, pp 101-14.

Wistow, G. and Harrison, S. (1998) 'Rationality and rhetoric: the contribution to social care policy making of Sir Roy Griffiths 1986-91', *Public Administration*, vol 76, no 4, pp 649-68.

Wood, B. (2000) *Patient power? The politics of patients' associations in Britain and America*, Buckingham: Open University Press.

Woods, K. (2002) 'Health policy and the NHS in the UK 1997-2002', in J. Adams and P. Robinson (eds) *Devolution in practice: Public policy differences within the UK*, London: Institute for Public Policy Research, pp 25-59.

Woods, K. (2004) 'Political devolution and the health services in Great Britain', *International Journal of Health Services*, vol 34, no 2, pp 323-39.

Wright, O. (2003) 'Television death led to 14,000 smear tests', *The Times*, 23 February, p 5.

Wyatt, M. (2002) 'Partnership in health and social care: the implications of government guidance in the 1990s in England with particular reference to voluntary organisations', *Policy & Politics*, vol 30, no 2, pp 167-82.

Yavchitz, A., Boutron, I., Befeta, A., Marroun, I., Charles, P., Mantz, J. and Ravaud, P. (2012) 'Misrepresentation of randomised controlled trials in press releases and news coverage: a cohort study', *PLoS Medicine*, vol 9, no 9, e1001308.

Ziglio, E., Hagard., S., and Brown, C. (2005) 'Health promotion development in Europe: barriers and new opportunities', in E. Scriven and S. Garman (eds) *Promoting health: Global perspectives*, Basingstoke: Palgrave, pp 229-38.

Index